Contemporary Topics in Radiation Medicine, Part I: Current Issues and Techniques

Editors

RAVI A. CHANDRA
LISA A. KACHNIC
CHARLES R. THOMAS Jr

HEMATOLOGY/ONCOLOGY CLINICS OF NORTH AMERICA

www.hemonc.theclinics.com

Consulting Editor
GEORGE P. CANELLOS

December 2019 • Volume 33 • Number 6

ELSEVIER

1600 John F. Kennedy Boulevard • Suite 1800 • Philadelphia, Pennsylvania, 19103-2899

http://www.theclinics.com

HEMATOLOGY/ONCOLOGY CLINICS OF NORTH AMERICA Volume 33, Number 6
December 2019 ISSN 0889-8588, ISBN 13: 978-0-323-68326-5

Editor: Stacy Eastman
Developmental Editor: Kristen Helm

Hematology/Oncology Clinics (ISSN 0889-8588) is published bimonthly by Elsevier Inc., 360 Park Avenue South, New York, NY 10010-1710. Months of issue are February, April, June, August, October, and December. Business and Editorial Offices: 1600 John F. Kennedy Blvd., Ste. 1800, Philadelphia, PA 19103–2899. Customer Service Office: 3251 Riverport Lane, Maryland Heights, MO 63043. Periodicals postage paid at New York, NY and at additional mailing offices. Subscription prices are $430.00 per year (domestic individuals), $830.00 per year (domestic institutions), $100.00 per year (domestic students/residents), $480.00 per year (Canadian individuals), $1028.00 per year (Canadian institutions) $547.00 per year (international individuals), $1028.00 per year (international institutions), and $255.00 per year (international and Canadian students/residents). International air speed delivery is included in all *Clinics* subscription prices. All prices are subject to change without notice. **POSTMASTER:** Send address changes to *Hematology/Oncology Clinics of North America*, Elsevier Health Sciences Division, Subscription Customer Service, 3251 Riverport Lane, Maryland Heights, MO 63043. Customer Service (orders, claims, online, change of address): Elsevier Health Sciences Division, Subscription **Customer Service, 3251 Riverport Lane, Maryland Heights, MO 63043. Tel: 1-800-654-2452 (U.S. and Canada); 314-447-8871 (outside U.S. and Canada). Fax: 314-447-8029. E-mail: journalscustomerservice-usa@elsevier.com (for print support); journalsonlinesupport-usa@elsevier.com (for online support)**.

Reprints. For copies of 100 or more, of articles in this publication, please contact the Commercial Reprints Department, Elsevier Inc., 360 Park Avenue South, New York, New York 10010-1710; Tel.: 212-633-3874, Fax: 212-633-3820, E-mail: reprints@elsevier.com.

Hematology/Oncology Clinics of North America is covered in *MEDLINE/PubMed (Index Medicus), EMBASE/ Excerpta Medica,* and *BIOSIS.*

Contributors

CONSULTING EDITOR

GEORGE P. CANELLOS, MD
William Rosenberg Professor of Medicine, Department of Medical Oncology, Dana-Farber Cancer Institute, Boston, Massachusetts, USA

EDITORS

RAVI A. CHANDRA, MD, PhD
Assistant Professor, Department of Radiation Medicine, Oregon Health & Science University, Portland, Oregon, USA

LISA A. KACHNIC, MD, FASTRO
Professor and Chair, Department of Radiation Oncology, Vagelos College of Physicians and Surgeons, Columbia University Irving Medical Center, New York, New York, USA

CHARLES R. THOMAS Jr, MD
Department of Radiation Medicine, Oregon Health & Science University, Portland, Oregon, USA

AUTHORS

STEPHEN ABEL, DO
Division of Radiation Oncology, Allegheny Health Network Cancer Institute, Pittsburgh, Pennsylvania, USA

VIJAY AGUSALA, BS, MBA
Medical Student, Department of Radiation Oncology, UT Southwestern Medical Center, Dallas, Texas, USA

ABIGAIL T. BERMAN, MD, MSCE
Department of Radiation Oncology, University of Pennsylvania, Philadelphia, Pennsylvania, USA

MARYANN BISHOP-JODOIN, MEd
Scientific Writer, Department of Radiation Oncology, University of Massachusetts Medical School, Worcester, Massachusetts, USA

JOSEPH CASTER, MD, PhD
Assistant Professor, Radiation Oncology, University of Iowa Carver College of Medicine, Iowa City, Iowa, USA

INDRIN J. CHETTY, PhD
Director, Physics Division, Department of Radiation Oncology, Henry Ford Cancer Institute, Henry Ford Health System, Detroit, Michigan, USA

DEBORAH E. CITRIN, MD
Senior Investigator, Radiation Oncology Branch, Center for Cancer Research, National Cancer Institute, Bethesda, Maryland, USA

CHRISTOPHER R. DEIG, MD
Radiation Medicine, Oregon Health & Science University, Portland, Oregon, USA

PHILLIP M. DEVLIN, MD, FACR, FASTRO, FFRRCSI(HON)
Chief, Division of Brachytherapy, Institute Physician, Dana Farber Cancer Institute, Associate Professor of Radiation Oncology, Harvard Medical School, Boston, Massachusetts, USA

GRETE MAY ENGESETH, MS
Department of Radiation Oncology, The University of Texas MD Anderson Cancer Center, Houston, Texas, USA

THOMAS J. FITZGERALD, MD
Chair, Department of Radiation Oncology, University of Massachusetts Medical School/ UMass Memorial Health Care, Worcester, Massachusetts, USA; Director of the Imaging and Radiation Oncology Core (IROC), Lincoln, Rhode Island, USA

CLIFTON DAVID FULLER, MD, PhD
Department of Radiation Oncology, The University of Texas MD Anderson Cancer Center, Houston, Texas, USA

STEPHEN J. GARDNER, MS
Director, QA and Safety, Physics, Department of Radiation Oncology, Henry Ford Cancer Institute, Henry Ford Health System, Detroit, Michigan, USA

AMARDEEP S. GREWAL, MD
Department of Radiation Oncology, University of Pennsylvania, Philadelphia, Pennsylvania, USA

MARY GRONBERG, MS
Department of Radiation Oncology, The University of Texas MD Anderson Cancer Center, Houston, Texas, USA

C. TILDEN HAGAN IV, BSE
Graduate Research Assistant, UNC/NCSU Joint Department of Biomedical Engineering, Laboratory of Nano- and Translational Medicine, Carolina Center for Cancer Nanotechnology Excellence, Carolina Institute of Nanomedicine, Lineberger Comprehensive Cancer Center, Department of Radiation Oncology, University of North Carolina at Chapel Hill, Chapel Hill, North Carolina, USA

RENJIE HE, PhD
Department of Radiation Oncology, The University of Texas MD Anderson Cancer Center, Houston, Texas, USA

CHRISTINE E. HILL-KAYSER, MD
Associate Professor, Department of Radiation Oncology, University of Pennsylvania, Philadelphia, Pennsylvania, USA

SOPHIA C. KAMRAN, MD
Department of Radiation Oncology, Massachusetts General Hospital, Harvard Medical School, Boston, Massachusetts, USA

AASHEESH KANWAR, MD
Radiation Medicine, Oregon Health & Science University, Portland, Oregon, USA

FLORENCE K. KEANE, MD
Department of Radiation Oncology, Massachusetts General Hospital, Harvard Medical School, Boston, Massachusetts, USA

JOSHUA KIM, PhD
Senior Staff Physicist, Department of Radiation Oncology, Henry Ford Cancer Institute, Henry Ford Health System, Detroit, Michigan, USA

MICHAEL J. LaRIVIERE, MD
Resident Physician, Department of Radiation Oncology, University of Pennsylvania, Philadelphia, Pennsylvania, USA

FRAN LAURIE, BS
Academic Administrator, Department of Radiation Oncology, University of Massachusetts Medical School, Worcester, Massachusetts, USA

SOYOUNG LEE, PhD
Division of Radiation Oncology, Allegheny Health Network Cancer Institute, Pittsburgh, Pennsylvania, USA

SICONG LI, DSc
University of Nebraska Medical Center, 987521 Nebraska Medical Center, Omaha, Nebraska, USA

ETHAN B. LUDMIR, MD
Department of Radiation Oncology, University of Texas MD Anderson Cancer Center, Houston, Texas, USA

ALEXANDER LUKEZ, BS
Student, University of Massachusetts Medical School, Worcester, Massachusetts, USA

BRIGID McDONALD, BS
Department of Radiation Oncology, The University of Texas MD Anderson Cancer Center, Houston, Texas, USA

JAMES M. METZ, MD
Professor and Chair, Department of Radiation Oncology, University of Pennsylvania, Philadelphia, Pennsylvania, USA

LAUREN O'LOUGHLIN, BS
Student, University of Massachusetts Medical School, Worcester, Massachusetts, USA

SOPHIE J. OTTER, MBBChir, MRCP, FRCR
Consultant Oncologist, Royal Surrey County Hospital, Guildford, United Kingdom

ALLISON SACHER, MD
Radiation Oncologist, Department of Radiation Oncology, University of Massachusetts Medical School/UMass Memorial Health Care, Worcester, Massachusetts, USA

PATRICIA MAE G. SANTOS, MD, MS
Resident Physician, Department of Medicine, Memorial Sloan Kettering Cancer Center, New York, New York, USA

CHENG B. SAW, PhD
Northeast Radiation Oncology Centers (NROC), Dunmore, Pennsylvania, USA

JONATHAN D. SCHOENFELD, MD, MPhil, MPH
Department of Radiation Oncology, Brigham and Women's Hospital/Dana-Farber Cancer Institute, Boston, Massachusetts, USA

SAMUEL R. SCHROEDER, MD, MBA
Resident, Department of Radiation Oncology, UT Southwestern Medical Center, Dallas, Texas, USA

DAVID J. SHER, MD, MPH
Associate Professor, Department of Radiation Oncology, UT Southwestern Medical Center, Dallas, Texas, USA

VISHWAJITH SRIDHARAN, MD, MBA
Harvard-MIT Division of Health Sciences and Technology, Harvard Medical School, Cambridge, Massachusetts, USA

ALEXANDRA J. STEWART, MD, MRCP, FRCR
Consultant Oncologist, Royal Surrey County Hospital, Guildford, United Kingdom

SONJA STIEB, MD
Department of Radiation Oncology, The University of Texas MD Anderson Cancer Center, Houston, Texas, USA

BO SUN, PhD
Research Associate, Laboratory of Nano- and Translational Medicine, Carolina Center for Cancer Nanotechnology Excellence, Carolina Institute of Nanomedicine, Lineberger Comprehensive Cancer Center, Department of Radiation Oncology, University of North Carolina at Chapel Hill, Chapel Hill, North Carolina, USA

REID F. THOMPSON, MD, PhD
Assistant Professor, Radiation Medicine, Oregon Health & Science University, Staff Physician, Division of Hospital & Specialty Medicine, VA Portland Healthcare System, Portland, Oregon, USA

VIVEK VERMA, MD
Division of Radiation Oncology, Allegheny Health Network Cancer Institute, Pittsburgh, Pennsylvania, USA

ANDREW Z. WANG, MD
Associate Professor, Laboratory of Nano- and Translational Medicine, Carolina Center for Cancer Nanotechnology Excellence, Carolina Institute of Nanomedicine, Lineberger Comprehensive Cancer Center, Department of Radiation Oncology, University of North Carolina Hospitals, University of North Carolina-Chapel Hill, Chapel Hill, North Carolina, USA

HENNING WILLERS, MD
Department of Radiation Oncology, Massachusetts General Hospital, Harvard Medical School, Boston, Massachusetts, USA

Contents

This article gives a tutorial on basic therapeutic medical physics. Medical health physics dealing with the issue of radiation protection for personnel and the public in the radiation environment is explained first. Next, we introduce the concept of absorbed dose related to energy deposition in tissues and then dosimetry instrumentation. Three-dimensional treatment planning systems that are now an integral component of modern radiation therapy are described. External beam radiation therapy, particle beam radiation therapy, and brachytherapy are briefly described. The change in quality assurance for contemporary radiation therapy program is highlighted.

Radiation biology has entered the era of precision oncology, and this article reviews time-tested factors that determine the effects of fractionated radiation therapy in a wide variety of tumor types and normal tissues: the association of tumor control with radiation dose, the importance of fractionation and overall treatment time, and the role of tumor hypoxia. Therapeutic gain can only be achieved if the increased tumor toxicity produced by biological treatment modifications is balanced against injury to early-responding and late-responding normal tissues. Developments in precision oncology and immuno-oncology will allow an emphasis on treatment individualization and predictive biomarker development.

Modern radiation therapy treatment planning and delivery is a complex process that relies on advanced imaging and computing technology as well as expertise from the medical team. The process begins with simulation imaging, in which three-dimensional computed tomography images (or magnetic resonance images in some cases) are used to characterize the patient anatomy. From there, the radiation oncologist delineates the relevant target/tumor volumes and normal tissue and communicates the goals for treatment planning. The planning process attempts to generate a radiation therapy treatment plan that will deliver a therapeutic dose of radiation to the tumor while sparing nearby normal tissue.

Imaging in radiation oncology has a wide range of applications. It is necessary not only for tumor staging and treatment response assessment after
therapy but also for the treatment planning process, including definition of
target and organs at risk, as well as treatment plan calculation. This article
provides a comprehensive overview of the main imaging modalities
currently used for target delineation and treatment planning and gives
insight into new and promising techniques.

Stereotactic radiation therapy (RT) involves the delivery of high dose-per-
fraction treatments to small intracranial (stereotactic radiosurgery [SRS])
and extracranial (stereotactic body radiotherapy [SBRT]) sites. SRS and
SBRT share several overarching principles that differentiate stereotactic
RT from conventionally fractionated radiation techniques. This review describes historical aspects of SRS/SBRT and definitions thereof, and a
comparison with more modern semantics. Key principles of the stereotactic radiotherapeutic modalities are discussed, followed by an overview of
the technical considerations involved. Lastly, the accepted appropriate
clinical indications for stereotactic RT are outlined, and the potential role
of stereotactic treatment in future oncologic management are also
discussed.

Proton therapy is a form of external beam radiotherapy that has several advantages over conventional photon (x-ray) radiotherapy. Protons are useful in 2 scenarios that apply to a large proportion of cancer patients: lack of
exit dose allows for delivery of a therapeutic radiation dose to tumors in
challenging anatomic locations, and reduction in integral dose (low-dose
bath) to normal tissues that may reduce the risk of late toxicities and secondary cancers. The emergence of smaller, more economically viable
single-room proton units has led to the expansion in use of this technology
across the world.

Brachytherapy involves the placement of radioactive sources within or
very close to the tumor. This placement allows a high dose of radiotherapy
to be delivered to the tumor while sparing the surrounding normal tissue.
The delivery of brachytherapy has changed markedly over the years,
with newer radioactive sources making delivery safer, image guidance
techniques allowing more accurate placement of sources, and advanced

planning systems allowing brachytherapy to be truly adaptive. This article explores the most modern techniques and current uses of brachytherapy in the treatment of gynecological, prostate, breast, rectal, and skin cancers.

Intentional and unintentional radiation exposures have a powerful impact on normal tissue function and can induce short-term and long-term injury to all cell systems. Radiation effects can lead to lifetime-defining health issues for a patient and can produce complications to all organ systems. Providers need to understand acute and late effects of radiation treatment and how the fingerprints of therapy can have an impact on health care in later life. This article reviews current knowledge concerning normal tissue tolerance with therapy.

Radiation therapy is one of the most commonly used treatments for cancer. Radiation modifiers are agents that alter tumor or normal tissue response to radiation, such as radiation sensitizers and radiation protectors. Radiation sensitizers target aspects of tumor molecular biology or physiology to enhance tumor cell killing after irradiation. Radioprotectors prevent damage of normal tissues selectively. Radiation modifiers remain largely investigational at present, with the promise that molecular characterization of tumors may enhance the capacity for successful clinical development moving forward. A variety of radiation modifiers are described.

Preclinical studies combining immunotherapy and radiation therapy have suggested promising synergy, prompting translation into clinical trials. Radiation has been shown to significantly alter the tumor microenvironment, cause immunogenic cell death, and potentiate anti–tumor immune responses. Several radiation parameters may modulate these effects. Clinical data to date have suggested that combination therapy is largely well tolerated, but additional study is warranted to better estimate both short-term and long-term risks of combination treatment and extend these data to new immunotherapy agents. Ensuring proper radiation access and quality is critical to the success of future trials.

Nanotechnology has made remarkable contributions to clinical oncology. Nanotherapeutics and diagnostic tools have distinctive characteristics which allow them superior abilities to deliver therapeutics and imaging agents for radiation oncology. Compared to solid biopsies and imaging, the analysis of circulating tumor cells (CTCs) offers a more rapid, real-time, and less invasive method to monitor the dynamic molecular profiles of tumors. The potential of CTCs to be translated as a novel cancer biomarker has been demonstrated in numerous clinical studies. This review will discuss clinical applications of nanomaterials in radiation oncology and the implication of CTCs in cancer detection and monitoring.

The integration of artificial intelligence in the radiation oncologist's workflow has multiple applications and significant potential. From the initial patient encounter, artificial intelligence may aid in pretreatment disease outcome and toxicity prediction. It may subsequently aid in treatment planning, and enhanced dose optimization. Artificial intelligence may also optimize the quality assurance process and support a higher level of safety, quality, and efficiency of care. This article describes components of the radiation consultation, planning, and treatment process and how the thoughtful integration of artificial intelligence may improve shared decision making, planning efficiency, planning quality, patient safety, and patient outcomes.

Patient-reported outcome and health-related quality of life scales have the potential to engage patients and providers, allowing for better communication and shared decision-making in oncology care. When monitored longitudinally, they facilitate earlier interventions that may help with symptom management and improve traditional outcome metrics, including survival. Their use in clinical trials has allowed for changes in guidelines in the management of various cancers. The voice and experience of the patient, captured by these scales, enable providers to better detail the journey patients can expect to experience during and after treatment.

The diagnosis and treatment of cancer places patients at risk for serious financial consequences, which are detrimental to overall health and well-being. The concept of financial toxicity (FT) describes monetary and health implications related to the financial burden of receiving care. To investigate this important area, the authors first explore aspects of the modern American health care insurance system that relate to cancer care. Then they summarize relevant literature across multiple domains of FT that include monetary, functional, and patient-reported measures. The authors conclude by making simple recommendations to begin addressing FT in clinical practice.

HEMATOLOGY/ONCOLOGY CLINICS OF NORTH AMERICA

SERIES OF RELATED INTEREST

Surgical Oncology Clinics of North America
https://www.surgonc.theclinics.com/

THE CLINICS ARE AVAILABLE ONLINE!
Access your subscription at:
www.theclinics.com

Preface

Current Issues and Techniques

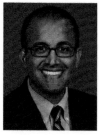
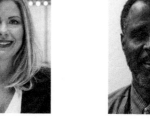

Ravi A. Chandra, MD, PhD   Lisa A. Kachnic, MD, FASTRO   Charles R. Thomas Jr, MD

Editors

Radiotherapy remains one of the most common, although misunderstood, tools in the oncology management arsenal, as up to two-thirds of all patients receive this modality at some point during their cancer continuum. Radiation Oncology is a rapidly evolving specialty, with substantial innovation in the technical and clinical aspects of radiation treatment over recent years. This two-part series aims to update practicing oncologists and associated care team members on many of the exciting changes that are taking place in this field.

In this issue of *Hematology/Oncology Clinics of North America*, we discuss the practical basis of radiation medicine as well as recent advances in radiation treatment and delivery. The contributors comprise the brightest minds within our specialty. Moreover, they have written each article with the expressed intent of educating non–radiation medicine clinicians on the topic at hand, with an eye toward the future.

We would like to thank all of our authors for their efforts in making this a successful endeavor. We would also like to acknowledge Kristen Helm, Stacy Eastman, and the team at Elsevier for their generous contributions of time, talent, expertise, and discipline to ensure an outstanding pair of issues of the *Hematology/Oncology Clinics of North America*.

Ravi A. Chandra, MD, PhD
Department of Radiation Medicine
Oregon Health & Science University
3181 SW Sam Jackson Park Road
Portland, OR 97239, USA

Hematol Oncol Clin N Am 33 (2019) xiii–xiv
https://doi.org/10.1016/j.hoc.2019.09.001
0889-8588/19/© 2019 Published by Elsevier Inc.

Lisa A. Kachnic, MD, FASTRO
Department of Radiation Oncology
Vagelos College of Physicians and Surgeons
Columbia University Irving Medical Center
622 West 168th Street
CHONY North, B Level, Room 11
New York, NY 10032, USA

Charles R. Thomas Jr, MD
Department of Radiation Medicine
Oregon Health & Science University
3181 SW Sam Jackson Park Road
Portland, OR 97239, USA

E-mail addresses:
chandrra@ohsu.edu (R.A. Chandra)
lak2187@cumc.columbia.edu (L.A. Kachnic)
thomasch@ohsu.edu (C.R. Thomas)

Basic Therapeutic Medical Physics

Cheng B. Saw, PhD[a],*, Sicong Li, DSc[b]

KEYWORDS

- Radiation protection • Absorbed dose • Treatment planning systems
- External beam radiation therapy • Particle beam therapy • Brachytherapy
- Quality assurance

KEY POINTS

- The basis of radiation therapy is the interaction of radiation with tissues and thereafter the deposition of energy (absorbed dose) causing biological effects.
- Various dosimetry instrumentations are accessible to characterize radiation beams, both for the calibration of the radiation therapy machines and in vivo measurements in patients.
- Radiation therapy processes are highly technical using equipment connected through digital networks to extract patient information, plan the radiation beams, and deliver the radiation dose accurately to the tumor volumes.
- Quality assurance and radiation protection are essential parts of radiation therapy to ensure safe and accurate delivery of radiation doses to patients using sophisticated machines.

INTRODUCTION

Radiation therapy is a technology-driven medical subspecialty. It is 1 of the 3 modalities used in the management of cancers besides chemotherapy and surgery. The medical applications of radiation began immediately after the discovery of the X-ray by Roentgen and radium by Curie. Radiation therapy has evolved through a number of innovations, including the development of artificially produced isotopes, the introduction of high-energy radiation therapy machines, the development of remote afterloading machines for brachytherapy, and the transformation to imaged-based radiation therapy. The transformation to image-based radiation therapy marks a shift in paradigm for radiation oncology practices and also the transition of radiation therapy into the electronic age.

Disclosure Statement: The authors have nothing to disclose.
[a] Northeast Radiation Oncology Centers (NROC), 1110 Meade Street, Dunmore, PA 18512, USA;
[b] University of Nebraska Medical Center, 987521 Nebraska Medical Center, Omaha, NE 68198, USA
* Corresponding author.
E-mail address: cheng.saw@aol.com

Hematol Oncol Clin N Am 33 (2019) 915–928
https://doi.org/10.1016/j.hoc.2019.08.009
0889-8588/19/© 2019 Elsevier Inc. All rights reserved.

A crucial entity of image-based radiation therapy is the 3-dimensional (3D) treatment planning system. It consists of a sophisticated software package that extracts patient data and tumor information from image datasets acquired using imaging modalities, designs treatment plans, and generates instructions for executions by dose delivery systems to treat the patients. The exquisite images in the image dataset allow clear delineation of the tumors and anatomic organs in 3 dimensions, making the radiation fields to focus on the tumors and spare the surrounding normal tissues. Because of the fast computing power and large computer storage space, the designing processes of the treatment plan can be complex and yet the treatment plan can be generated within days. Modern treatment techniques cannot be implemented without the use of the 3D treatment planning systems. The 3D treatment planning system is also capable of managing temporal effects caused by periodic motion, such as respiratory movements.

The advancement of radiation medicine has been attributed to the participation of research physicists with interest in radiation. These research physicists, called radiation physicists, can be found in research laboratories, national laboratories, nuclear plants, and hospitals. With the expanded use of radiation, the term "radiation physics" has been subdivided into specialized fields. Health physics deals with the issue of radiation exposure to personnel and the public in the radiation environment. Medical physics refers to the field of physics as applied to medicine. With the profound influence of radiation medicine, medical physicists are generally responsible for the radiation-producing equipment and the technical aspects of the use of the equipment to support patient care. The term "radiation oncology physics" or "therapeutic medical physics" refers to the physics as applied to radiation oncology or radiation therapy. Therapeutic medical physics concentrates on the following:

a. The physical aspects of therapeutic application of radiation.
b. The equipment used in radiation production, applications, measurements, and evaluation.
c. The quality control of each step in the application of radiation to patients.
d. Providing consults to the radiation oncology team.

RADIATION PROTECTION

Associated with the medical use of radiation is the concern of radiation that can harm humans. In the past, radiation protection was concerned with the exposures to personnel and medical staff. These concerns were linked to high exposures from radionuclides of radium-226, radon-222, cobalt-60, and cesium-137. These radionuclides emit high-energy gamma rays and had high exposures to personnel and medical staff performing the medical procedures, such as in source preloading technique. The development of afterloading techniques has reduced the exposure levels significantly by having the radiation sources brought to the patient for treatment after the medical procedures. These radionuclides are now rarely used clinically. High-activity cobalt-60 and cesium-137 sources in teletherapy units are moved mechanically into positions to treat the patients. These sources can jam and require repair, giving exposures to the physicists or service engineers in addition to the patients and therapists. Today medical linear accelerators are the primary radiation therapy machines where there is no source per se, and the machine can be simply turned off for repairs.

The exposure limits are dictated by the state and federal regulatory guidelines. Generally these guidelines in the United States were adopted from the National Council on Radiation Protection and Measurements recommendations.[1] The dose-limiting recommendations are summarized in **Table 1**. The equivalent dose expresses the exposure to a tissue type or an organ. The effective dose is the whole body exposure derived by summing the weighted doses to various organs. The SI unit of equivalent dose and effective dose is the Sievert (Sv). It is the product of the biological factor and the absorbed dose expressed in Gray (Gy). In the medical environment, the biological factor can be taken as one. The traditional unit of equivalent dose and effective dose is the rem (radiation equivalent man). One Sievert is equal to 100 rem.

ABSORBED DOSE

When a high-energy photon beam traverses through a medium, the atoms are excited and ionized. The excitation and ionization in tissues cause biological effects in radiation therapy. As a result of the ionization, kinetic energies are released and electrons with a range of energies are ejected from the atoms. The ejected electrons undergo further interactions through excitations and ionizations, and thereafter deposit their energies to the medium downstream. The amount of energy transferred to the electrons at the point of the initial interaction is called "kerma," an acronym for kinetic energy released in a medium per unit mass. The second stage of the energy-transfer process is called "absorbed dose." Not all the energy transferred to the medium at the point of initial interaction is absorbed. Some of the energy is radiated away as bremsstrahlung, and the remaining is called "collision kerma." The absorbed dose

Table 1 Dose-limiting recommendations	
Types of Exposure	**Dose Limit, mSv**
Occupational exposures	
Effective dose limits	
Annual	50
Cumulative	10× age
Equivalent dose annual limits for tissues and organs	
Lens of eye	150
Skin, hand and feet	500
Public exposures (annual)	
Effective dose limit, continuous or frequent exposure	1
Effective dose limit, infrequent exposure	5
Effective dose limits for tissues and organs	
Lens of eye	15
Skin, hand and feet	50
Education and training exposures (annual)	
Effective dose limit	1
Equivalent dose limits for tissues and organs	
Lens of eye	15
Skin, hand and feet	50
Embryo-fetus exposures (monthly)	
Equivalent dose limit	0.5
Negligible individual dose (annual)	0.01

(With permission of the National Council on Radiation Protection and Measurements, http://NCRPonline.org.)

is the energy retained in the medium along the path of the electrons. If the electron track has an appreciable length, the transfer of energy (kerma) and the absorption of energy (absorbed dose) take place at separate locations.

When a photon beam impinges on a medium, the initial ionization of atoms takes place at the surface of the medium. The energy is directly transferred to the ejected electrons, and so kerma has a maximum value at the surface. Then kerma decreases as a function of depth because the photon beam intensity (fluence) decreases resulting from the beam absorption and scatter. On the other hand, absorbed dose is initially low at the medium surface and increases to a maximum and thereafter decreases as a function of depth into the medium. The region from the surface to the depth of maximum dose is called the "buildup region." The position of the maximum absorbed dose is called "point of equilibrium," and the region beyond the maximum dose is the region of transient electronic equilibrium. True electronic equilibrium does not exist because kerma is continuously decreasing, creating fewer energetic electrons in the forward direction. Therefore, the absorbed dose curve is always higher than the collision kerma curve beyond the depth of maximum dose, as shown in **Fig. 1**.

The absorbed dose in air (or in free space) has been used as follows:

a. To characterize the output of a radiation-producing machine
b. To perform tumor dose calculations involving tissue-air-ratios and backscatter factors
c. To calculate dosimetry of photon beams

As described, the absorbed dose has been equated to the collision kerma under equilibrium condition. Under such condition, the collision kerma in air is merely the total kinetic energies transferred to air to produce ion pairs. The collection of charge per unit mass is the exposure, X. The absorbed dose is related to the exposure as

$$D(air) = X \cdot (W/e),$$

where (W/e) is the energy expended in producing an ion pair and has a value of 33.97 eV per ion pair or 33.97 J/C.

The absorbed dose in a medium can be determined by examining the fluence in air and the fluence in the medium. The ratio of these values is called the attenuation factor, A. The next parameter is the relative mass absorption coefficients that relate the absorption characteristic in air and the medium. This factor is called the f-factor or the roentgen-to-rad factor, f. The generalized equation is given as follows:

$$D(medium) = f \cdot X \cdot A.$$

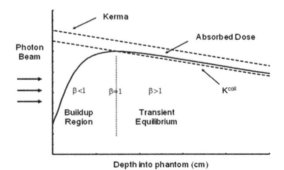

Fig. 1. Relationship between kerma and absorbed dose.

The determination of absorbed dose in a medium through exposure has some practical challenges, in particular for high-energy photon beams. The dosimetry system has to be very large to account for the length of the electron tracks. The second concern is the concept of exposure being defined for photons only. The conceptual approach for the determination of absorbed dose in a medium was based on the Bragg-Gray Cavity theory.[2] This theory or principle states that the absorbed dose at a point in the medium is related to the ionization of a gas-filled cavity at the same point. The relationship is established through the ratio of the mean unrestricted mass collision stopping powers $[S/\mu]$ of the medium to the gas and given as follows:

$$D(medium) = J(W/e)[S/\mu],$$

where J is the charge collected per unit mass of gas.

DOSIMETRY SYSTEMS

Radiation dosimetry or simply dosimetry refers to the subject matter of measuring absorbed dose. This term is loosely used to include other dosimetric quantities, such as exposure, equivalent dose, kerma, and their time derivatives. The mechanisms of detecting radiation are based on the physical interaction of radiation with matter.[3] The detectors called radiation dosimeters or simple dosimeters will have a radiation-sensitive volume to interact with the radiation. If the sensitive volume consists of air, the physical interactions are ionizations resulting in producing ion pairs. If the dosimeter is connected to a reader, the whole arrangement is called a dosimetry system. For example, an ionization chamber connected to an electrometer constitutes an ionization system. If the dosimetry system is based on calculations from the first principle of interactions, the dosimetry system is called absolute dosimetry system, otherwise it is a relative dosimetry system. A relative dosimetry system uses a calibration curve (relating the responses to absorbed dose) measured in a known field to determine the absorbed dose. The commonly used dosimeters are as follows:

a. Ion chambers
b. Diodes
c. Metallic-oxide-semiconductor field-effect transistor (MOSFET)
d. Thermoluminescence detectors (TLD)
e. Optically simulated luminescence detectors (OSLD)

Diodes and MOSFET are solid state or semiconductor detectors. TLD and OSLD are luminescence materials. Because of the need to understand the radiation dose pattern in 3 dimensions, gel dosimetry is being investigated.

A useful dosimetry system must exhibit certain desirable characteristics among which are the following:

a. Good response
b. Sufficient sensitivity to detect minimal radiation
c. Excellent precision and accuracy
d. Independence of dose rate
e. Energy independence for the measurements of a variety of beam qualities
f. Excellent spatial resolution
g. Convenient of use.

Linear response proportional to the amount of imparting radiation is preferred for easy interpolation, otherwise correction factors must be applied for a nonlinear response dosimetry system. The independence of dose rate requires that the integrated responses be the same regardless of the dose rates used. Although a detector has a finite size, the physical dimension should be sufficiently small to approximate to a point dose measurement. Examples of small dosimeters are the TLD and pinpoint microchamber.

The most widely used dosimetry system in radiation therapy is the ion chamber and electrometer system. This dosimetry system is used to calibrate radiation therapy machines in accordance the American Association of Physicists in Medicine (AAPM) reference dosimetry protocol commonly referred to as TG-51 dosimetry protocol.[4] This dosimetry system must be calibrated at an accredited dosimetry calibrated laboratory (ADCL) traceable to the National Standard every 2 years. In addition, it is used for relative dosimetry, for example, measuring the following:

a. The percent depth dose
b. Doses in the buildup region
c. Penumbra doses
d. Output factors

An ion chamber consists of an outer shell that defines the sensitive volume and an inner central electrode; however, the outer shell must be designed such that the ionization collected in the chamber is not influenced by its physical size and physical density of the medium surrounding the collecting volume. The central electrode acts as a terminal for the collection of charge and the electrode is adjusted so the chamber is effectively air-equivalent. The dosimetry using this system is described as follows:

$$D = M \cdot k_Q \cdot N_D \,,$$

where M is the corrected measurement, k_Q is the quality conversion factor, and N_D is the ADCL coefficient that converts ionization measurements into absorbed dose. The measurements must be corrected for measuring conditions such as the following:

a. Temperature and pressure
b. Ion-combination
c. Polarization
d. Electrometer accuracy

OSLDs are commonly used in clinics today. The operational principle is similar to TLD. The certain crystalline material embedded in TLD and OSLD is capable of storing a minute amount of energy deposited (energy traps) by radiation. When the crystal is heated, it emits a certain amount of light that is proportional to the amount of radiation absorbed in the TLD. Instead of heating, a stimulated emission process is used to determine the amount of radiation absorbed in the OSLD. The OSLD dosimeter is a chip of carbon-doped aluminum oxide (Al_2O_3:C). Unlike TLD, no preparation of the OSLD, such as annealing or batching, is needed.

TREATMENT PLANNING SYSTEMS

Radiation therapy procedure has changed from mechanical-based to imaged-based technology. The procedure for a patient undergoing radiation therapy consists of the following:

a. Patient simulation
b. Treatment planning
c. Patient dose verification

d. Target localization
e. Radiation dose delivery

In the past, the patient simulation involved an immobilization system to hold the patient in position for both the simulation and treatments. Then radiation beam entry called beam ports were defined, and treatment planning parameters such as patient body contour and interfield distances were manually collected. The treatment planning process consists of digitizing the manually collected patient data and then running the radiation dose calculations. At the radiation therapy machine before radiation dose delivery, the setup parameters from the treatment planning report were manually checked and confirmed using radiographs. In addition, the machine parameters were double checked before radiation dose delivery.

The introduction of a 3D treatment planning system (TPS) signaled the shift of paradigm for radiation oncology into image-based radiation therapy. The TPS has been considered the "brain" of modern radiation therapy procedure. It contains a 3D dose calculation algorithm based on the convolution techniques or Monte Carlo method to generate the radiation dose distribution. The patient simulation consists of immobilizing the patient and then simply scanning the region of interest using a helical computed tomography (CT) scanner. If the target is anticipated to move, gating technique called 4DCT scanning can be implemented to record the internal tumor motion. The patient is released immediately. The visit time for the patient is therefore very short compared with the traditional method. The image dataset is downloaded through the network using DICOM protocols (an international standard for digital data transmission) into the treatment planning system and the treatment planning parameters, such as the body contour, are extracted automatically after a virtual patient is constructed by the TPS. The dose planner (medical dosimetrist or physicist) can take as long as needed to generate a high-quality treatment plan.

The treatment planning processes involve 4 steps, as outlined in **Fig. 2**. The first step is downloading the CT image dataset and preparing the image data set for treatment planning (planning image dataset). This involves the following:

a. Selecting appropriate Hounsfield unit conversion to electron density curve
b. Replacing CT couch with the treatment couch
c. Defining laser points

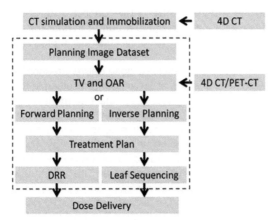

Fig. 2. A typical treatment planning workflow. Tasks within the dotted plots are performed by the TPS. TV, target volume.

d. Setting the original on the image dataset

e. Extracting patient body contour

f. Constructing a virtual patient

Next, the outlines or contours of the target volume and organs at risk (OARs) are drawn. Before contouring, the image dataset is evaluated for target motion. If the tumor is not visible on the CT image dataset, coregistration with other imaging modalities, such as PET or MRI, whereby the tumors are visible, may be required to define the target volume. After the target and OARs are defined, the prescription dose and other treatment concerns are discussed. The treatment planning process proceeds in 2 ways called forward planning and inverse planning. In forward planning, the radiation fields are placed based on the dose planner experience and knowledge to obtain a quality treatment plan. On the other hand, the inverse planning requires inputs of the desired doses on the target volume and dose limits to the OARs and then allows the computer to search for an optimal treatment plan that satisfies these dose constraints. Because the target volume and OARs are competing doses, the dose planner must decide and adjust the priority of each of these structures and repeat the process until an acceptable treatment plan is obtained.

After the planning, the TPS creates the digitally reconstructed radiographs (DRRs) for the verification of OAR sparing and target localization at the treatment machine before radiation dose delivery. The DRRs behave like radiographs of the patient taken by an x-ray machine with the same source to patient distances. In addition to creating DRRs, the TPS also must breakdown the treatment plan (leaf sequencing) in such a way that it can be delivered by a radiation therapy machine through a verification and record system.

The design of a treatment plan can be very complex. A 3D planning software package permits the implementation of conformal radiation therapy (CRT), intensity-modulated radiation therapy (IMRT), and volumetric modulated arc therapy (VMAT). In CRT planning, the radiation fields are designed so that the radiation dose conforms to the target volume.[5] In IMRT planning, the radiation fields are modulated so that the target volume is covered with the prescription dose and OARs are spared as needed.[6] In VMAT planning, conformal arcs are modulated as the machine gantry rotates around the patient. The VMAT treatment technique is elegant in producing radiation dose to conform to the target volume and minimize the radiation dose to OARs, as well as shorten the dose delivery times compared with IMRT. **Fig. 3** shows a sample dose distribution in the treatment of prostate cancer. The optimized target dose coverage and isodose lines that can curve around to spare the rectum and bladder are attributed to the use of inverse planning and the implementation of the IMRT treatment technique.

Focal irradiation refers to the specialized dose delivery technique in which multiple narrow radiation beams are directed at focal points resulting in the formation of very small but concentrated high-dose regions for the treatment of small lesions. In the past, this treatment technique was limited to a few medical centers, but today it can be implemented in a larger number of facilities using modern medical linear accelerators because of the advanced technology in radiation therapy. The initial application of this technique was the irradiation of intracranial lesions in a single fraction without regard for the radiobiological impact of the treatment. The focal irradiation of intracranial lesions given in a few fractions is called stereotactic radiosurgery or simply radiosurgery.[7] If the treatment is fractionated, it is called stereotactic radiation therapy. If the lesion is outside the brain, the focal irradiation is called stereotactic body radiation therapy (SBRT) or stereotactic ablative therapy (SABR).[8] **Fig. 4** shows a sample of

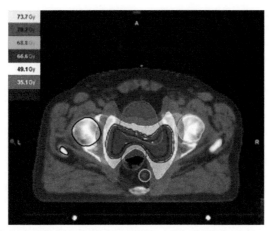

Fig. 3. Complex dose distribution in the treatment of prostate bed.

dose distribution in the treatment of lung lesion using SBRT technique. The high-dose region is very small and the dose conformation to the target volume spares most of the lungs. Failure to understand the principle of focal irradiation technique can lead to increased skin or normal tissue toxicities.[9]

EXTERNAL BEAM RADIATION THERAPY

External beam radiation therapy refers to the delivery of radiation dose from a radiation source external to the patient. In the past, this form of radiation dose delivery was called teletherapy to signify that the source was at a distance from the patient. The radiation source was originally produced in orthovoltage machines. Approximately

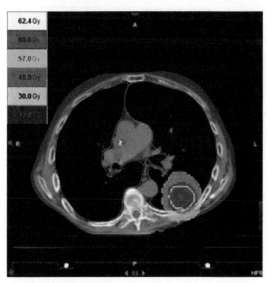

Fig. 4. Conformal high-dose region for the treatment of lung lesion using SBRT treatment technique.

1950, there was development of accelerator technology leading to the production of high-energy therapy machines and radionuclide teletherapy machines. The use of cobalt-60 and cesium-137 teletherapy has declined over the years. Early accelerators such as Van de Graaff and Betatrons had been decommissioned except medical linear accelerators.

The medical linear accelerator produces photon beams by accelerating electron beam to strike a target. The electron beam, in the form of pulses, is injected in phase with the microwave power into the waveguide. An electron pulse in phase can be conceptually explained as a person surfing on the sea wave. If the surfing is in phase with the wave, the person would be accelerated. Microwave power is supplied by either a magnetron or a klystron. Once the electron pulses reach a certain kinetic energy, the pulse of electron beam is stirred to strike a target. The emitted photon beam is collimated using the primary collimator and then the secondary collimators. Instead of secondary collimators, medical linear accelerators have a multileaf collimation system that is driven by a microprocessor to shape and modulate the traversing photon beam to deliver radiation dose to the tumors. The photon beam entry can be oriented around the patient by rotating the machine gantry. Flexibility also involves the use of collimator rotation and treatment couch rotation. Contemporary medical linear accelerators, as shown in **Fig. 5**, have improved mechanical tolerances to within ±1 mm and image-guidance radiation therapy (IGRT) systems to perform precise targeting and accurate radiation dose delivery.

The alignment of the patient to the radiation beam is performed using IGRT technology. The imaging system integrated into the treatment machine is called on-board imaging system. There are 2 types of imaging techniques called kV-kV imaging and cone-beam computed tomography (CBCT). In the kV-kV imaging technique, 2 orthogonal radiographs are taken and compared with the DRRs from the TPS. On

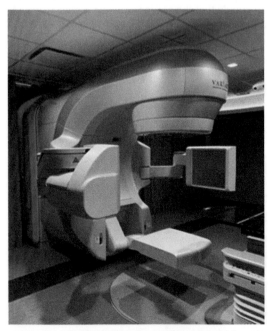

Fig. 5. Contemporary medical linear accelerator with on-board imaging system for IGRT. (*Courtesy of* Varian Medical Systems, Palo Alto, CA.)

the other hand, a CBCT requires radiographs to be taken around the patient and reconstructed in the axial, coronal, and sagittal views. The CBCT images are coregistered with those exported from the TPS and the deviations are used to align the patient. This methodology has resulted in the precise localization of the target in modern radiation therapy. Other methods of patient alignment have been used, including in-room CT, ultrasound-based system, optical surface monitoring system, and Calypso extracranial tracking system.

Although most of the dose delivery systems in the radiation therapy facility are medical linear accelerators, there are other types of dose delivery systems. The helical tomotherapy was designed to perform IMRT. It consists of a small linear accelerator mounted on a rotating gantry delivering radiation dose to the patient as the patient moves through the gantry like a helical CT scanner. The helical tomotherapy is an efficient machine in performing extended length treatment. The Cyberknife is another dose delivery system consisting of a small linear accelerator mounted on a robotic arm. The robotic arm moves the irradiation source to strategic locations around the patient to deliver the radiation dose in non-coplanar fashion, using the optimal delivery angles in a 3D space. Such arrangement is well suited to perform focal irradiation. The Gamma Knife system consists of 192 cobalt sources arranged in a hemispheric fashion around the patient's head to treat intracranial lesions. With the advancement of technology, it is anticipated that future dose delivery systems will be highly automated and simplify radiation dose delivery processes.

Particle Beam Radiation Therapy

The use of charged-particle beams in radiation therapy is increasing. The law governing the interactions of charged-particle beams with matter is the long-range Coulomb force. The interaction generally does not involve direct hits of the orbital electrons or the atomic nuclei. Although the chance of interaction with orbital electrons is small, it dominates the energy transfer for the range of energies in charged-particle beam therapy. When a collision occurs, it causes the excitation and ionization of atoms. The rate of energy transfer increases as the particles slow down as the inverse square of the velocity. At very low energies or low velocity, most of the energy is deposited at the end of the range through nucleic interactions with oxygen and carbon, the principal constituents of tissues. This abrupt energy transfer to a small area in tissue leads to the observation of a dose enhancement peak called the Bragg Peak. In principle, the particle energy can be adjusted such that the Bragg Peak occurs within the target volume space. This is the impetus of proton beam radiation therapy to optimize the radiation dose delivery. Because the target volume has a large physical size, a series of different proton beam energies is used so that the systematic sum covers the target volume. This process is called spread out Bragg Peak. Conceptually, a single field can be used for the treatment and hence limit doses to normal tissue. This concept is very appealing, especially in the treatment of childhood cancers. However, with the level of sophistication offered, intensity-modulated particle beam therapy is often used. Besides protons, heavier nuclei like carbon-13 have been used in radiation therapy. In addition to localization, a heavier particle beam has higher Relative Biological Effectiveness, which is an advantage for the treatment of radioresistant tumors.

Brachytherapy

Brachytherapy is a treatment modality in which the radiation source is placed near or directly into the tumors. Because the dose falls off from a radiation source as an inverse square of the distance, the radiation dose is highly conformal to the tumors and spares the normal tissues. A limitation of brachytherapy has been the accessibility of the tumor or target volume. Brachytherapy is classified as low-dose rate (LDR), medium-dose rate, and high-dose rate (HDR). We think of LDR brachytherapy as the treatment in days, whereas for HDR brachytherapy, the treatment is in minutes. Another distinction in brachytherapy is temporary and permanent implants. In temporary implants, the sources are removed after the treatment, whereas in permanent implants the sources are left in the patient to decay. Contemporary temporary brachytherapy is performed using remote afterloading systems in particular using HDR remote afterloading systems. The remote afterloading technology allows the radiation source to be inserted into the patient remotely and perform the medical procedure in a shielded room thereby eliminating the radiation exposure to the personnel and medical staff.

The brachytherapy procedure involves inserting catheters or applicators into the patient typically in an operating room. These catheters or applicators provide pathways for loading and holding radiation sources. After the insertion, the patient is scanned using an imaging modality, typically CT helical scanner, to define the location of the catheters and/applicators. The image dataset is downloaded into a TPS in which the target volume and OARs are delineated. The catheters or applicators are constructed for source position definition called dwell positions. The dwell positions are then activated (dwell times) to create the dose distribution. Once the treatment plan is accepted, the description of the dwell position and dwell times is exported and retrieved by the remote afterloading system for radiation dose delivery. The advantages of HDR brachytherapy are as follows:

a. The optimization of dose patterns
b. Short treatment times in the order of a few minutes
c. Outpatient treatment
d. Reduced radiation hazards

Radioactive sources used in permanent implants have lower photon energies, as listed in **Table 2**. Hence, it is ease to handle for radiation protection, such as wearing gloves and a lead apron. The implant procedure is typically performed in an operating room, and as such is performed in a limited number of facilities.

QUALITY ASSURANCE

Quality assurance (QA) in radiation therapy stresses on the ability of the therapeutic procedures to deliver the prescribed dose to the target volume allowing a variation no more than ±5%.[10] The uncertainties associated with these therapeutic procedures were assessed and tolerance levels were assigned to comply with the stated constraints as published in AAPM Report No. 13.[11] This AAPM Report deals only with the physical aspects of radiation therapy, namely instrumentation and equipment.

Table 2
Radionuclides used in brachytherapy

Radionuclides	Energy, MeV	Half-Life	Applications
Cesium-131	0.030	9.7 d	Permanent
Cobalt-60	1.25	5.27 y	High-dose rate
Iodine-125	0.028	59.5 d	Permanent
Iridium-192	0.38	73.8 d	High-dose rate
Palladium-103	0.021	17.0 d	Permanent

As radiation therapy matures, the QA is not only limited to the physical aspects but should also include the clinical aspects of patient care. This was discussed in the AAPM Report No. 46 published in 1994 and also the need on continuing quality improvement indices.[12]

Since the publication of AAPM Report No. 46, radiation therapy has undergone a shift in paradigm into imaged-based technology. Hence, some routine radiation therapy procedures are no longer considered to be routine in the new image-based radiation therapy era. The radiation oncology community had expressed concerns that the technological advancements in radiation therapy have been so rapid that safeguards and QA are not keeping pace. This led AAPM and American Society of Radiation Oncology to hold a joint symposium on QA in 2007. The emphasis from the symposium was to transform from prescriptive-based to risk assessment-based in the design of the QA procedures.

DISCUSSION

Radiation therapy is a constantly evolving medical subspecialty. Besides external beam radiation therapy, particle beam therapy, and brachytherapy, there are on-going innovations for the therapeutic use of radiation as well as other physics-related programs. Concurrent, adjuvant, or neoadjuvant radiation therapy in combination with chemotherapy is an example of on-going innovation program. Intraoperative radiation therapy involves the irradiation of the tumor bed at the time of surgery and requires the cooperation of the surgical and radiation oncology team. Photodynamic therapy is the use of optical frequency to trigger introduced chemical agent in tissues to cause ablative effects. Hyperthermia is the use of heat in combination with chemotherapy and/or radiation to treat radioresistant tumors. Internal radionuclide therapy is the use of radionuclides for systemic treatment. High-intensity focused ultrasound is a recent and noninvasive innovation that uses ultrasound and imaging to treat prostate cancer. Artificial intelligence, either machine learning or deep learning, is being investigated in radiation therapy. Therapeutic medical physics is not limited to radiation therapy technology but all types of technologies to ensure their safe and efficient application to support patient care.

SUMMARY

The interaction of radiation with tissues and thereafter energy deposition (absorbed dose) causing biological effects is the basis of radiation therapy. There are a number of dosimeters available to measure radiation doses. Contemporary radiation therapy is highly automated using a series of imaging, computing, and dose delivery equipment connected through the digital networks. Three-dimensional TPSs offer the ability to generate complex treatment plans and break down into executable instructions for the radiation dose delivery systems to deliver the prescribed doses. Because radiation therapy processes are highly technical and complex, QA and radiation protection are essential to support safe and optimal patient treatments.

REFERENCES

1. NCRP report no. 116. Limitation of exposure to ionization radiation. Bethesda (MD): National Council on Radiation Protection and Measurements; 1993.
2. John HE, Cunningham JR. The physics of radiology. 4th edition. Springfield (IL): Charles C Thomas Publisher; 1983 [Chapter 7].

3. Saw CB. Foundation of radiological physics. Omaha (NE): C.B.Saw Publishing, LLC; 2004.
4. Almond PR, Biggs PJ, Coursey BM, et al. AAPM report no. 67. AAPM's TG51 protocol for clinical reference dosimetry of high-energy photon and electron beams. Med Phy 1999;26:1847–70.
5. Fraass BA. The development of conformal radiation therapy. Med Phy 1995;22: 1911–21.
6. Purdy JA. The development of intensity-modulated radiation therapy. In: Sternick ES, editor. The theory & practice of intensity modulated radiation therapy. Madison (WI): Advanced Medical Publishing; 1997. p. 51–73.
7. AAPM report no. 54. Stereotactic radiosurgery. Woodbury (NY): American Institute of Physics, Inc.; 1995.
8. Benedict SH, Yenice KM, Followill D, et al. AAPM report no. 101. Stereotactic body radiation therapy: the report of AAPM Task Group 101. Med Phy 2010;37: 4078–101.
9. Hoppe BS, Laser B, Kowalski AV, et al. Acute skin toxicity following stereotactic body radiation therapy for stage I non-small-cell lung cancer: who's at risk. Int J Radiat Oncol Biol Phys 2008;72:1283–6.
10. ICRU report no. 24. Determination of absorbed dose in a patient irradiated by beams of X or gamma rays in Radiotherapy procedures. Washington (DC): International Commission on Radiation Units and Measurements; 1976.
11. AAPM report no. 13. Physical aspects of quality assurance in radiation therapy. New York: American Institute of Physics, Inc.; 1984.
12. Kutcher GJ, Coia L, Gillin M, et al. AAPM report no. 46. Comprehensive QA for radiation oncology: report of AAPM Radiation Therapy Committee Task Group 40. Med Phy 1994;21:581–618.

Toward a New Framework for Clinical Radiation Biology

Henning Willers, MD*, Florence K. Keane, MD, Sophia C. Kamran, MD

KEYWORDS

- Radiation biology • Ionizing radiation • Fractionation • Biomarkers
- Precision radiation medicine • Immuno-oncology

KEY POINTS

- Time-tested factors that inform fractionated radiation therapy include the relationship between local tumor control and radiation dose as well as the importance of fractionation and overall treatment time.
- Technological advances provide opportunities for developing predictive tumor and normal tissue biomarkers that will enhance therapeutic gain in individual patients.
- Immunostimulatory and immunosuppressive effects of radiation are increasingly appreciated and will affect patient management in multiple ways.
- Developments in precision oncology and immuno-oncology pave the way toward a new framework for radiation biology that emphasizes treatment individualization and predictive biomarker development.

INTRODUCTION TO CLINICAL RADIATION BIOLOGY

Over the past century, experimental insights into biological responses to ionizing radiation (IR) in conjunction with medical physics advances, clinical studies, and clinical empiricism have shaped the way IR is delivered in the treatment of cancers.[1] A critical contribution of radiation biology to clinical practice has provided a rational basis for IR dosing, dose fractionation, and treatment duration to maximize local control (LC) of tumors while limiting injury to normal tissues. Historically, the framework of the so-called Rs has been used to explain the effects of curative radiation therapy (RT) on tumors and normal tissues (**Fig. 1**A). However, a deepening understanding of the hallmarks

Disclosure: Dr. Willers has received funding from National Cancer Institute (Grant number U01CA220714).
Department of Radiation Oncology, Massachusetts General Hospital, Harvard Medical School, 55 Fruit Street, Boston, MA 02114, USA
* Corresponding author.
E-mail address: hwillers@partners.org
twitter: @henningwillers (H.W.); @KatieKeaneMD (F.K.K.); @sophia_kamran (S.C.K.)

Hematol Oncol Clin N Am 33 (2019) 929–945
https://doi.org/10.1016/j.hoc.2019.07.001
0889-8588/19/© 2019 Elsevier Inc. All rights reserved.

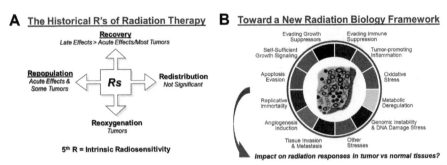

Fig. 1. Clinical radiation biology concepts. (*A*) Classic Rs of fractionated radiation therapy.[1] (*B*) Hallmarks of cancer, which may provide a basis for a better understanding and prediction of RT effects in individual tumors and patients. ([*B*] *Adapted from* Hanahan D, Weinberg RA. Hallmarks of cancer: the next generation. Cell 2011;144(5):646-674; with permission.)

of cancer requires a reassessment of the factors that determine biological responses to IR (**Fig. 1B**).[2] Essential features of any new clinical radiation biology framework will have to include an appreciation of intertumoral and interpatient heterogeneity, the resulting need to establish tumor biomarkers to predict RT outcomes, and a realization of the immune-specific effects of RT.[3,4]

This article discusses time-tested biological concepts underlying the clinical application of RT, adapted from an earlier review.[1] It considers the evolving importance of the precision radiation medicine concept that is beginning to affect clinical practice as well as the exciting interactions of IR with antitumor immune responses. The complexity of this rapidly expanding field and space constraints require us to use simplifications for didactic purposes; some of these may represent our own biases. The authors also apologize to the many investigators whose work we are unable to cite.

DNA DAMAGE INDUCTION AND REPAIR
Radiation Damage to DNA

Damage to DNA is the principal mechanism by which IR injures cells and tissues.[1] The creation of DNA double-strand breaks (DSBs) represents the most important damage that, if not adequately repaired, may directly or indirectly lead to cell death. Photon-based IR deposits its energy mostly in spurs, regions about twice the diameter of the DNA double helix. Damage sites are therefore complex (clustered lesions). For example, a DSB may be accompanied by extensive base damage, which is difficult for the cell to repair accurately. DSBs can produce many types of chromosomal aberrations and rearrangements. Lethal aberrations are those that cause cells to die when attempting mitosis. Alternatively, lethally damaged cells may continue to divide a limited number of times before undergoing mitotic or apoptotic death or finally ceasing to divide. Because IR often makes cells lose their proliferative capacity rather than causing immediate cell death, radiation biologists prefer the term cell inactivation rather than killing.

Double-strand Break Repair

The two principal DSB repair pathways are homologous recombination repair (HRR) and nonhomologous end joining (NHEJ), which use separate as well as overlapping protein complexes. The study of these pathways has been a rapidly evolving field over the past 2 decades.[5–8] Defects in HRR or NHEJ result in inaccurately repaired or unrepaired DSBs, leading to genomic alterations in the surviving cells that can promote malignant transformation. At the same time, DSB repair may affect tumor radiosensitivity and sensitivity to dose fractionation (discussed later).

RADIATION DOSE-RESPONSE RELATIONSHIPS
Clonogenic and Cancer Stem Cells

Clonogenic tumor cells have historically been defined as cells that have the capacity to produce an expanding family of daughter cells and form colonies following irradiation in an in vitro assay or give rise to a recurrent tumor in in vivo models. To what extent clonogenic cells resemble cancer stem cells (CSCs) is poorly understood but the terms have been used interchangeably.[9,10] To control a tumor, all CSCs have to be inactivated as only one surviving CSC can give rise to a recurrence. At first approximation, cell inactivation by IR is both random and logarithmic.[1] The success of treatment is determined by the fraction of tumors without any surviving CSCs. As a result, logarithmic cell inactivation translates into a sigmoid dose-response curve (**Fig. 2**A). In many patients, a dose high enough for tumor eradication cannot be delivered without unacceptable injury to surrounding normal tissues. **Fig. 2**B illustrates how local tumor control probability (TCP) decreases with increasing tumor volume, which correlates with a higher number of CSCs. Similarly, clinical data suggest that TCP declines with increasing tumor volume.[11,12]

Tumor Control Probability Curves

In clinical practice, TCP curves for a patient population are presumed to be flatter than in individual patients because of interpatient and intertumoral heterogeneity (**Fig. 2**C).[1]

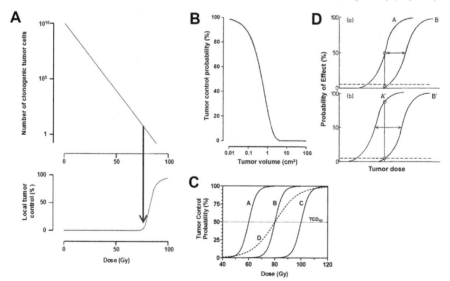

Fig. 2. Dose-response relationships. (A) Linear increase in dose produces exponential tumor cell inactivation, which translates into LC as a function of Poisson statistics. (B) The relationship between the number of clonogenic tumor cells/CSCs and IR dose dictates the decline in LC with increasing tumor volume. (C) Hypothetical clinical dose-response curves. A–C, Individual tumors. (D) Composite curve; TCD50, dose required to control 50% of tumors. (D) Therapeutic ratio. A, Probability of effect on tumor (eg, LC). B, Probability of normal tissue complications (eg, late effects). (Adapted from Willers H, Held KD. Introduction to clinical radiation biology. Hematol Oncol Clin North Am 2006;20(1):7; with permission.)

The more heterogeneous a patient population is, the flatter the dose-response curve becomes and the more difficult it is to detect an improvement in treatment outcome with increasing dose. Factors that cause a flattening of the curve include differences in tumor size (number of CSCs), DSB repair capacity, and hypoxia. Therefore, it is not possible to apply the dose-response findings observed in a population (curve D) to a given patient whose individual dose-response curve is unknown (curves A, B, or C). To allow predictions for an individual patient from a dose-response relationship observed in a clinical study population, it is crucial to make that patient population as homogenous as possible, which results in a steeper composite curve; for example, by limiting the range of tumor volumes or excluding likely incurable tumors. Alternatively, predictive biomarkers may guide in the identification of individual curves or subsets (discussed later).[13]

THERAPEUTIC RATIO
Tumor Versus Normal Tissue Effects

The goal of RT is to achieve maximal LC while limiting injury to surrounding normal tissues and the patient.[1] Early-responding or acute-responding normal tissues are typically those that have a high cell turnover rate (eg, skin, mucosa). These tissues express damage usually within weeks of RT. By contrast, late-responding normal tissues are slowly turning over or not proliferating and express damage after months and years (eg, kidney, spinal cord). To inactivate all CSCs that could give rise to a recurrence, acute side effects of a certain severity are often accepted. However, the risk of serious late complications must be minimized in surviving patients.

Improving the Therapeutic Ratio

Both tumor effect and normal tissue complications need to be carefully considered.[1] In **Fig. 2**D, tumor dose is plotted against TCP (curve A) and dose-limiting late normal tissue complications (curve B). The delivery of a curative dose is generally associated with a certain risk of complications. Increasing the tumor dose beyond the dose indicated on curve A may result in an unacceptable risk. To improve the therapeutic ratio, curves A and B need to be separated from each other; that is, the effect on the tumor needs to be enhanced (curve A shifts left, as shown), or complications need to be reduced (B shifts right), or both. This outcome may be achieved by making RT delivery more precise or biologically modifying RT.

THE R OF RECOVERY
Split-dose Recovery

Fractionation means that the total dose is divided into several daily treatments of a specific size. Fractionation with 5 daily treatments per week of 1.8 to 2 Gy has evolved empirically in many countries.[1] This approach has been found to spare late-responding normal tissues relative to tumors and, over a several-week treatment course, limit acute toxicity just enough to facilitate the delivery of tumoricidal total doses. Together with the technical ability to focus the dose on the tumor through multiple beams or arcs, fractionation effects form the basis of the ability of RT to eradicate tumors without prohibitive toxicity (**Fig. 3**A).

The sparing of late-responding normal tissues by fractionation can be described by the recovery of cells from a certain damage type between fractions. In this concept, each of these damages are by themselves sublethal, but when 2 of them interact they become lethal. As illustrated in **Fig. 3**B, sublethal damage caused by an earlier fraction cannot interact with a later fraction if repaired in time. Somewhat surprisingly,

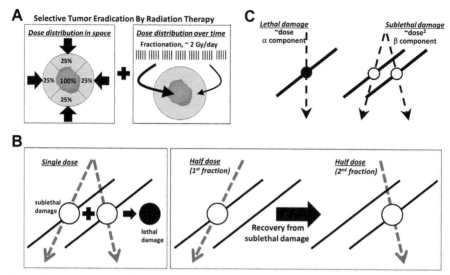

Fig. 3. Importance of radiation dose fractionation. (*A*) Success of RT is based on physical dose conformality and fractionation. (*B*) Lethal and sublethal IR damage as predicted from the linear-quadratic formalism.[1] (*C*) Cell/tissue sparing caused by split-dose recovery. In this example, the sublethal damage caused by delivery of half the dose cannot interact with sublethal damage produced by the second to form lethal damage because of recovery during the interfraction time interval.

the molecular basis of this split-dose recovery remains incompletely understood.[14–16] A compelling hypothesis is that certain types of DSBs when produced in the G0/1 phase of the cell cycle (in which late-responding normal tissues mostly reside) are particularly prone to forming lethal chromosomal aberrations. These aberrations may be caused by unscheduled NHEJ, which generates DNA rearrangements through misrejoining of DSB ends when these are in close proximity. Thus, reducing dose/fraction decreases the probability of DSBs coinciding and subsequent misrejoining.

Fractionation Sensitivity of Normal Tissues and Tumors

Importantly, there exists a consistent difference between early-responding and late-responding normal tissues in their sensitivity to fraction size. Late-responding tissues universally have a greater ability to recover from sublethal damage during fractionated exposure than do early-responding tissues.[1] This different fractionation effect is described by the α/β ratio, which is derived from the linear-quadratic (LQ) formulism used to fit IR survival data. The α component corresponds to lethal IR-induced lesions, which is proportional to the fractional dose, whereas the β component corresponds to sublethal lesions and is thus proportional to fractional dose squared (**Fig. 3C**). The α/β ratio for early-responding tissues is high, ~7 to 20 Gy, with 10 Gy often used as a typical value, because the contribution of sublethal damage to overall cell kill is small (small β). By contrast, late-responding tissues have an average α/β of ~3 Gy, reflecting a greater contribution of β. In clinical practice, α/β ratios and biologically effective doses derived from these values are often used to guide RT fractionation.

Historically, it has been assumed that most tumors respond to fractionation like early-responding normal tissues, with an $\alpha/\beta = 10$ Gy.[1] However, it has become clear that this is a major oversimplification. Several cancer types, such as breast and

Table 1
Cancers α/β values likely not a generic 10 Gy but highly variable

Cancer Type	α/β (Gy)[17–22,b]	Discussion
Adenocarcinomas		
Prostatic	1.2–2.7	—
Breast	2.2–4.6	—
Esophageal cancer	4.9	—
NSCLC[a]	3.9, 8.2	Variable values reported, including >50 Gy, heterogeneity?
Rectal	2.7–11.1	—
Squamous Cell Cancers		
Head/neck	<10–30	Mostly >10 Gy, heterogeneity?
Cervical	10–53	—
Other Examples		
Melanoma	0.6–2.5	Mechanism for low α/β despite fast growth rate unknown
Meningioma	~3.5	Low α/β consistent with typically very slow growth rate
Bladder	13–24	—
SCLC	>>10	Lack of shoulder in vitro suggests very high or infinite α/β

Abbreviations: NSCLC, non–small cell lung cancer; SCLC, small cell lung cancer.
[a] Non–small cell lung cancer contains a mix of histologies, predominantly adenocarcinoma.
[b] Values selected to highlight variability and difference from oversimplified average 10-Gy value.

prostatic adenocarcinoma, have α/β values less than 10 Gy (**Table 1**).[17–22] Even within a given cancer type there is likely considerable variation in α/β. For example, slow-growing lepidic lung adenocarcinomas might have an α/β less than 10 Gy, whereas the α/β of much faster growing squamous cell cancers and small cell lung cancers (SCLCs) are greater than or equal to 20 Gy. Other factors, such as hypoxia and repopulation, affect α/β ratio as well. Predictive biomarkers are urgently needed to stratify tumors according to their α/β.

The low α/β of some tumors have inspired efforts to hypofractionate RT (>2 Gy/fraction). Highly conformal RT delivery approaches ensure that late-responding normal tissues in proximity to the tumor, which also have a low α/β ratio, are only partly exposed to biologically high doses. Importantly, the fractionation sensitivity associated with partial organ irradiation is poorly understood but it seems that much higher maximum doses can be delivered than would be predicted from LQ estimates. In contrast, the use of hyperfractionation (<1.8 Gy/fraction twice a day) to spare late-responding normal tissues has decreased over the past decade.

THE R OF REPOPULATION
Accelerated Repopulation

The time over which the total dose is delivered becomes important if there is repopulation of stem cells within the irradiated tissue or tumor during a multiweek treatment course (**Fig. 4**).[1] During RT, the doubling time of the CSC fraction may become as short as 4 to 5 days compared with often several months before RT. This accelerated CSC repopulation can compensate for ~0.6 to 1 Gy/d in some tumor types, such as

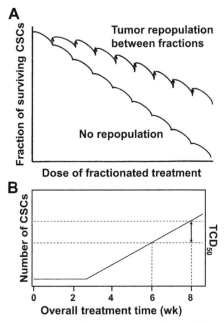

Fig. 4. Tumor cell repopulation during fractionated radiation therapy and the importance of overall treatment time. (*A*) Effect of fractionated IR on clonogenic cell survival with/ without tumor cell repopulation between the fractions. Repopulation increases cell survival. (*B*) The impact of overall treatment time on outcome. Because tumor cells may proliferate rapidly during treatment after a ~3-week lag time, treatment prolongation greater than 6 weeks is associated with an increase in the number of CSCs that need to be inactivated and correspondingly with an increased total dose required to achieve a certain probability of LC. (*Adapted from* Willers H, Held KD. Introduction to clinical radiation biology. Hematol Oncol Clin North Am 2006;20(1):17; with permission.)

head and neck squamous cell cancers (HNSCCs). This kind of dose loss may reduce TCP by ~1%/d.

Repopulation is thought to be an adaptive response to the cytotoxic effects of IR and is likely caused by several poorly understood factors.[10,23] Also, because of the lack of reliable CSC markers, it is currently not possible to detect the fraction of CSCs undergoing accelerated repopulation in a tumor. Thus, although a tumor may initially respond to RT, as shown by radiographic shrinkage, the CSC subpopulation within that tumor may already be rapidly proliferating, thereby offsetting the delivered dose. Clinical and experimental data suggest that accelerated tumor cell repopulation may commence after a lag period of 3 to 4 weeks.[1]

Overall Treatment Time in Clinical Practice

It is unlikely that all tumors of a given histology respond to RT with accelerated repopulation. There is still a lack of clinically tested biomarkers to predict which individual tumors have the potential for accelerated repopulation and which do not.[10] It follows that the overall treatment time should be kept as short as possible for all tumors that have the capacity for accelerated repopulation, such as HNSCC, lung and cervical squamous cancers, and SCLC.[1] This recommendation implies that RT should start on a Monday and not on a Friday to avoid the 2 additional weekend days. In case of unplanned treatment interruptions, several RT adjustments are available to deliver the total dose within the originally prescribed overall time, including treating twice a day, treating on weekends, or increasing total dose (while respecting normal tissue tolerance).

Similar to tumors, an accelerated repopulation response of hierarchical early-responding normal tissues can offset dose as well. Shortening the RT course thus not only improves the tumor effect but also increases acute toxicity, such as mucositis and esophagitis, because early-responding tissues have less time to regenerate. By contrast, treatment duration is not thought to affect slowly proliferating or nonproliferating late-responding normal tissues. However, some exceptions do apply; see Ref.[1]

Radiation Therapy Combined with Chemotherapy

The role of overall treatment time and the importance of accelerated tumor cell repopulation are complicated by the administration of chemotherapy. There are data suggesting that overall treatment time can be less important with concurrent chemotherapy.[24–28] For example, standard fractionated RT over 7 weeks was inferior to a 6-week accelerated course in HNSCC.[29] However, in a repeat of that trial with concurrent cisplatin (3 and 2 concurrent cycles, respectively), there was no difference in outcome.[24] This finding suggests either absence of accelerated repopulation in the presence of chemotherapy or that repopulation occurring during the 1-week differential was offset by the extra cycle of cisplatin in the 7-week arm. In contrast, in the treatment of SCLC with concurrent chemoradiotherapy, the duration of RT remains important, and $\sim$1 Gy/d seems to be needed to compensate for the tumor-sparing effect of treatment prolongation.[28,30] This finding is consistent with the notion that chemotherapeutic agents may not suppress or counterbalance accelerated tumor cell proliferation.[1]

Altered Fractionation

Insights into the importance of fraction size and treatment time generated a variety of altered fractionation schemes that were applied successfully in the clinic. However, these twice-a-day or 3-times-a-day regimens have fallen largely out of favor.[1] Examples of accelerated treatment courses in current clinical practice include (1) twice-a-day regimens (eg, 45 Gy, 1.5 Gy twice a day, 3 weeks, for SCLC[28]); (2) Saturday treatments (eg, $\sim$66 Gy, 2 Gy QD, <6 weeks, for HNSCC in Denmark[31]); (3) hypofractionated RT approaches (facilitated by technologies such as intensity-modulated RT[32]).

THE R OF REOXYGENATION

Cells irradiated in the absence of oxygen are 2-fold to 3-fold more IR resistant than well-oxygenated cells.[1] The mechanism underlying the oxygen effect is not entirely clear but may involve the production of irreparable damage by reaction of molecular oxygen with IR-induced DNA radicals. Variable levels of hypoxia exist in tumors with likely different degrees of associated radioresistance. Radiobiological hypoxia conferring full IR resistance is expected at oxygen concentrations of $\sim$0.1% and lower.[33] In experimental tumors, hypoxic fractions of $\sim$15% are frequently measured with a range of 0% to 50%; similar levels may also be applicable to human tumors.[1]

Hypoxic cells limit the response of tumors to high single doses that preferentially kill well-oxygenated cells, thereby leaving hypoxic cells behind. If this occurs during fractionated RT, the fraction of hypoxic cells slowly increases, thereby increasing the radioresistance of the tumor. However, it is thought that the process of reoxygenation returns the high proportion of hypoxic cells, created immediately after each dose fraction, back toward the level that existed before the delivery of that fraction. If reoxygenation is complete during the time interval between the fractions, hypoxic cells are expected to have little influence on the outcome of treatment. Very short overall treatment times may limit reoxygenation and cause hypoxia to negatively affect treatment outcomes, as has been discussed for stereotactic therapy regimens.[34] Detection and biomarkers of tumor hypoxia as well as therapeutic approaches to overcome hypoxia have recently been reviewed.[33,35]

RADIATION THERAPY IN THE ERA OF PRECISION ONCOLOGY
Precision Radiation Medicine

The concept of precision oncology is expected to transform all aspects of cancer management in the future.[36] Its overarching theme is that management is individualized and tailored to each patient and tumor.[37] A personalized approach can incorporate a variety of genomic, epigenetic, transcriptomic, proteomic, metabolomics, and other patient-specific and tumor-specific factors (**Fig. 5**). Although biologically personalized treatment has been studied for decades in radiation oncology, precision radiation medicine has failed to make a clinical impact to date.[3,4] However, the advent of genomic tumor profiling is expected to provide predictive and prognostic biomarkers that can guide RT individualization.[37]

Tumor Heterogeneity and Predictive Biomarkers

With the advent of next-generation sequencing, gene expression profiling, and experimental studies of tumor sensitivity/resistance, it is now appreciated that there are numerous effects of RT on tumor cells and the microenvironment that are incompletely

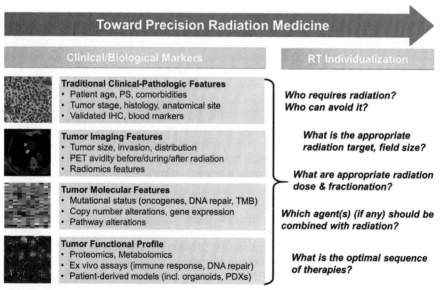

Fig. 5. Opportunities for applying precision medicine tools to guide radiation oncology. IHC, immunohistochemistry; PDX, patient-derived xenografts; PS, performance status; TMB, tumor mutational burden. (*Adapted from* Kamran SC, Lennerz JK, Margolis C, et al. Genomic evolution and acquired resistance to preoperative chemoradiation therapy (CRT) in rectal cancer. J Clin Oncol 2018;36:supplement 4S;abstract 613; with permission.)

understood; many of these may be genomically driven.[37] Studying genomic biomarkers for RT is complex for several reasons. RT is often delivered together with cytotoxic chemotherapy or other systemic agents; hence, it can be difficult to deduce tumor response/resistance effects for RT alone. Furthermore, in large public databases, such as The Cancer Genome Atlas, many sequenced disease states and settings do not include patients who received RT or details of delivered RT.

Methodologies to Identify Candidate Tumor Biomarkers for Radiation Sensitivity/Resistance

Gene expression patterns in tumor samples have been studied with the goal of identifying a signature of IR sensitivity/resistance. Torres-Roca and colleagues[38–40] have identified and extensively verified a 10-gene radiosensitivity index signature that was originally derived using a panel of cancer cell lines. This gene signature was validated in separate clinical cohorts with different tumor types and further evaluated in conjunction with radiobiological estimates to derive a genomics-adjusted radiation dose.[40] Another example is the OncotypeDx test, a gene expression signature for breast cancer genes related to estrogen receptor signaling and cell proliferation. This test has been studied with respect to LC after RT.[41] Separately, an RT-directed gene expression–based assay has been validated for the postprostatectomy setting.[42]

Modern sequencing techniques have facilitated genomic analyses on small amounts of formalin-fixed paraffin-embedded tumor tissue as well as deeply sequenced post-RT samples that may have little, if any, tumor cells left for potential discovery. Using this technology, studies have compared patient-matched pre-RT and post-RT tumors to obtain insight into clonal evolution in response to treatment and understand mechanisms of radioresistance.[43–46] For example, whole-exome sequencing before and after chemoradiotherapy showed that co-occurring *KRAS/ TP53* mutations in rectal cancers conferred a poor response, confirming the radioresistance associated with this genotype.[43,44,47]

Minimally invasive techniques such as circulating tumor DNA (ctDNA) or circulating tumor cells (CTCs) to monitor disease status in response to treatment have paved the way to study dynamic tumoral evolution and tumor heterogeneity without needing multiple tissue biopsies. One study found that, among patients with localized lung cancer who experienced a recurrence after definitive treatment, ctDNA was present in the first posttreatment blood sample, and this presence preceded any other indicators of recurrence by ~5 months.[48] Another study established a blood-based CTC signature in patients with localized and metastatic prostate cancer.[49]

In addition, the use of genomics is not limited to predicting tumor sensitivities but can also be applied to normal tissue toxicity. Of particular interest are single gene polymorphisms and gene expression signatures, validation of which will require large collaborative efforts.[50]

DNA Repair Biomarkers

DNA damage stress, altered DNA repair, and genomic instability constitute hallmarks of cancer that can affect the response to DNA-damaging agents.[5,51,52] However, whether DNA repair alterations affect the sensitivity of cancers to RT remains largely unknown. Genetic or epigenetic HRR defects seem to be common in a variety of cancers.[6,51] In vitro, defective HRR (eg, caused by *BRCA*1/2 mutations) is clearly associated with radiosensitivity.[53] Unexpectedly, this does not readily translate into improved outcomes clinically, and the reasons behind this discrepancy remain unclear.[54] In contrast with HRR, functional NHEJ defects seem to be less frequent in cancers. *ATM*, which may have roles in both HRR and NHEJ, confers pronounced in vitro radiosensitivity when defective, and monoallelic *ATM* mutations in human tumors may cause clinical radiosensitivity.[55] Other examples of clinically relevant DNA damage response (DDR) biomarkers in bladder cancer include overexpression of MRE11 for RT sensitivity and mutations in *ERCC2* for chemosensitivity and potentially also chemoradiosensitivity.[56–58]

The identification of functionally relevant genomic alterations in DDR genes is challenging for several reasons, including the large number of DDR genes, alterations in multiple genes within the same pathway, and difficulties determining functionally important mutations or changes in genes expression levels.[51] Thus, gene expression signatures specific for DDR defects, such as the Recombination Proficiency Score, constitute an attractive alternative.[59] Functional precision radiation medicine represents an alternative or complementary approach. Here, nuclear accumulations of DDR proteins visualized microscopically in tumor biopsies could be used as functional biomarkers to determine DDR pathway status.[60] Potential future directions for biomarker development in radiation oncology are summarized in **Fig. 6**.

RADIATION THERAPY IN THE ERA OF IMMUNO-ONCOLOGY
Arrival of Immunotherapy

Over the past 10 years, immunotherapy has revolutionized the management of advanced cancers. Immune checkpoint inhibitors (ICIs), immune cell therapy, and vaccine-based treatments are in use in multiple tumor types. Interest in combining RT and immunotherapy was initially driven in part by reports of the abscopal effect; that is, the effect of RT at a distance from an irradiated target. A pivotal case report in a patient with metastatic melanoma treated with ipilimumab and RT[61] correlated disease response with levels of peripheral immune cells and antibody titers against a melanoma antigen. Many subsequent studies have reported encouraging results with the combination of RT and ICI in metastatic cancers.[62–65]

Effects of Radiation Therapy on the Immune System

RT has both immunostimulatory and immunosuppressive effects that are independent of systemic therapy. Ongoing clinical trials are largely based on the potential for RT to

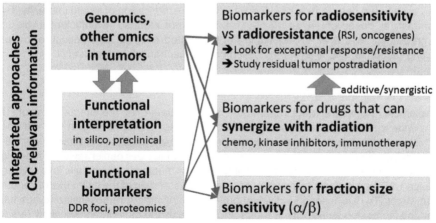

Fig. 6. Areas of need to develop tumor biomarkers to guide radiation oncology. Chemo, chemotherapy; CSC, cancer stem cells; DDR, DNA damage response; RSI, Radiosensitivity Index.

induce a systemic immune response by converting the irradiated target into an in situ vaccine.[66] The impact of RT on the immune system is multifactorial and includes induction of immunogenic cell death, altered expression of cytokines, and changes in the tumor microenvironment.[67–69] RT induces several effects on tumor cells, including upregulation of transcription factors and surface molecules.[70,71] By inducing immunogenic cell death and tumor antigen release, RT promotes antigen cross-presentation by dendritic cells, leading to activation and proliferation of tumor-specific T cells.[72,73] RT has also been associated with an increase in tumor-infiltrating lymphocytes,[74] likely caused by changes in the vascular endothelium and increased expression of chemokines. This proliferation of lymphocytes in turn allows potentiation of the immune response beyond the local area of RT. In addition, phenotypic changes in cells that survive RT can modulate susceptibility to an immune response; for example, RT can alter expression of PD-L1 (programmed death ligand 1) on tumor cells.[75]

It is becoming increasingly likely that the therapeutic effects of RT at least in part rely on the presence of an intact immune system. In support of this notion, in a murine model of fibrosarcoma, the dose required to control 50% of tumors increased significantly in immunosuppressed animals.[76] Additional preclinical studies have similarly shown a lack of response to RT, even with theoretically ablative doses, in immunodeficient states.[77,78]

RT can also lead to immunosuppression; for example, through lymphopenia, which has been associated with reduced survival in multiple cancer types.[79–81] RT can further cause a relative increase in regulatory T-cell populations and activation of transforming growth factor beta,[67,72,82] which can lead to downregulation of the immune response. Studies have therefore focused on the combination of RT and ICI to overcome RT-induced immunosuppression and maximize response.

Optimization of the Synergy of Radiation Therapy and Immune Checkpoint Inhibitors

The optimal dose, fractionation, and timing of RT related to ICI are of great interest. Preclinical studies suggest that abscopal response relies in part on fractionation. For example, in a mammary carcinoma model, only 8 Gy $\times$ 3 in combination with anti–cytotoxic T-lymphocyte–associated protein 4 (CTLA4) treatment led to a tumor response outside the RT field.[83] In contrast, 20 to 30 Gy $\times$ 1 did not induce any abscopal responses. This finding correlated with upregulation of Trex1, a DNA exonuclease, and associated degradation of cytosolic DNA and suppression of innate immunity. By contrast, at doses of $\sim$8 to 12 Gy, Trex1 was not induced at sufficient levels to degrade cytosolic DNA.[83] Sequencing of RT related to ICI is also critical for maximizing response, and likely varies based on the mechanism of a given ICI.

SUMMARY

This article reviews the most important factors that determine the effectiveness of RT in a wide variety of tumor types and normal tissues. Therapeutic gain can only be achieved if the increased tumor toxicity produced by biological treatment modifications is balanced against injury to normal tissues. Since our earlier review,[1] the field has now firmly entered the era of precision radiation medicine, which calls for a revised clinical radiation biology framework. A better understanding of the hallmarks of cancer that affect RT responses in individual patients, with/without radiosensitizing agents, and the increasing availability of tumor and normal tissue biomarkers will allow radiation oncologists to maximize therapeutic gain by individualizing therapies. In addition, although RT has historically been viewed as a purely local therapy, increased understanding of its immunostimulatory and immunosuppressive effects and the advent of ICI have led to an appreciation of the systemic effects of RT. Thus, although in many instances RT must remain an unselective physical tool to sterilize the last surviving, dormant, and drug-resistant CSCs that pose an obstacle to cure, in other settings RT may set up the tumor microenvironment to complete this task.

REFERENCES

1. Willers H, Held KD. Introduction to clinical radiation biology. Hematol Oncol Clin North Am 2006;20(1):1–24.
2. Hanahan D, Weinberg RA. Hallmarks of cancer: the next generation. Cell 2011; 144(5):646–74.
3. Kirsch DG, Diehn M, Kesarwala AH, et al. The future of radiobiology. J Natl Cancer Inst 2018;110(4):329–40.
4. Baumann M, Krause M, Overgaard J, et al. Radiation oncology in the era of precision medicine. Nat Rev Cancer 2016;16(4):234–49.
5. Ma J, Setton J, Lee NY, et al. The therapeutic significance of mutational signatures from DNA repair deficiency in cancer. Nat Commun 2018;9(1):3292.
6. Willers H, Pfäffle HN, Zou L. Targeting homologous recombination repair in cancer. Academic Press, Elsevier; 2012.
7. Pannunzio NR, Watanabe G, Lieber MR. Nonhomologous DNA end-joining for repair of DNA double-strand breaks. J Biol Chem 2018;293(27):10512–23.
8. Willers H, Dahm-Daphi J, Powell SN. Repair of radiation damage to DNA. Br J Cancer 2004;90(7):1297–301.
9. Willers H, Azzoli CG, Santivasi WL, et al. Basic mechanisms of therapeutic resistance to radiation and chemotherapy in lung cancer. Cancer J 2013;19(3):200–7.
10. Krause M, Yaromina A, Eicheler W, et al. Cancer stem cells: targets and potential biomarkers for radiotherapy. Clin Cancer Res 2011;17(23):7224–9.
11. Dubben HH, Thames HD, Beck-Bornholdt HP. Tumor volume: a basic and specific response predictor in radiotherapy. Radiother Oncol 1998;47(2):167–74.
12. Alexander BM, Othus M, Caglar HB, et al. Tumor volume is a prognostic factor in non-small-cell lung cancer treated with chemoradiotherapy. Int J Radiat Oncol Biol Phys 2011;79(5):1381–7.
13. Krause M, Dubrovska A, Linge A, et al. Cancer stem cells: Radioresistance, prediction of radiotherapy outcome and specific targets for combined treatments. Adv Drug Deliv Rev 2017;109:63–73.
14. Liu M, Lee S, Liu B, et al. Ku-dependent non-homologous end-joining as the major pathway contributes to sublethal damage repair in mammalian cells. Int J Radiat Biol 2015;91(11):867–71.
15. Somaiah N, Yarnold J, Lagerqvist A, et al. Homologous recombination mediates cellular resistance and fraction size sensitivity to radiation therapy. Radiother Oncol 2013;108(1):155–61.
16. Utsumi H, Elkind MM. Requirement for repair of DNA double-strand breaks by homologous recombination in split-dose recovery. Radiat Res 2001;155(5):680–6.
17. Bentzen SM, Overgaard J, Thames HD, et al. Clinical radiobiology of malignant melanoma. Radiother Oncol 1989;16(3):169–82.
18. Geh JI, Bond SJ, Bentzen SM, et al. Systematic overview of preoperative (neoadjuvant) chemoradiotherapy trials in oesophageal cancer: evidence of a radiation and chemotherapy dose response. Radiother Oncol 2006;78(3):236–44.
19. Thames HD, Bentzen SM, Turesson I, et al. Time-dose factors in radiotherapy: a review of the human data. Radiother Oncol 1990;19(3):219–35.

20. Vogelius IR, Bentzen SM. Dose response and fractionation sensitivity of prostate cancer after external beam radiation therapy: a meta-analysis of randomized trials. Int J Radiat Oncol Biol Phys 2018;100(4):858–65.

21. START Trialists' Group, Bentzen SM, Agrawal RK, Aird EG, et al. The UK Standardisation of Breast Radiotherapy (START) Trial A of radiotherapy hypofractionation for treatment of early breast cancer: a randomised trial. Lancet Oncol 2008; 9(4):331–41.

22. van Leeuwen CM, Oei AL, Crezee J, et al. The alfa and beta of tumours: a review of parameters of the linear-quadratic model, derived from clinical radiotherapy studies. Radiat Oncol 2018;13(1):96.

23. Huang Q, Li F, Liu X, et al. Caspase 3-mediated stimulation of tumor cell repopulation during cancer radiotherapy. Nat Med 2011;17(7):860–6.

24. Nguyen-Tan PF, Zhang Q, Ang KK, et al. Randomized phase III trial to test accelerated versus standard fractionation in combination with concurrent cisplatin for head and neck carcinomas in the Radiation Therapy Oncology Group 0129 trial: long-term report of efficacy and toxicity. J Clin Oncol 2014;32(34):3858–66.

25. Bourhis J, Sire C, Graff P, et al. Concomitant chemoradiotherapy versus acceleration of radiotherapy with or without concomitant chemotherapy in locally advanced head and neck carcinoma (GORTEC 99-02): an open-label phase 3 randomised trial. Lancet Oncol 2012;13(2):145–53.

26. Meade S, Sanghera P, McConkey C, et al. Revising the radiobiological model of synchronous chemotherapy in head-and-neck cancer: a new analysis examining reduced weighting of accelerated repopulation. Int J Radiat Oncol Biol Phys 2013;86(1):157–63.

27. Machtay M, Hsu C, Komaki R, et al. Effect of overall treatment time on outcomes after concurrent chemoradiation for locally advanced non-small-cell lung carcinoma: analysis of the Radiation Therapy Oncology Group (RTOG) experience. Int J Radiat Oncol Biol Phys 2005;63(3):667–71.

28. Turrisi AT 3rd, Kim K, Blum R, et al. Twice-daily compared with once-daily thoracic radiotherapy in limited small-cell lung cancer treated concurrently with cisplatin and etoposide. N Engl J Med 1999;340(4):265–71.

29. Fu KK, Pajak TF, Trotti A, et al. A Radiation Therapy Oncology Group (RTOG) phase III randomized study to compare hyperfractionation and two variants of accelerated fractionation to standard fractionation radiotherapy for head and neck squamous cell carcinomas: first report of RTOG 9003. Int J Radiat Oncol Biol Phys 2000;48(1):7–16.

30. Faivre-Finn C, Snee M, Ashcroft L, et al. Concurrent once-daily versus twice-daily chemoradiotherapy in patients with limited-stage small-cell lung cancer (CONVERT): an open-label, phase 3, randomised, superiority trial. Lancet Oncol 2017;18(8):1116–25.

31. Overgaard J, Hansen HS, Specht L, et al. Five compared with six fractions per week of conventional radiotherapy of squamous-cell carcinoma of head and neck: DAHANCA 6 and 7 randomised controlled trial. Lancet 2003;362(9388): 933–40.

32. Bakst RL, Lee N, Pfister DG, et al. Hypofractionated dose-painting intensity modulated radiation therapy with chemotherapy for nasopharyngeal carcinoma: a prospective trial. Int J Radiat Oncol Biol Phys 2011;80(1):148–53.

33. Hammond EM, Asselin MC, Forster D, et al. The meaning, measurement and modification of hypoxia in the laboratory and the clinic. Clin Oncol (R Coll Radiol) 2014;26(5):277–88.

34. Brown JM, Carlson DJ, Brenner DJ. The tumor radiobiology of SRS and SBRT: are more than the 5 Rs involved? Int J Radiat Oncol Biol Phys 2014;88(2):254–62.

35. Hill RP, Bristow RG, Fyles A, et al. Hypoxia and Predicting Radiation Response. Semin Radiat Oncol 2015;25(4):260–72.

36. Hall WA, Bergom C, Thompson RF, et al. Precision Oncology and genomically guided radiation therapy: a report from the American Society for Radiation Oncology/American Association of Physicists in Medicine/National Cancer Institute Precision Medicine Conference. Int J Radiat Oncol Biol Phys 2018;101(2): 274–84.

37. Kamran SC, Mouw KW. Applying Precision Oncology Principles in Radiation Oncology. JCO Precis Oncol 2018;1–23. https://doi.org/10.1200/PO.18.00034.

38. Eschrich SA, Pramana J, Zhang H, et al. A gene expression model of intrinsic tumor radiosensitivity: prediction of response and prognosis after chemoradiation. Int J Radiat Oncol Biol Phys 2009;75(2):489–96.

39. Hall JS, Iype R, Senra J, et al. Investigation of radiosensitivity gene signatures in cancer cell lines. PLoS One 2014;9(1):e86329.

40. Scott JG, Berglund A, Schell MJ, et al. A genome-based model for adjusting radiotherapy dose (GARD): a retrospective, cohort-based study. Lancet Oncol 2017;18(2):202–11.

41. Mamounas EP, Tang G, Fisher B, et al. Association between the 21-gene recurrence score assay and risk of locoregional recurrence in node-negative, estrogen receptor-positive breast cancer: results from NSABP B-14 and NSABP B-20. J Clin Oncol 2010;28(10):1677–83.

42. Zhao SG, Chang SL, Spratt DE, et al. Development and validation of a 24-gene predictor of response to postoperative radiotherapy in prostate cancer: a matched, retrospective analysis. Lancet Oncol 2016;17(11):1612–20.

43. Hong TS, Wo JY, Borger DR, et al. Phase II study of proton-based stereotactic body radiation therapy for liver metastases: importance of tumor genotype. J Natl Cancer Inst 2017;109(9):1–8.

44. Kamran SC, Lennerz JK, Margolis CA, et al. Integrative Molecular Characterization of Resistance to Neoadjuvant Chemoradiation in Rectal Cancer. Clin Cancer Res 2019. [Epub ahead of print].

45. Mouw KW, Cleary JM, Reardon B, et al. Genomic evolution after chemoradiotherapy in anal squamous cell carcinoma. Clin Cancer Res 2017;23(12):3214–22.

46. Sakai K, Kazama S, Nagai Y, et al. Chemoradiation provides a physiological selective pressure that increases the expansion of aberrant TP53 tumor variants in residual rectal cancerous regions. Oncotarget 2014;5(20):9641–9.

47. Wang M, Han J, Marcar L, et al. Radiation resistance in KRAS-mutated lung cancer is enabled by stem-like properties mediated by an osteopontin-EGFR pathway. Cancer Res 2017;77(8):2018–28.

48. Chaudhuri AA, Chabon JJ, Lovejoy AF, et al. Early detection of molecular residual disease in localized lung cancer by circulating tumor DNA profiling. Cancer Discov 2017;7(12):1394–403.

49. Miyamoto DT, Lee RJ, Kalinich M, et al. An RNA-based digital circulating tumor cell signature is predictive of drug response and early dissemination in prostate cancer. Cancer Discov 2018;8(3):288–303.

50. Herskind C, Talbot CJ, Kerns SL, et al. Radiogenomics: a systems biology approach to understanding genetic risk factors for radiotherapy toxicity? Cancer Lett 2016;382(1):95–109.

51. Pearl LH, Schierz AC, Ward SE, et al. Therapeutic opportunities within the DNA damage response. Nat Rev Cancer 2015;15(3):166–80.

52. Jackson SP, Helleday T. DNA REPAIR. Drugging DNA repair. Science 2016; 352(6290):1178–9.

53. Kan C, Zhang J. BRCA1 mutation: a predictive marker for radiation therapy? Int J Radiat Oncol Biol Phys 2015;93(2):281–93.

54. Castro E, Goh C, Leongamornlert D, et al. Effect of BRCA mutations on metastatic relapse and cause-specific survival after radical treatment for localised prostate cancer. Eur Urol 2015;68(2):186–93.

55. Ma J, Setton J, Morris L, et al. Genomic analysis of exceptional responders to radiotherapy reveals somatic mutations in ATM. Oncotarget 2017;8(6):10312–23.

56. Liu D, Plimack ER, Hoffman-Censits J, et al. Clinical validation of chemotherapy response biomarker ERCC2 in muscle-invasive urothelial bladder carcinoma. JAMA Oncol 2016;2(8):1094–6.

57. Van Allen EM, Mouw KW, Kim P, et al. Somatic ERCC2 mutations correlate with cisplatin sensitivity in muscle-invasive urothelial carcinoma. Cancer Discov 2014;4(10):1140–53.

58. Choudhury A, Nelson LD, Teo MT, et al. MRE11 expression is predictive of cause-specific survival following radical radiotherapy for muscle-invasive bladder cancer. Cancer Res 2010;70(18):7017–26.

59. Pitroda SP, Pashtan IM, Logan HL, et al. DNA repair pathway gene expression score correlates with repair proficiency and tumor sensitivity to chemotherapy. Sci Transl Med 2014;6(229):229ra42.

60. Willers H, Gheorghiu L, Liu Q, et al. DNA damage response assessments in human tumor samples provide functional biomarkers of radiosensitivity. Semin Radiat Oncol 2015;25(4):237–50.

61. Postow MA, Callahan MK, Barker CA, et al. Immunologic correlates of the abscopal effect in a patient with melanoma. N Engl J Med 2012;366(10):925–31.

62. Luke JJ, Lemons JM, Karrison TG, et al. Safety and clinical activity of pembrolizumab and multisite stereotactic body radiotherapy in patients with advanced solid tumors. J Clin Oncol 2018;36(16):1611–8.

63. Tang C, Welsh JW, de Groot P, et al. Ipilimumab with stereotactic ablative radiation therapy: phase I results and immunologic correlates from peripheral T cells. Clin Cancer Res 2017;23(6):1388–96.

64. Golden EB, Chhabra A, Chachoua A, et al. Local radiotherapy and granulocyte-macrophage colony-stimulating factor to generate abscopal responses in patients with metastatic solid tumours: a proof-of-principle trial. Lancet Oncol 2015;16(7):795–803.

65. Twyman-Saint Victor C, Rech AJ, Maity A, et al. Radiation and dual checkpoint blockade activate non-redundant immune mechanisms in cancer. Nature 2015; 520(7547):373–7.

66. Vanpouille-Box C, Pilones KA, Wennerberg E, et al. In situ vaccination by radiotherapy to improve responses to anti-CTLA-4 treatment. Vaccine 2015;33(51): 7415–22.

67. Klopp AH, Spaeth EL, Dembinski JL, et al. Tumor irradiation increases the recruitment of circulating mesenchymal stem cells into the tumor microenvironment. Cancer Res 2007;67(24):11687–95.

68. Gerber SA, Sedlacek AL, Cron KR, et al. IFN-gamma mediates the antitumor effects of radiation therapy in a murine colon tumor. Am J Pathol 2013;182(6): 2345–54.

69. Golden EB, Pellicciotta I, Demaria S, et al. The convergence of radiation and immunogenic cell death signaling pathways. Front Oncol 2012;2:88.

70. Germano G, Lamba S, Rospo G, et al. Inactivation of DNA repair triggers neoantigen generation and impairs tumour growth. Nature 2017;552(7683):116–20.
71. Reits EA, Hodge JW, Herberts CA, et al. Radiation modulates the peptide repertoire, enhances MHC class I expression, and induces successful antitumor immunotherapy. J Exp Med 2006;203(5):1259–71.
72. Sharabi AB, Nirschl CJ, Kochel CM, et al. Stereotactic radiation therapy augments antigen-specific PD-1-mediated antitumor immune responses via cross-presentation of tumor antigen. Cancer Immunol Res 2015;3(4):345–55.
73. Gameiro SR, Jammeh ML, Wattenberg MM, et al. Radiation-induced immunogenic modulation of tumor enhances antigen processing and calreticulin exposure, resulting in enhanced T-cell killing. Oncotarget 2014;5(2):403–16.
74. Matsumura S, Wang B, Kawashima N, et al. Radiation-induced CXCL16 release by breast cancer cells attracts effector T cells. J Immunol 2008;181(5):3099–107.
75. Parikh F, Duluc D, Imai N, et al. Chemoradiotherapy-induced upregulation of PD-1 antagonizes immunity to HPV-related oropharyngeal cancer. Cancer Res 2014; 74(24):7205–16.
76. Stone HB, Peters LJ, Milas L. Effect of host immune capability on radiocurability and subsequent transplantability of a murine fibrosarcoma. J Natl Cancer Inst 1979;63(5):1229–35.
77. Lee Y, Auh SL, Wang Y, et al. Therapeutic effects of ablative radiation on local tumor require CD8+ T cells: changing strategies for cancer treatment. Blood 2009; 114(3):589–95.
78. Lugade AA, Moran JP, Gerber SA, et al. Local radiation therapy of B16 melanoma tumors increases the generation of tumor antigen-specific effector cells that traffic to the tumor. J Immunol 2005;174(12):7516–23.
79. Grossman SA, Ye X, Lesser G, et al. Immunosuppression in patients with high-grade gliomas treated with radiation and temozolomide. Clin Cancer Res 2011; 17(16):5473–80.
80. Wild AT, Ye X, Ellsworth SG, et al. The association between chemoradiation-related lymphopenia and clinical outcomes in patients with locally advanced pancreatic adenocarcinoma. Am J Clin Oncol 2015;38(3):259–65.
81. Ellsworth SG. Field size effects on the risk and severity of treatment-induced lymphopenia in patients undergoing radiation therapy for solid tumors. Adv Radiat Oncol 2018;3(4):512–9.
82. Bouquet F, Pal A, Pilones KA, et al. TGFbeta1 inhibition increases the radiosensitivity of breast cancer cells in vitro and promotes tumor control by radiation in vivo. Clin Cancer Res 2011;17(21):6754–65.
83. Vanpouille-Box C, Alard A, Aryankalayil MJ, et al. DNA exonuclease Trex1 regulates radiotherapy-induced tumour immunogenicity. Nat Commun 2017;8:15618.

Modern Radiation Therapy Planning and Delivery

Stephen J. Gardner, MS*, Joshua Kim, PhD, Indrin J. Chetty, PhD

KEYWORDS

- Radiation therapy • Treatment planning • Image-guided radiation therapy
- MRI-guided radiation therapy • Intensity-modulated radiation therapy
- Volumetric-modulated radiation therapy

KEY POINTS

- Radiation therapy treatment planning uses three-dimensional imaging to generate high-quality treatment plans that deliver doses to the target while sparing normal tissue.
- Image-guided radiation therapy allows precise targeting of the tumor, including imaging before and during the treatment procedure.
- Magnetic resonance–guided radiation therapy provides further soft tissue visualization and therefore offers increased ability for online adaptive radiation therapy when combined with a linear accelerator.

COMPUTED TOMOGRAPHY–BASED RADIATION THERAPY TREATMENT PLANNING
Simulation and Imaging

Put simply, the goal of radiation therapy is to maximize the therapeutic ratio; to maximize the delivered dose to the target (tumor) and minimize dose to normal tissue. The process for individual radiation oncology patients begins at the simulation appointment. The term simulation refers to the intent of this process: to simulate the treatment geometry for treatment planning purposes with the goal of providing an individualized treatment plan that is both precise and accurate. To generate the treatment plan for each patient, data must be acquired; the data in this case are three-dimensional (3D) imaging. The current standard for 3D imaging in radiation oncology simulation is computed tomography (CT). There are 2 significant factors that make CT images essential for radiotherapy planning: (1) the CT images inherently contain electron density information, which is vital for dose calculation with heterogeneity corrections;

Disclosure: Henry Ford Health System holds research agreements with Varian Medical Systems and Philips Healthcare.
Department of Radiation Oncology, Henry Ford Cancer Institute, Henry Ford Hospital, 2799 W. Grand boulevard, Detroit, MI 48202, USA
* Corresponding author.
E-mail address: sgardne8@hfhs.org

and (2) the CT images are geometrically robust, which is vital for the accurate targeting of tumors during treatment planning and treatment delivery.

Computed tomography imaging

Conceptually, the process of CT image acquisition involves taking many planar radiograph images (projections) and then combining them via an image reconstruction technique to obtain a 3D image set. This 3D image set is typically composed of several two-dimensional (2D) views in the axial plane separated by the slice thickness. The first-generation CT scanner was developed by Sir Godfrey Hounsfield in 1967. Since that initial innovation, the improvements in this technology have been remarkable: multiple generations of CT scanners were developed in the last 40 years or more.[1] The current CT scanners have multiple detector rows within the array (up to 320 slices), are capable of generating images of any body site, with in-plane resolution up to 1024 × 1024 matrix size, with images acquired within a matter of seconds. Advancements in detectors, computational power, and electronics have largely driven these improvements. In addition, reconstruction improvements (namely, iterative reconstruction algorithms and metal artifact reduction; **Fig. 1**) have allowed further improvement to images on the image reconstruction/software end.[2,3]

Patient organ motion

The description of CT earlier did not consider the impact of internal organ motion during image acquisition. However, when generating a geometrically robust treatment plan for patients, clinicians must consider the effects of internal organ motion on the image acquisition process (and, therefore, also the treatment planning and treatment delivery process). During normal body function, many types of motion, both regular and irregular, occur as patients attempt to remain still during an imaging or treatment procedure. Most radiation therapy–related investigation has focused on respiratory motion resulting from the movement of tissues in the thorax and upper abdomen during breathing. The effects of respiratory motion can even extend to the pelvis.[4] The motion of the heart during the cardiac cycle is another source of motion in the thorax. Although the respiratory and cardiac motion is a regular source of organ motion, other types of movement are irregular. For example, movement associated with the digestive process in the abdomen and pelvis can cause displacement of organs and tissues. Further, the bladder experiences differential filling and can also cause organ and tissue displacement. There are therefore many sources of internal organ motion that pose a challenge for accurate targeting in radiation therapy, and this motion must be managed properly to ensure accurate targeting of tumors with radiation therapy (**Fig. 2**).

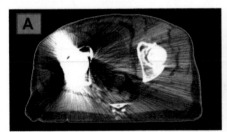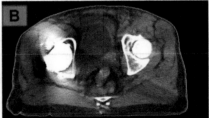

Fig. 1. Comparison of images of a patient with a prosthetic hip implant. (*A*) The uncorrected axial view. (*B*) Improved image quality and visualization using metal artifact reduction in the image reconstruction process.

Patient positioning and immobilization

A typical radiation therapy treatment course can span anywhere from 1 to more than 44 fractions of daily treatment. During the entire course of therapy, the aim is to achieve the same patient positioning on a daily basis. Thus, there is a need to position the patient in a way that meets a minimum need for comfort (to ensure feasibility) but also to immobilize the patient in such a way to ensure consistency of setup. These two parameters (immobilization and patient comfort) are often at odds with one another, and therefore must be optimized with the overall treatment goal in mind.

Respiration-correlated computed tomography

Because of the advancements in CT image acquisition efficiency, the temporal resolution of the CT image acquisition allows correlation with the respiratory cycle.[5] In this way, a surrogate for the respiratory cycle can be correlated with the images during the CT image, creating a time stamp for each image. The external respiratory surrogate data can be used to separate the respiratory cycle into bins (phases) and the image acquisition includes intentional oversampling. In the most common method of four-dimensional (4D)-CT acquisition, the images are retrospectively binned according to their time stamp and placed in a phase within the respiratory cycle (the typical convention is to separate the respiratory cycle into 10 phases). The end result is a group of CT images that depict the anatomy throughout the respiratory cycle.

Contouring and Targeting

Once all relevant imaging has been acquired, the next step in the radiation therapy process involves delineation of relevant organs and tissues on the planning image; in most cases, the planning image is the simulation CT image set. This process of delineation of structures (contouring) is performed by the radiation oncologist and is essential for guiding the downstream treatment planning and treatment delivery. The process of contouring performed on the patient's CT image allows the complete customization of the radiation therapy planning and delivery for each patient.

In general, radiation oncologists delineate the gross tumor volume (GTV), defined by the ICRU (International Commission on Radiation Units and Measurements) as the

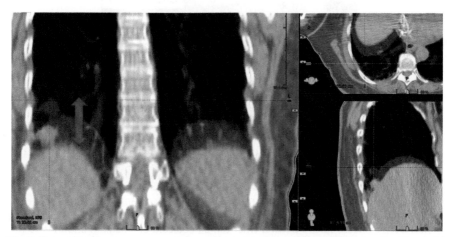

Fig. 2. Example of tumor movement caused by respiratory motion. This image is a blend of 2 four-dimensional CT phases, showing end inhale and end exhale for a patient with lung cancer. The tumor motion in the superior-inferior direction is approximately 2.5 cm.

"gross palpable or visible/demonstrable extent and location of malignant growth."[6] From there, the clinical target volume (CTV) is defined, representing the GTV and any subclinical microscopic malignant disease that needs to be eliminated. The CTV is an expansion of the GTV and represents the true target: the goal of radiation therapy is treat the entire CTV. However, as discussed earlier, the effects of internal organ motion cannot be ignored. Thus, for patients in whom the motion of the CTV must be explicitly managed, the internal target volume (ITV) is defined, which represents the CTV with an internal margin for motion.[7] If necessary, radiation oncologists typically use the 4D-CT image to delineate the full extent of tumor motion to create the ITV contour. Practically, the ITV is defined most often for treatment of thoracic tumors and some upper abdominal tumors as well. The ITV accounts for expected internal organ motion, but it does not account for variations in setup throughout the treatment course. The planning target volume (PTV) is an expansion of the CTV (or ITV) and is created to account for both the internal margin and setup margin. Conceptually, the PTV is covered with the prescribed radiation dose so that there is adequate assurance (eg, >95% probability) of covering the CTV with the prescribed radiation dose for each fraction over the course of treatment. **Fig. 3** provides an example of GTV-CTV-PTV and organs-at-risk (OAR) contouring. In addition to target structures, radiation oncologists delineate OAR. These structures depend on the treatment site. For example, in prostate cancer, typical OAR include the bladder, rectum, small bowel, penile bulb, and femoral heads. For lung cancer, typical OAR include the normal lung, heart,

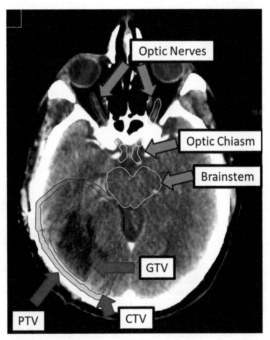

Fig. 3. Axial image of a patient being treated for a primary brain tumor after resection. Note the expansion of the GTV (representing the resection cavity) to the CTV (to account for microscopic disease spread beyond what can be detected on imaging) and then to the PTV (to account for geometric uncertainty). Also, several organs-at-risk contours are shown: brainstem, optic chiasm, and optic nerves. Note the proximity of the PTV to the brainstem; this captures the necessity for both advanced imaging and planning techniques.

esophagus, and spinal cord. Overall, the contoured structures provide instruction to the treatment planner regarding which areas to target and which to avoid. Therefore, the goal of treatment planning is to optimize these two parameters with a treatment plan that is physically deliverable.

During the contouring phase, additional image data from complementary modalities may be used to aid in the visualization and delineation of the target and OAR; most commonly, MRI and PET are used through image registration to the planning CT image. More information on the use of MRI is provided later. Although MRI commonly provides anatomic information, the use of PET imaging gives physiologic (or functional) information. The most common PET radiotracer is ^{18}F-fluorodeoxyglucose (FDG), which has been evaluated for use in radiotherapy planning for a variety of disease sites, including cervix,[8] head and neck (MK Garg, J Glanzman, S Kalnicki, presented at the Seminars in Nuclear Medicine, 2012, unpublished), lymphoma,[9] non–small cell lung cancer,[10] and esophageal cancers.[11] Overall, FDG-PET is widely used in radiation oncology and is useful in the diagnosis, staging, and assessment of tumor response to treatment. In addition to FDG-PET, other radiotracers have been used to provide characterization of the tumor, including ^{18}F-fluoromisonidazole to detect tumor hypoxia[12] and ^{68}Ga–prostate-specific membrane antigen to detect prostate cancer.[13]

Treatment Planning Strategies

A typical radiation therapy treatment plan is delivered on a linear accelerator. These machines use high-powered x-rays that are focused by multiple forms of collimation, including multileaf collimators (MLCs), to shape the radiation beam. The MLC has the ability to dynamically shape the edge of the beam as well as modulate the intensity of the fluence with the beam aperture.

Three-dimensional conformal radiation therapy

During 3D conformal radiation therapy (CRT) planning, static beam angles are chosen to best deliver dose to the tumor and spare surrounding normal tissue. In addition, the MLC shapes are defined to cover the target adequately. This style of planning often uses simple geometry and the planning style is forward planned. That is, the treatment planner modifies the beam characteristics (beam shape, beam angle, beam energy) to obtain a desired dose distribution.

Intensity-modulated radiation therapy and volumetric-modulated radiation therapy

Although 3D-CRT planning involves the modification of the beam characteristics to achieve a desired dose distribution, intensity-modulated radiation therapy (IMRT)/volumetric-modulated radiation therapy (VMAT) planning starts with a desired dose distribution with the goal of determining beam characteristics that achieve this desired dose distribution. This process is often called inverse planning, because the process is inverted relative to 3D-CRT planning. When IMRT/VMAT planning is performed properly, the system is able to achieve superior dose distributions compared with forward-planned 3D-CRT planning for many commonly treated disease sites. In particular, the inverse-planning approach is able to provide conformal dose distributions for both concave and convex target geometries. In general, the inverse-planning process requires the treatment planner to create a set of dosimetric constraints for the target and OAR; these constraints represent the desired dose distribution for the optimization algorithm. There are some differences between IMRT and VMAT; namely, VMAT involves continuous delivery as the linear accelerator rotates around the patient, whereas IMRT involves static delivery and the linear accelerator rotates between beam deliveries. Further comparing 3D-

CRT planning with the IMRT/VMAT approach, note that the inverse-planning approach also involves more beam angles (whether in the form of static gantry angles or using arc delivery). The additional beam angles, along with the optimization of beam shape and beam intensity within each field, are the main factors that allow improvements in plan quality for inverse planning relative to traditional 3D-CRT planning.

Treatment plan evaluation

For each planning style, the radiation dose is calculated on the CT image set, which allows qualitative visual review of the dose level to the target structures as well as OAR structures. Further, the dose distribution can be quantitatively verified through the use of the dose volume histogram , which displays the dose level for a given volume of a structure. During the review of the treatment plan, radiation oncologists keep a close eye on the shape of the dose distribution relative to the target and OAR, the location of areas of high dose level (so-called hot spots) and low dose level (cold spots), any potential areas of undercoverage of the target, and other aspects of the plan. After the radiation oncologist has reviewed and approved the treatment plan, the treatment planner and radiation physicist ensure that the plan meets relevant hospital criteria through the use of checklists and other quality-assurance tools. The treatment plan goes through a redundant series of checks before the plan is first treated.

IMAGE-GUIDED RADIATION THERAPY

Although the goal of treatment planning is to maximize the therapeutic ratio (maximize dose to the target and minimize dose to healthy tissues) by optimization of planned dose on the patient model (derived from simulation CT images), the purpose of image-guided radiation therapy (IGRT) is to ensure that radiation is accurately delivered to the patient in accordance with the treatment plan. It can be envisioned that it is not always straightforward to deliver the planned dose distribution as was intended because of uncertainties associated in setting up the patient, motion caused by respiration and other factors, and so forth. Note that the treatment plan is optimized on a static set of images of the patient (or patient model), whereas the treatment is delivered to a live patient. The objective then of IGRT is to incorporate information gleaned from images acquired before or during treatment, and to incorporate this information to modify the patient setup so as to most accurately target the tumor. Information gleaned from daily imaging can be used to better optimize planning margins, with the potential to reduce planning margins to minimize dose to surrounding healthy tissues.[14] In its most general sense, IGRT applies to any imaging data that are included at the time of patient treatment to improve patient setup and hence target localization accuracy. The techniques available for image guidance range from simple planar radiographs (which have been used for many years, since the inception of radiation therapy) to volumetric imaging using radiographs, and more recently MRI (discussed later) and PET.

In general, image-guided delivery systems can be classified as radiograph-based, optical/surface-guided, infrared (IR) camera–based, ultrasonography (US)-based, fiducial marker–based, combination systems, and emerging systems (eg, MRI and PET). A brief review of each of these general types of image-guidance systems is provided here.

Radiographic Imaging

Perhaps the first application of image guidance was related to the use of planar radiographs captured using film cassettes to assess the accuracy of the patient setup.

Planar imaging (eg, using film) is better able to localize the high-contrast structures, such as bony anatomy; bones are more pronounced even with megavoltage radiographs but to a much lesser degree than kilovoltage radiographs, because the Compton interaction type is dominant in the megavoltage energy range. Compton scatter degrades image contrast because of the lack of attenuation or absorption of x-rays. In contrast, kilovoltage radiographs have much better contrast because the photoelectric effect, in which the x-ray is entirely attenuated/absorbed, is more prevalent in the kilovoltage energy range. With megavoltage radiographs, despite the limited contrast, clinicians are able to visualize bony structures, which is reasonably accurate for localization of tumors in regions that are rigid (eg, head/neck, brain, spine). In such regions, a correspondence can be made between the tumor location and surrounding bony anatomy during treatment planning, which can be compared with that observed during planar radiograph imaging during patient setup. However, planar imaging is less useful for localizing tumors and surrounding soft tissue in regions where patient motion (caused by nonrigid body anatomy and/or respiratory-induced motion) is prevalent. Examples include the upper and lower thorax, gastrointestinal tract, pelvis and genitourinary system. The development of volumetric imaging systems in the treatment room through the invention of cone-beam CT (CBCT) imagers on a linear accelerator in 2002 represented a significant advancement in radiation therapy.[15] This development enabled, for the first time, the ability to visualize the tumor and normal tissues in 3D on the linear accelerator. When setting up a patient, acquisition of 3D imaging of the tumor and surrounding organs allows clinicians to more accurately correlate the treatment anatomy to the planned treatment anatomy, and thereby shift the patient with a greater degree of precision to hit the target and avoid normal tissues relative to planar (2D) radiographs, especially in treatment sites where the tumor is affected by respiratory-induced motion. In such situations, alignment of the tumor (or soft tissue) between the treatment and planning CT scans using CBCT facilitates more accurate positioning of the moving tumor relative to 2D radiograph imaging. Another in-room CT technique comprises a CT scanner placed on rails in the treatment room, at the opposite end of the linear accelerator couch.[16] This CT-on-rails system allows patients to be scanned with a diagnostic-quality CT scanner immediately before treatment, and information can be fused to the planning CT images. However, patient repositioning is required for treatment on the linear accelerator. Overall, volumetric imaging during patient setup and/or treatment using CBCT-based image guidance has improved the accuracy of target localization, which has subsequently led to the use of smaller planning margins (for CTV-to-PTV expansion)[17,18] and consequently greater sparing of healthy tissues.

Optical Imaging

Optical imaging allows monitoring of the patient during treatment (intrafraction motion) without the need for ionizing radiation. Surface-based image guidance is typically performed using optical images acquired from a set of mounted cameras to acquire an optical image of the patient surface, which is compared with that from simulation to set up the patient.[19,20] Surface-based systems are able to monitor subtle patient movements during treatment; thresholds can be defined and radiation delivery automatically halted if movement is beyond the limit. At present the commercially available products include AlignRT (VisionRT, London, United Kingdom), C-Rad Sentinel (C-RAD AB, Uppsala, Sweden), and IDENTIFY/HumediQ (Varian Medical Systems, Palo Alto, CA), all with the ability to perform rapid surface imaging of patients during a radiotherapy treatment. These devices generate 3D models of the patient surface using photogrammetry. The AlignRT system uses 2 cameras for stereotactic imaging, whereas the C-Rad Sentinel system scans using a line scanning mode with a single camera and laser system. The IDENTIFY system uses a DICOM (Digital Imaging and Communications in Medicine) surface generated from automated DICOM-RT (radiation therapy) import, and the patient is positioned based on the DICOM-RT structure set. These devices are calibrated relative to the room isocenter. For planning CT-based alignment, a reference radiation therapy structure set is acquired, which includes the reference 3D model of the patient surface and its geometric relationship to the room isocenter. Surface-based systems can be used for motion management and are applied in the clinic in a variety of treatment settings,[19–22] including breast, prostate, brain, and thorax. Other details on optical imaging/surface-guided systems are available elsewhere,[23] including the American Association of Physicists in Medicine (AAPM) Task Group Report No. 147.[24] Optical tracking of surface-based surrogates is optimal when there is good correlation between tumor motion and the surface-based surrogate or in cases in which the body surface is closely related to tumor location, such as for patients with breast cancer. However, tracking of surface-based surrogates of tumor motion may be problematic in some situations in which there is poor correlation between movement of the external patient surface and motion of the tumor.

Infrared Imaging

Infrared imaging systems are most often independent devices that are coupled with linear accelerators to enhance image-guided capabilities. The ExacTrac X-Ray 6-D stereotactic IGRT system (BrainLAB AG, Feldkirchen, Germany) uses a combination of IR-based localization and kilovoltage radiographic imaging to position patients and perform online positioning corrections. The system consists of an IR-based localization system (ExacTrac) for initial patient setup and precise control of couch movement, using a robotic couch, and a radiographic kilovoltage radiograph imaging system (X-Ray 6-D) for position verification and readjustment based on internal anatomy or implanted fiducial markers. The IR system can be used to monitor a patient's respiration and provide a signal to the linear accelerator for tracking and gating of the treatment beam. Couch translations and rotations determined by the imaging component are guided by the IR system, based on markers (IR reflectors) attached either to the couch or to the patient. Detailed review and clinical application of the ExacTrac technology are provided elsewhere.[24–26] Other IR camera–based systems include the Varian RPM system, in which an IR reflective block positioned on the patient surface is imaged by IR cameras and can be used to monitor the patient's respiratory trace as a surrogate for tumor motion in the thorax and abdomen. This signal is electronically coupled to the linear accelerator and can be used to gate the radiation beam.[23,24] The CyberKnife system (Accuray, Sunnyvale, CA) also uses IR imaging via IR reflectors and cameras for patient localization as well as target tracking.[23,24]

Ultrasonography Imaging

In-room US is an image-guidance platform initiated almost exclusively for the prostate,[27] and was later applied for abdominal and breast sites.[28,29] A US probe is used to acquire 3D treatment images, which are fused to those acquired during simulation for optimizing the patient setup. Newer applications include the ability to track the prostate in real time by placing the US probe in the vicinity of the perineum during treatment. Commercially available models, including BATCAM/Nomos (Best Medical International, Springfield, VA) and Clarity/RESTITU (Elekta, Stockholm, Sweden), provide 3D imaging information. The BATCAM system acquires 3D information via real-time, intersecting 2D planar images. The Clarity system acquires a 3D volumetric data set by sweeping of the US probe through multiple planes while the system acquires static frames to be interpolated into a 3D volume. In addition to assessment of interfraction motion, US-IGRT has been reported to allow a real-time assessment of respiratory-induced intrafraction motion immediately before treatment start.[28] Applications on the use of US-guided extracranial radiosurgery have also been proposed.[30] US-guided imaging has been reported to have several benefits, including being a minimally invasive, nonionizing approach; affording good soft tissue visualization; and the ability to characterize respiratory-induced motion immediately before start of treatment.[23,31,32] However, this technique has also been reported to have high interuser variability, and has been shown to depend on training and user expertise, and US probe pressure.[23,32] It may also be limited for imaging of tumors situated behind bony structures.[23]

Fiducial Marker–Based Imaging

Marker-based systems typically consist of gold seeds (or other markers, a few millimeters in length) or transponders that are implanted into the tumor to create fiducial points that are visible via imaging in the treatment room. Radiograph imaging can be used to locate these markers and hence visualization of the tumor is possible during the treatment.[33] Electromagnetic transponders via the Calypso system (Varian Medical Systems, Palo Alto, CA) track the tumor in manner similar to GPS (global positioning system) monitoring and have become a popular option for localization of prostate[34] and, more recently, lung tumors.[35] Location of the tumor is monitored in real time by tracking of the coordinates of 2 or more electromagnetic transponders implanted within the tumor. Although fiducial markers enable direct monitoring of the tumor, implantation of these devices is invasive, with associated risk of infection and pneumothorax (in the case of lung tumors).

Combination Approaches and Emerging Technologies

Combination image-guided systems refer to linear accelerators that incorporate 2 or more of the approaches defined earlier. For instance, a linear accelerator may be equipped with ancillary camera systems for surface-based monitoring, and at the same time offer kilovoltage and megavoltage radiograph imaging, and the ability to track electromagnetic transponders implanted within the tumor. Redundancy of independent imaging modalities is made possible with combination systems.[14] Tracking of PET-based tracer information in the treatment room using emission imaging represents a technology in development. This concept involves radiation delivered along PET lines of response by a fast-rotating ring therapy unit consisting of a linear accelerator and PET detectors.[36] A newly developed technology, the RefleXion system (RefleXion, Hayward, CA), incorporates a ring-based PET detector that detects the emission of a radioactive tracer delivered to the patient.[37,38] This technology claims the ability to image biological activity within the tumor in real time. It invokes the concept of biologically guided radiation therapy,[39] in which biological information, such as tumor hypoxia, can be used to tailor higher dose levels to more radioresistant regions of the tumor. In addition, the use of MRI in the treatment room, the next focus in this article, is a rapidly emerging technology.

In summary, there is a vast array of imaging tools in the treatment room for accurate targeting of the tumor and avoidance of normal tissues. It is important that each image-guidance system be evaluated to determine uncertainties in localization accuracy. These uncertainties should be folded back into the planning phase, ultimately to create treatment plans that are robust to these delivery inaccuracies.[18]

MAGNETIC RESONANCE–GUIDED RADIATION THERAPY
Offline MRI Guidance

MRI has become an essential tool for informing clinical decision making and guidance of radiotherapy treatments. CT uses ionizing radiation projected through the body at different angles to generate a series of projection images that are used to reconstruct a map of linear attenuation values of the object, whereas MRI instead places an object within an external magnetic field and uses precisely timed radiofrequency pulses to excite precessing magnetic dipoles in order to generate a signal whose intensity depends on the magnetization within the various voxels of the body. By varying the timing of the applied excitations, the signal intensity of the tissues within the body will also vary based on, among many other things, magnetic relaxation properties, tissue composition, and flow characteristics within the tissue. This property has resulted in the ability of MRI to provide excellent soft tissue contrast that enables easy visualization of structures and tissue boundaries that are difficult or impossible to distinguish in CT images. These advantages of MRI have prompted many centers to install dedicated MRI units within their own departments that have been modified for the needs of radiation oncology rather than relying on diagnostic MRI units, which are often inconveniently located relative to radiation oncology departments and require working around their busy diagnostic schedules. Although open-bore magnetic resonance (MR) systems were used early on because they overcame some of the limitations imposed by the smaller bore size of closed-bore systems at the time,[40,41] newer closed-bore MRI units have been introduced with wider bores (70 cm) and flat table-tops that can be more readily incorporated into radiation oncology centers because the patient can be set up within the bore in their treatment positions using their immobilization devices. Laser positioning systems can also be added within the MR vault to accommodate radiotherapy simulation needs.

Anatomic MRI as an adjunct to computed tomography

Historically, MRI has been implemented as an adjunct to CT in order to combine the simple correlation between CT intensity values and electron density information and geometric integrity of CT images with the excellent soft tissue contrast of MR images. MR images from either diagnostic MRI scanners or radiotherapy-dedicated MR simulation units are registered to the patient's CT simulation image, and a CT-MR fusion is then used during contouring of the patient's target and OAR volumes (**Fig. 4**). Several studies have shown the superiority of MRI for visualization and contouring of both tumor and OARs or for reducing interobserver variability in many sites, including prostate,[42] rectum,[43] cervical,[44] breast,[45] and brain.[46] MRI has long been used in this way for stereotactic radiosurgery to identify lesions that would have been indistinguishable from surrounding soft tissue if CT were the only available modality.[47] One disadvantage to this approach is the introduction of systematic errors that arise from the inherent uncertainties in registration of the MR to the CT.[48]

Functional MRI as an adjunct to computed tomography

In addition to anatomic information, research into functional MRI (fMRI) has sought to use metabolic, pathologic, and physiologic information obtained from MR images to identify particular areas of interest in order to deliver focused treatment to those areas as well as to potentially evaluate tumor response to radiotherapy. fMRI sequences can be studied separately or in combination and many are currently under investigation for their use in radiotherapy. Diffusion-weighting imaging, which studies the restriction of random brownian motion of water molecules in tumors, has been studied for its utility in staging, target delineation, and treatment response.[49,50] Dynamic contrast-

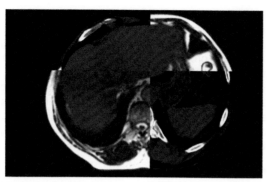

Fig. 4. Diagnostic MR image (*bottom left, top right*) viewed in a split window with the treatment planning CT (*top left, bottom right*) for contouring where the contrast between the lesion and healthy liver appears more clearly on MRI.

enhanced MRI identifies the properties of the vasculature, such as vessel permeability, which is useful in monitoring tumor response.[49–51] MR spectroscopic imaging can be used to characterize the chemical composition within a given image voxel in order to identify cancer biomarkers.[52]

MRI-Only Treatment Planning

Given the significant benefits of MRI and the drawbacks of coregistering MR and CT images, there has been significant interest in developing an MR-only simulation workflow. However, there are significant obstacles in MRI that must be overcome for the further development of these strategies, many of which are discussed here.

Spatial integrity

Geometric distortions in MRI are in 2 categories: system-specific distortions and patient-specific distortions. The 2 major components of system-specific distortion are inhomogeneity of the main magnetic field and nonlinearity in the magnetic field produced by spatial gradient coils. These components are inherent to the particularities of the individual magnet and are typically corrected for in postprocessing implemented by the manufacturer of the system. Of the two, the dominant source of distortion is gradient nonlinearity. Price and colleagues[53] showed that the amount of residual distortion after vendor corrections in a 1.0-T vertical MR scanner caused by gradient nonlinearity can exceed 3 mm within 15 cm from the isocenter, but that this can be reduced to less than 1 mm across the field of view after postvendor applied corrections. Significant distortions may also arise from patient-specific sources, such as chemical shift artifacts[54] and magnetic susceptibility,[55] which are difficult to correct for because of the transient nature of intrapatient and interpatient magnetic properties.

Motion

Because of the length of time required for MRI, motion artifacts can be a significant issue, particularly in the lung and abdomen. Efforts have been made to reduce the length and number of sequences required for radiotherapy needs. However, fast sequences often come with increased geometric distortion. Motion management strategies such as implementation of breath-hold techniques may be beneficial in order to reduce motion artifacts to an acceptable level for certain disease sites.

Electron density information

MR intensity values lack any intrinsic relationship to the electron density values that are essential for inhomogeneity corrections in modern dose calculation algorithms. Several methods have been proposed for using MR images to generate a "synthetic" CT image with intensity values that can be easily converted into electron density values and that can be used to generate digitally reconstructed radiographs. These methods can broadly be classified into 3 groups: methods that assign a bulk density value to all voxels within a set of segmented regions,[56] methods that convert MR-image voxel intensity values directly to CT values,[57–59] and methods that generate an atlas that can be deformed to a patient-specific MR image.[60,61]

Online MRI Guidance

Recently, MR-guided radiation therapy (MRgRT) treatment machines have been introduced, which use MRI as the primary modality for IGRT. The first clinically implemented MRgRT system (ViewRay MRIdian, Cleveland, OH) combined a split-magnet 0.35-T MR scanner with 3 cobalt-60 heads located within the central gap.[62] Various designs have been introduced to overcome the technical challenges of operating a linear accelerator within the magnetic field of an MRI unit. Proposed designs have ranged from an MR-on-rails system, in which an MRI scanner enters and exits the linear accelerator vault via a rail system much like the CT-on-rails concept, to systems that fully combine a linear accelerator and superconducting magnet.[63] The ViewRay MRIdian design with a linear accelerator replacing the cobalt-60 heads was the first MR–linear accelerator system to be approved by the US Food and Drug Administration (FDA), whereas the Elekta Unity (AB, Sweden), which uses a 1.5-T MRI scanner, has also recently gained FDA approval.[64] These units not only take advantage of the excellent soft tissue contrast for patient localization but can also be used to continuously monitor the target or OARs during treatment delivery. This feature is particularly useful in patients with highly mobile tumors (eg, abdominal lesions), for which the information can be used in motion management strategies such as automatically gated breath-hold techniques. Reported allowable scan times range from 17 seconds to roughly 3 minutes for the ViewRay system, with treatment time from patient setup to completion of patient treatment averaging approximately 30 minutes for conventional fractionations and averaging roughly 45 minutes for stereotactic body radiation therapy deliveries.

Adaptive magnetic resonance–based planning

One additional advantage of a combined MR–linear accelerator system is its utility for daily adaptive radiotherapy (ART). ART is the process of adapting a patient's plan to observed changes in the anatomy of the patient throughout the course of treatment. On-board MRI makes it feasible to observe daily variations in the soft tissue structures, particularly in the abdomen, allowing daily modifications to either escalate dose to the target while maintaining constant toxicity to normal structures or reduce dose to OARs.

SUMMARY AND FUTURE DIRECTIONS

Modern radiation therapy treatment planning and delivery is a complex process that relies on advanced imaging and computing technology as well as expertise from the medical team. The process begins with simulation imaging, in which 3D CT images (or MR images in some cases) are used to characterize the patient anatomy. From there, the radiation oncologist delineates the relevant target/tumor volumes and normal tissue and communicates the goals for treatment planning. The planning process attempts to generate a radiation therapy treatment plan that will deliver a therapeutic dose of radiation to the tumor while sparing nearby normal tissue. Various planning techniques are available for modern treatment planning and can be used as determined by the needs of each patient. IGRT has allowed further precision in the targeting of tumors in radiation therapy. In addition, the use of MRI in radiation therapy has provided further advances in soft tissue visualization and adaptive radiation therapy. Future innovations are likely to include further integration of advanced imaging techniques (including advanced MRI image acquisition sequences and novel PET radiotracers) into the routine clinical workflow, with the downstream potential to shape the dose distribution to maximize the biological effect of radiotherapy treatment.

REFERENCES

1. Bushberg JT, Boone JM. The essential physics of medical imaging. Philadelphia: Lippincott Williams & Wilkins; 2011.
2. Glide-Hurst C, Chen D, Zhong H, et al. Changes realized from extended bit-depth and metal artifact reduction in CT. Med Phys 2013;40(6Part1):061711.
3. Hara AK, Paden RG, Silva AC, et al. Iterative reconstruction technique for reducing body radiation dose at CT: feasibility study. AJR Am J Roentgenol 2009;193(3):764–71.
4. Malone S, Crook JM, Kendal WS. Respiratory-induced prostate motion: quantification and characterization. Int J Radiat Oncol Biol Phys 2000;48(1):105–9.
5. Ford E, Mageras G, Yorke E, et al. Respiration-correlated spiral CT: a method of measuring respiratory-induced anatomic motion for radiation treatment planning. Med Phys 2003;30(1):88–97.
6. Prescribing I. Recording and reporting photon beam therapy. ICRU Rep 1993;50.
7. Wambersie A. ICRU report 62, prescribing, recording and reporting photon beam therapy (supplement to ICRU Report 50). ICRU News 1999.
8. Dolezelova H, Slampa P, Ondrova B, et al. The impact of PET with 18FDG in radiotherapy treatment planning and in the prediction in patients with cervix carcinoma: results of pilot study. Neoplasma 2008;55(5):437–41.
9. Terezakis SA, Hunt MA, Kowalski A, et al. [18F] FDG-positron emission tomography coregistration with computed tomography scans for radiation treatment planning of lymphoma and hematologic malignancies. Int J Radiat Oncol Biol Phys 2011;81(3):615–22.
10. Greco C, Rosenzweig K, Cascini GL, et al. Current status of PET/CT for tumour volume definition in radiotherapy treatment planning for non-small cell lung cancer (NSCLC). Lung Cancer 2007;57(2):125–34.
11. Jimenez-Jimenez E, Mateos P, Aymar N, et al. Radiotherapy volume delineation using 18F-FDG-PET/CT modifies gross node volume in patients with oesophageal cancer. Clin Transl Oncol 2018;20(11):1460–6.
12. Hendrickson K, Phillips M, Smith W, et al. Hypoxia imaging with [F-18] FMISO-PET in head and neck cancer: potential for guiding intensity modulated radiation therapy in overcoming hypoxia-induced treatment resistance. Radiother Oncol 2011;101(3):369–75.
13. van Leeuwen PJ, Stricker P, Hruby G, et al. 68Ga-PSMA has a high detection rate of prostate cancer recurrence outside the prostatic fossa in patients being considered for salvage radiation treatment. BJU Int 2016;117(5):732–9.

14. Mayyas E, Chetty IJ, Chetvertkov M, et al. Evaluation of multiple image-based modalities for image-guided radiation therapy (IGRT) of prostate carcinoma: a prospective study. Med Phys 2013;40(4):041707.
15. Jaffray DA, Siewerdsen JH, Wong JW, et al. Flat-panel cone-beam computed tomography for image-guided radiation therapy. Int J Radiat Oncol Biol Phys 2002; 53(5):1337–49.
16. Cheng CW, Wong J, Grimm L, et al. Commissioning and clinical implementation of a sliding gantry CT scanner installed in an existing treatment room and early clinical experience for precise tumor localization [published online ahead of print 2003/06/11]. Am J Clin Oncol 2003;26(3):e28–36.
17. Bissonnette JP, Purdie TG, Higgins JA, et al. Cone-beam computed tomographic image guidance for lung cancer radiation therapy [published online ahead of print 2008/12/20]. Int J Radiat Oncol Biol Phys 2009;73(3):927–34.
18. Mageras GS, Mechalakos J. Planning in the IGRT context: closing the loop [published online ahead of print 2007/10/02]. Semin Radiat Oncol 2007;17(4):268–77.
19. Bert C, Metheany KG, Doppke KP, et al. Clinical experience with a 3D surface patient setup system for alignment of partial-breast irradiation patients. Int J Radiat Oncol Biol Phys 2006;64(4):1265–74.
20. Krengli M, Gaiano S, Mones E, et al. Reproducibility of patient setup by surface image registration system in conformal radiotherapy of prostate cancer. Radiat Oncol 2009;4:9.
21. Gierga DP, Riboldi M, Turcotte JC, et al. Comparison of target registration errors for multiple image-guided techniques in accelerated partial breast irradiation. Int J Radiat Oncol Biol Phys 2008;70(4):1239–46.
22. Schoffel PJ, Harms W, Sroka-Perez G, et al. Accuracy of a commercial optical 3D surface imaging system for realignment of patients for radiotherapy of the thorax. Phys Med Biol 2007;52(13):3949–63.
23. De Los Santos J, Popple R, Agazaryan N, et al. Image guided radiation therapy (IGRT) technologies for radiation therapy localization and delivery [published online ahead of print 2013/05/15]. Int J Radiat Oncol Biol Phys 2013;87(1):33–45.
24. Willoughby T, Lehmann J, Bencomo JA, et al. Quality assurance for nonradiographic radiotherapy localization and positioning systems: Report of Task Group 147. Med Phys 2012;39(4):1728–47.
25. Huang Y, Zhao B, Chetty IJ, et al. Targeting accuracy of image-guided radiosurgery for intracranial lesions a comparison across multiple linear accelerator platforms. Technol Cancer Res Treat 2016;15(2):243–8.
26. Yin F-F, Zhu J, Yan H, et al. Dosimetric characteristics of Novalis shaped beam surgery unit. Med Phys 2002;29(8):1729–38.
27. Boda-Heggemann J, Kohler FM, Kupper B, et al. Accuracy of ultrasound-based (BAT) prostate-repositioning: a three-dimensional on-line fiducial-based assessment with cone-beam computed tomography [published online ahead of print 2008/03/04]. Int J Radiat Oncol Biol Phys 2008;70(4):1247–55.
28. Fuss M, Salter BJ, Cavanaugh SX, et al. Daily ultrasound-based image-guided targeting for radiotherapy of upper abdominal malignancies. Int J Radiat Oncol Biol Phys 2004;59(4):1245–56.
29. Warszawski A, Baumann R, Karstens JH. Sonographic guidance for electron boost planning after breast-conserving surgery. J Clin Ultrasound 2004;32(7): 333–7.
30. Meeks SL, Buatti JM, Bouchet LG, et al. Ultrasound-guided extracranial radiosurgery: technique and application. Int J Radiat Oncol Biol Phys 2003;55(4): 1092–101.

31. Fuss M, Wong A, Fuller CD, et al. Image-guided intensity-modulated radiotherapy for pancreatic carcinoma. Gastrointest Cancer Res 2007;1(1):2–11.
32. Molloy JA, Chan G, Markovic A, et al. Quality assurance of U.S.-guided external beam radiotherapy for prostate cancer: Report of AAPM Task Group 154. Med Phys 2011;38(2):857–71.
33. Schiffner DC, Gottschalk AR, Lometti M, et al. Daily electronic portal imaging of implanted gold seed fiducials in patients undergoing radiotherapy after radical prostatectomy [published online ahead of print 2007/01/24]. Int J Radiat Oncol Biol Phys 2007;67(2):610–9.
34. Kupelian P, Willoughby T, Mahadevan A, et al. Multi-institutional clinical experience with the Calypso System in localization and continuous, real-time monitoring of the prostate gland during external radiotherapy [published online ahead of print 2006/12/26]. Int J Radiat Oncol Biol Phys 2007;67(4):1088–98.
35. Shah AP, Kupelian PA, Waghorn BJ, et al. Real-time tumor tracking in the lung using an electromagnetic tracking system [published online ahead of print 2013/03/26]. Int J Radiat Oncol Biol Phys 2013;86(3):477–83.
36. Fan Q, Nanduri A, Yang J, et al. Toward a planning scheme for emission guided radiation therapy (EGRT): FDG based tumor tracking in a metastatic breast cancer patient [published online ahead of print 2013/08/10]. Med Phys 2013;40(8):081708.
37. Mazin S, Nanduri A, Pelc N. SU-GG-J-03: emission guided radiation therapy system: a feasibility study. Med Phys 2010;37(6Part9):3145.
38. Yang J, Yamamoto T, Thielemans K, et al. 156: a feasibility study for real-time tumor tracking using positron emission tomography (PET). Med Phys 2011;38(6Part9):3479.
39. Ling CC, Humm J, Larson S, et al. Towards multidimensional radiotherapy (MD-CRT): biological imaging and biological conformality [published online ahead of print 2000/06/06]. Int J Radiat Oncol Biol Phys 2000;47(3):551–60.
40. Glide-Hurst CK, Wen N, Hearshen D, et al. Initial clinical experience with a radiation oncology dedicated open 1.0T MR-simulation. J Appl Clin Med Phys 2017;16(2):218–40.
41. Mah D, Steckner M, Palacio E, et al. Characteristics and quality assurance of a dedicated open 0.23 T MRI for radiation therapy simulation. Med Phys 2002;29(11):2541–7.
42. Villeirs GM, Van Vaerenbergh K, Vakaet L, et al. Interobserver delineation variation using CT versus combined CT + MRI in intensity-modulated radiotherapy for prostate cancer. Strahlenther Onkol 2005;181(7):424–30.
43. O'Neill BDP, Salerno G, Thomas K, et al. MR vs CT imaging: low rectal cancer tumour delineation for three-dimensional conformal radiotherapy. Br J Radiol 2009;82(978):509–13.
44. Mitchell DG, Snyder B, Coakley F, et al. Early invasive cervical cancer: Tumor delineation by magnetic resonance imaging, computed tomography, and clinical examination, verified by pathologic results, in the ACRIN 6651/GOG 183 intergroup study. J Clin Oncol 2006;24(36):5687–94.
45. Den Hartogh MD, Philippens MEP, van Dam IE, et al. MRI and CT imaging for preoperative target volume delineation in breast-conserving therapy. Radiat Oncol 2014;9(1):1–9.
46. Cattaneo GM, Reni M, Rizzo G, et al. Target delineation in post-operative radiotherapy of brain gliomas: Interobserver variability and impact of image registration of MR(pre-operative) images on treatment planning CT scans. Radiother Oncol 2005;75(2):217–23.

47. Jansen EPM, Dewit LGH, Van Herk M, et al. Target volumes in radiotherapy for high-grade malignant glioma of the brain. Radiother Oncol 2000;56(2):151–6.

48. Jonsson JH, Karlsson MG, Karlsson M, et al. Radiation Oncology 2010 Jonsson. 2010. 1–8.

49. Tsien C, Cao Y, Chenevert T. Clinical applications for diffusion MRI in radiotherapy. Semin Radiat Oncol 2014;24(3):218–26.

50. Van Der Heide UA, Korporaal JG, Groenendaal G, et al. Functional MRI for tumor delineation in prostate radiation therapy. Imaging Med 2011;3(2):219–31.

51. Guo W, Luo D, Chen X, et al. Dynamic contrast-enhanced magnetic resonance imaging for pretreatment prediction of early chemo-radiotherapy response in larynx and hypopharynx carcinoma. Oncotarget 2017;8(20):33836–43.

52. Posse S, Otazo R, Dager SR, et al. MR spectroscopic imaging: Principles and recent advances. J Magn Reson Imaging 2013;37(6):1301–25.

53. Price RG, Kadbi M, Kim J, et al. Characterization and correction of gradient nonlinearity induced distortion on a 1.0 T open bore MR-SIM. Med Phys 2015; 42(10):5955–60.

54. Weygand J, Fuller CD, Ibbott GS, et al. Spatial precision in magnetic resonance imaging–guided radiation therapy: the role of geometric distortion. Int J Radiat Oncol Biol Phys 2016;95(4):1304–16.

55. Wang H, Balter J, Cao Y. Patient-induced susceptibility effect on geometric distortion of clinical brain MRI for radiation treatment planning on a 3T scanner. Phys Med Biol 2013;58(3):465–77.

56. Aliaksandr K, Katherine M, Gert M, et al. Comparison of bulk electron density and voxel-based electron density treatment planning. J Appl Clin Med Phys 2011; 12(4):97–104.

57. Balter JM, Feng M, Cao Y, et al. Investigation of a method for generating synthetic CT models from MRI scans of the head and neck for radiation therapy. Phys Med Biol 2013;58(23):8419–35.

58. Johansson A, Karlsson M, Nyholm T. CT substitute derived from MRI sequences with ultrashort echo time. Med Phys 2011;38(5):2708–14.

59. Kim J, Glide-Hurst C, Doemer A, et al. Implementation of a novel algorithm for generating synthetic CT images from magnetic resonance imaging data sets for prostate cancer radiation therapy. Int J Radiat Oncol Biol Phys 2015;91(1): 39–47.

60. Emami H, Dong M, Nejad-Davarani SP, et al. Generating synthetic CTs from magnetic resonance images using generative adversarial networks. Med Phys 2018; 45(8):3627–36.

61. Han X. MR-based synthetic CT generation using a deep convolutional neural network method. Med Phys 2017;44(4):1408–19.

62. Mutic S, Dempsey JF. The ViewRay system : magnetic resonance-guided and controlled radiotherapy. Semin Radiat Oncol 2014;24(3):196–9.

63. Das IJ, McGee KP, Tyagi N, et al. Role and future of MRI in radiation oncology. Br J Radiol 2018;92(1094):20180505.

64. Tijssen RH, Philippens ME, Paulson ES, et al. MRI commissioning of 1.5 T MR-linac systems–a multi-institutional study. Radiother Oncol 2019;132:114–20.

Imaging for Target Delineation and Treatment Planning in Radiation Oncology
Current and Emerging Techniques

Sonja Stieb, MD, Brigid McDonald, BS, Mary Gronberg, MS,
Grete May Engeseth, MS, Renjie He, PhD,
Clifton David Fuller, MD, PhD*

KEYWORDS

- CT • MRI • PET • Functional imaging • Target delineation • Treatment planning
- Radiation oncology

KEY POINTS

- Computed tomography (CT) is still the state-of-the-art imaging method for target delineation and treatment planning in radiation oncology.
- Four-dimensional CT, dynamic contrast-enhanced CT, and dual-energy CT can be used to account for motion artifacts and to increase tissue contrast.
- Functional MRI and PET are promising imaging techniques to improve accuracy of target delineation.

INTRODUCTION

Radiation treatment has improved not only with technical advances in the treatment delivery machines but also to great extent by the implementation of new imaging modalities and advanced image sequences.

In radiation oncology, imaging is not exclusively used for diagnosis and tumor response assessment. It also plays an important role in the delineation of target volumes and organs at risk (OARs) as well as in treatment planning. Physician contouring is performed according to the recommendations made by the International Commission on Radiation Units and Measurements (ICRU Report 62 and 78).[1,2] According to the ICRU, the gross tumor volume (GTV) is the visible or clinical demonstrable

Disclosure: See last page of article.
Department of Radiation Oncology, The University of Texas MD Anderson Cancer Center, 1515 Holcombe Boulevard, Houston, TX 77030, USA
* Corresponding author.
E-mail address: CDFuller@mdanderson.org

Hematol Oncol Clin N Am 33 (2019) 963–975
https://doi.org/10.1016/j.hoc.2019.08.008
0889-8588/19/© 2019 Elsevier Inc. All rights reserved.

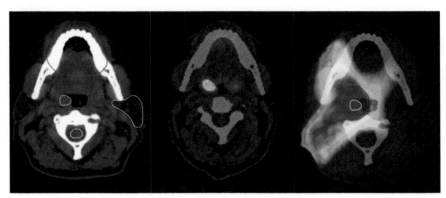

Fig. 1. A patient with T2 tonsil cancer of the right side receiving intensity-modulated radiotherapy with 66 Gy. (*Left*) Axial slice of planning computed tomography (CT) with tumor shown by light green. OARs: orange/cyan, parotid glands; light blue, part of the submandibular gland; yellow, spinal cord. (*Middle*) Corresponding slice of PET/CT with highly 18F-fluorodeoxyglucose (FDG)–active primary tumor (window level PET, 0.5–10 standardized uptake value); (*Right*) Treatment plan with gross tumor volume (GTV; indicates tumor) in green, clinical target volume (GTV + subclinical disease) in lilac, and planning target volume (CTV + geometric expansion) in red. High-dose area highlighted in orange/red.

location and extent of the tumor. The clinical target volume (CTV) is the tissue volume that contains the GTV and/or subclinical malignant disease. The planning target volume is a geometric volume generated by adding a margin to the CTV to account for treatment-related uncertainties such as setup errors and organ motion (**Fig. 1**).

For treatment planning, most radiation treatment centers are equipped with dedicated computed tomography (CT) scanners that are specifically designed for radiotherapy. CT enables accurate dose calculation in treatment planning systems by using the relative attenuation of a series of radiographs to calculate the absorbed dose to tissue.[3]

In addition to CT, MRI has become increasingly important, given the advantages of enhanced soft tissue contrast and no radiation dose. Newer approaches with the combined MRI linear accelerator (MR-Linac) enable - similar to cone-beam CT - improved accuracy of patient positioning compared with on-board radiographs, as well as real-time MRI during radiotherapy to track motion-induced target variability.[4] MRI is also of great importance for target definition, especially in cases in which CT provides poor imaging contrast between the tumor and surrounding tissues.

This article provides a comprehensive overview of the main imaging modalities currently used in radiation oncology as well as new and promising techniques for target delineation and treatment planning.

CT APPROACHES

Before receiving radiation therapy, each patient undergoes CT simulation, which is primarily driven by the necessity of CT for dose calculation.[5,6] Because CT is used for simulation and treatment planning, it is the primary image set used for contouring.

A major advantage of CT imaging is its fast acquisition time, which minimizes motion artifacts from breathing or swallowing.[7,8] CT is exceptionally effective at visualizing high-Z materials (eg, bone) and has uniform distortion across the acquisition field. However, the utility of CT is limited by its poor visualization of soft tissue, which causes difficulties in distinguishing between tumors and the healthy surrounding tissues. To account for this, complimentary imaging that adds anatomic and functional information, such as MRI, is often fused with the primary CT imaging.

Nevertheless, target volume definition is considered the largest uncertainty in modern radiotherapy.[9] Both imaging-related factors (ie, modality, technique, and interpretation) and patient-related factors (ie, organ motion and voluntary motion) can influence the accuracy of target definitions and are considered to contribute to both intrainstitutional and interinstitutional observer variations.[9–11] Substantial interobserver variations have been found for all treatment sites and all target volumes relevant to radiotherapy planning, of which some had significant impact on target dose coverage and OAR doses (**Fig. 2**).[12] Likewise, large interobserver and interinstitutional contouring differences were found in a multicenter Radiation Therapy Oncology Group study of structure delineation for breast cancer on CT. They reported variations in contoured volumes with standard deviations of up to 60%, and also dosimetric consequences for OARs.[13] Errors in target definitions are systematic in nature, thus the effect remains constant during the treatment course and may, in worst-case scenarios, lead to underdosage of the target and poorer local control and survival outcomes.[14,15]

Efforts to reduce observer variations in target definitions include improved imaging techniques, the use of contouring guidelines and atlases, standardization of training, autocontouring, and peer review. The use of written guidelines has been found to significantly improve consistency in target delineation and, in some situations, to reduce doses to OARs.[16] Guidelines exist for tumor and nodal contouring on CT and are available through the Radiation Therapy Oncology Group Core Laboratory for numerous treatment sites, including lung,[17] breast,[18] head and neck,[19] and prostate.[20]

Training interventions have also led to significant improvements in interobserver variability; target delineation courses have been shown to result in both smaller and more homogeneous target volumes among radiation oncologists.[21] Training and teaching that includes anatomic lessons followed by contouring practice with individual feedback is considered most successful.[16]

Further improvement in target delineation can be achieved by a clinical peer review process on radiation treatment plans, including information on patients' disease characteristics, diagnostic imaging review, and clinical and visual inspection of the patient.[22] Although contouring guidelines have led to improved standardization in target delineation, the contributions of technological innovations in CT have further improved target delineation accuracy through improved tumor/normal-tissue contrast and motion management. In a new technique called four-dimensional (4D) CT, a series of three-dimensional (3D) CT images are correlated with the patient's breathing cycle over time to produce a motion model of the tumor. 4D-CT simulation is now the standard of care at many hospitals for patients with lung, esophageal, and liver tumors because of improvements in motion management during radiation treatment, which ultimately improves tumor localization and reduces normal tissue doses.[23]

4D-CT can be used in several ways to improve motion management. If the scan indicates a small range of motion of the tumor through the breathing cycle, then the physician may elect to treat the patient free breathing and account for the motion during treatment planning by expanding the CTV to create the internal target volume (ITV). The motion margin is typically determined by population-based studies. However, with 4D-CT, the physician can define a patient-specific ITV that includes the full range of motion of the tumor. This patient-specific ITV approach is used in combination with

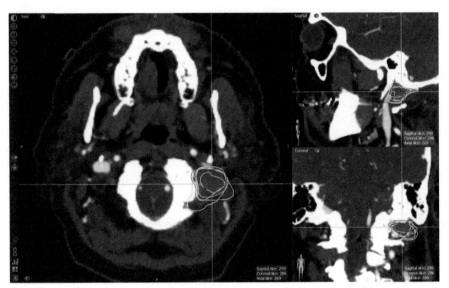

Fig. 2. The difference in contouring by radiation oncologists of a left skull base metastasis on 60-keV dual-energy CT. (*Left*) Axial slice, (*upper right*) sagittal view, (*lower right*) coronal view.

free breathing treatment for small ranges of motion indicated by 4D-CT imaging. However, if 4D-CT imaging indicates substantial motion, then strategies to reduce motion effects, such as breath hold and phase-based respiratory gating,[24,25] are needed. Comparison studies of 4D-CT motion management versus conventional 3D-CT have shown improved target coverage and subsequent reduced normal tissue dose.[26,27]

Other approaches for improving the accuracy of tumor delineation with CT are contrast administration and dual-energy (DE) CT. CT target delineation relies on inherent differences in the density and attenuation of tumors relative to surrounding soft tissue. However, when tumors such as liver tumors have similar attenuation characteristics to the surrounding tissues, intravenous (IV) contrast can be used to enhance the tumor visibility.[28] Differences in the uptake, retention, and washout of IV contrast can be helpful for identifying malignant disease. The combination of baseline CT imaging without contrast and subsequent imaging over time with IV contrast, called dynamic contrast-enhanced (DCE) CT,[29] can further increase tissue contrast and reduce target delineation variation in liver tumors.[30] In addition, for treatment sites where both organ motion and low tumor/healthy-tissue contrast is an issue (eg, in esophageal cancers), improvement in target definition may be achieved by using contrast-enhanced 4D-CT scans.[31]

DE-CT uses both low-energy (typically 80 kVp) and high-energy (typically 140 kVp) x-rays. Tissue attenuation depends not only on material characteristics but also on photon energy. Having 2 data points rather than 1 can improve the identification of tissue composition.[32] Although DE-CT is mainly used for diagnostic applications, its use is becoming more common in radiotherapy departments.[33] DE-CT offers the advantage of improved image quality through superior material separation and metal artifact reduction.[34,35] The subsequent impact on dose calculation accuracy, particularly in brachytherapy,[36] proton therapy,[37] and tumor delineation accuracy,[38,39] is being investigated.

MRI APPROACHES

For target delineation, MRI is primarily used in cases in which CT does not reveal sufficient contrast between the tumor and surrounding structures, such as for primary brain tumors and cerebral metastases. In this case, all contouring can be performed on a coregistered magnetic resonance (MR) image and transferred to the planning CT. In other disease sites, such as head and neck cancers, target delineation can also be performed primarily on MRI with adaptation on CT, as long as the patient setup is reproduced accurately enough to allow rigid registration between the CT and MR or a dedicate deformable image registration tool is available (**Fig. 3**).

The additional information from MRI can lead to a change in volume of the targets. In cases of brain tumors, MRI led to larger volumes,[40] whereas for the prostate bed reduced volumes with MRI were reported.[41] No difference in volume was reported when using MRI or CT for delineation for pharyngolaryngeal tumors,[42] lung cancer,[43] and the lumpectomy cavity of the breast.[44] However, even in cases of nonsignificant differences in target volume, a significant difference can appear regarding the outline of the structures. Interobserver comparisons have revealed higher similarity in contouring the lumpectomy cavity in breast cancer on MRI than on CT.[44] However, higher interobserver agreement was reported for CT than MRI and delineation of prostate bed[41] and lung cancer.[43] No difference was found in head and neck cancer[45] and brain tumors.[40]

Another approach to using MRI for target volume definition is with artificial intelligence, such as machine learning and deep learning,[46] but these methods require further validation and should only be used as guidance for physicians in target delineation.

Although so far only the standard MR sequences such as T1-weighted, T2-weighted, and T1-weighted postcontrast imaging are routinely used for delineation, other promising sequences, such as diffusion-weighted imaging (DWI), are under investigation. Delineation on DWI was shown to correlate better with microscopic tumor extent than the contours drawn on CT and standard MR sequences in patients with laryngeal cancer.[47] The addition of this sequence led to an adaptation of the target volume in 73% of patients with locally advanced cervical cancer[48] and to a larger target volume in patients with head and neck cancer compared with CT, PET, T2-weighted MRI, or a combination.[49]

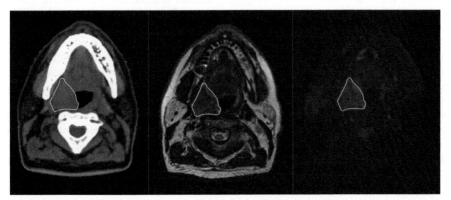

Fig. 3. A patient with T4 tonsil cancer of the right side (tumor delineated in *green*). (*Left*) Poor image contrast between tumor and surrounding tissue on CT; (*middle*) improved image contrast on T2-weighted MRI; (*right*) diffusion-weighted MRI for the same patient.

Furthermore, many groups have been involved in the application of MRI radiomics features extracted from various MRI sequences and have explored using these features as surrogates of a noninvasive predictive tool to guide diagnosis, tumor phenotyping, and therapy outcome across different disease sites. MRI radiomics models have been investigated to differentiate between benign and malignant disease and tumor grading in central nervous system,[50] liver,[51] prostate,[52,53] bladder,[54] and across other organ sites.[55,56] However, this method needs further validation before it can be applied clinically.

PET/CT AND SPECT/CT APPROACHES

PET and single-photon emission computed tomography (SPECT) are functional imaging techniques that are commonly leveraged in radiation oncology to differentiate between tumor and healthy tissues. They are typically combined with simultaneous CT to produce images that contain both anatomic and functional information, whereas only few centers so far offer combined PET/MR. PET/CT and SPECT/CT have been shown to improve lesion contrast and detectability and tumor staging accuracy compared with PET, SPECT, or CT alone,[57–59] which is particularly useful for target volume definition when there is poor contrast between the tumor and surrounding tissues on CT or MR.[60]

The most common PET radiotracer is 18F-fluorodeoxyglucose (18F-FDG), which is widely used for target delineation in many types of cancers, including head and neck cancer, lung cancer, and lymphoma, and can lead to significant adaptation of the treatment volumes.[61] For example, Prathipati and colleagues[62] compared target volumes for non–small cell lung cancer generated based on contrast-enhanced CT versus PET/CT and found that the primary volume was increased and decreased for 39% and 50% of patients with the addition of PET, respectively. Further, additional involved lymph nodes were identified for 27% of patients, which suggests that PET/CT allows more accurate detection and targeting of malignant masses and better sparing of noncancerous tissues.

However, 18F-FDG is a poor radiotracer for non–glucose-avid tumors such as low-grade prostate cancers and thyroid cancers.[63] In addition, there tends to be high uptake of 18F-FDG in benign lesions with increased glucose metabolism, such as acute inflammatory lesions and postsurgical scar tissue, resulting in a high rate of false-positives with 18F-FDG–PET/CT imaging.[64] Certain organs, such as the brain and heart, also require large amounts of glucose to meet their high metabolic demands, so the uptake of 18F-FDG in these organs can mask nearby lesions.

To overcome some of the shortcomings of 18F-FDG, a host of other positron-emitting radiotracers have been developed and evaluated for detection of cancerous masses, including 11C-choline. Choline is an effective radiotracer for identifying locally recurrent disease after radical prostatectomy[65,66] and for detecting lymph node involvement[67] or distant metastases. The addition of PET compared with CT alone can have a major impact on target volume or prescription dose, which changed in 56% of patients, as described by Alongi and colleagues.[68] However, major drawbacks of choline include the short physical half-life of 11C (20 minutes), which limits its use to institutions that have their own cyclotrons, as well as a reduced detection accuracy for microcarcinomas and micrometastases.

An emerging alternative to 11C-choline for prostate cancer is prostate-specific membrane antigen radiolabeled with 68Ga. Although its half-life is roughly 3 times longer than that of 11C (68 minutes), it is still inconvenient for transport among facilities. Nonetheless, 68Ga can be produced using a generator composed of the parent isotope 68Ge, which can be maintained in a hospital and eluted to obtain 68Ga as needed.[69]

Another emerging radiotracer is 18F-fluoroethyl-tyrosine (FET), which is used for brain cancer. Because of the brain's high metabolism of glucose, 18F-FDG is taken up by healthy brain cells, often masking malignant tissues in the brain in conventional 18F-FDG–PET imaging.[70] In a meta-analysis of 5 studies, 18F-FET–PET showed a pooled sensitivity and specificity of 0.94 and 0.88, respectively, compared with 0.38 and 0.86, respectively, for 18F-FDG–PET in patients with primary brain tumors.[71]

PET is considered a quantitative imaging modality, measuring the tracer activity in each pixel. Quantitative accuracy requires the raw voxel values to be corrected for photon attenuation in the patient, physical decay of the radionuclide, dead-time losses in the detector, and scatter and random coincidences.[6] The uptake of PET radiotracers can be quantified using the standardized uptake value (SUV), which characterizes the measured activity in a voxel as a fraction of the total administered activity.[72] However, SUV values can be affected by many factors, including reconstruction algorithms, partial volume effects, radiotracer distribution times, accuracy of patient body mass, and activity of radiotracer leftover in the syringe after injection, and are at best semiquantitative.[6,73]

The relative SUV of the tumor and nearby organs is used to differentiate malignant from healthy tissues, but visualization of the borders of high-uptake regions largely depends on the observer and the window/level settings used to view the PET/CT image.[74] To address this interobserver variability, many clinics use autosegmentation techniques based on threshold SUV values to define tumor boundaries. Even so, there are various thresholding methods used, including defining any voxels with SUV greater than 2.5 as tumor,[75] isocontouring based on a given percentage of maximum tumor SUV,[76] and thresholding based on the signal/background ratio,[77] whereas the reference tissue can vary as well. Schinagl and colleagues[78] compared contours generated by each of these methods with manually drawn contours based on visual interpretation of PET/CT for head and neck cancers. They observed significant variation in target volume and overlap fraction among all segmentation approaches. They also found that the SUV greater than 2.5 threshold, which is the most commonly used threshold value for lung cancer delineation, grossly overestimated the target volume in 45% of head and neck cases. This result was attributed to the high uptake of 18F-FDG in the muscular tissue in the head and neck compared with the low 18F-FDG uptake in healthy lung tissue. This example shows that thresholding methods that may work reasonably well for one disease site may not simply be extrapolated to other tumor sites without proper validation.

Similarly, caution should be exercised when extending the concept of SUV to radiopharmaceuticals other than 18F-FDG. Several studies have shown a significant difference in SUV values for emerging radiopharmaceuticals compared with 18F-FDG,[79,80] suggesting that SUV values cannot be reliably compared between different radiotracers because of differences in tracer metabolism.

Although autosegmentation of tumor volumes based on SUV values can speed up the segmentation process and provide a less subjective definition of tumor volumes, all contours used for radiation therapy planning should be reviewed and modified as appropriate based on an experienced radiation oncologist's clinical judgment.

In addition to defining the GTV for radiation planning purposes, PET/CT can be used to identify tumor subregions based on differential radiotracer uptake. In a process known as dose painting, different doses can be applied to subregions thought to be at a higher or lower risk of recurrence in order to increase the probability of long-term survival while decreasing the probability of radiation-induced side effects.

Several feasibility studies have shown the potential of this treatment method in head and neck cancers,[81–83] although further investigation and long-term follow-up are needed before dose painting can become the standard of care.

DISCLOSURE

S. Stieb is funded by the Swiss Cancer League (Switzerland) (BIL KLS-4300-08-2017), G.M. Engeseth by the Bergen Forskningsstiftlelse (Norway). C.D. Fuller received funding from the National Institutes of Health (NIH, United States)/National Institute for Dental and Craniofacial Research Award (1R01DE025248-01/R56DE025248) and Academic-Industrial Partnership Award (R01 DE028290), the National Science Foundation (NSF, United States), Division of Mathematical Sciences (United States), Joint National Institutes of Health (NIH)/NSF Initiative on Quantitative Approaches to Biomedical Big Data (QuBBD) grant (NSF 1557679), the NIH Big Data to Knowledge (BD2K) Program of the National Cancer Institute (NCI, United States) Early Stage Development of Technologies in Biomedical Computing, Informatics, and Big Data Science Award (1R01CA214825), the NCI Early Phase Clinical Trials in Imaging and Image-Guided Interventions Program (1R01CA218148), the NIH/NCI Cancer Center Support Grant (CCSG) Pilot Research Program Award from the University of Texas MD Anderson CCSG Radiation Oncology and Cancer Imaging Program (P30CA016672), the NIH/NCI Head and Neck Specialized Programs of Research Excellence (SPORE) Developmental Research Program Award (P50 CA097007), and the National Institute of Biomedical Imaging and Bioengineering (NIBIB) Research Education Program (R25EB025787). C.D. Fuller has received direct industry grant support, speaking honoraria, and travel funding from Elekta AB.

REFERENCES

1. Prescribing, Recording, and Reporting Photon-Beam Intensity-Modulated Radiation Therapy (IMRT): Contents. Journal of the International Commission on Radiation Units and Measurements 2016;10(1).
2. Landberg T, Chavaudra J, Dobbs J, et al. Report 62. Journal of the International Commission on Radiation Units and Measurements 2016;32(1).
3. Saw CB, Loper A, Komanduri K, et al. Determination of CT-to-density conversion relationship for image-based treatment planning systems. Med Dosim 2005; 30(3):145–8.
4. Kontaxis C, Bol GH, Stemkens B, et al. Towards fast online intrafraction replanning for free-breathing stereotactic body radiation therapy with the MR-linac. Phys Med Biol 2017;62(18):7233–48.
5. Khan FM, Gibbons JP, Sperduto PW. Khan's Treatment Planning in Radiation Oncology. Lippincott Williams & Wilkins; 2016.
6. Bushberg J, Seibert J, Leidholdt E, et al. The Essential Physics of Medical Imaging. In: Wolters Kluwer Health. 2011.
7. Pelc NJ. Recent and future directions in CT imaging. Ann Biomed Eng 2014; 42(2):260–8.
8. Barrett JF, Keat N. Artifacts in CT: recognition and avoidance. Radiographics 2004;24(6):1679–91.
9. Njeh CF. Tumor delineation: the weakest link in the search for accuracy in radiotherapy. J Med Phys 2008;33(4):136–40.
10. Rasch C, Steenbakkers R, van Herk M. Target definition in prostate, head, and neck. Semin Radiat Oncol 2005;15(3):136–45.

11. Chang ATY, Tan LT, Duke S, et al. Challenges for quality assurance of target volume delineation in clinical trials. Front Oncol 2017;7:221.

12. Vinod SK, Min M, Jameson MG, et al. A review of interventions to reduce interobserver variability in volume delineation in radiation oncology. J Med Imaging Radiat Oncol 2016;60(3):393–406.

13. Li XA, Tai A, Arthur DW, et al. Variability of target and normal structure delineation for breast cancer radiotherapy: an RTOG Multi-Institutional and Multi-observer Study. Int J Radiat Oncol Biol Phys 2009;73(3):944–51.

14. Chen AM, Chin R, Beron P, et al. Inadequate target volume delineation and localregional recurrence after intensity-modulated radiotherapy for human papillomavirus-positive oropharynx cancer. Radiother Oncol 2017;123(3):412–8.

15. Peters LJ, O'Sullivan B, Giralt J, et al. Critical impact of radiotherapy protocol compliance and quality in the treatment of advanced head and neck cancer: results from TROG 02.02. J Clin Oncol 2010;28(18):2996–3001.

16. Vinod SK, Jameson MG, Min M, et al. Uncertainties in volume delineation in radiation oncology: a systematic review and recommendations for future studies. Radiother Oncol 2016;121(2):169–79.

17. Nestle U, De Ruysscher D, Ricardi U, et al. ESTRO ACROP guidelines for target volume definition in the treatment of locally advanced non-small cell lung cancer. Radiother Oncol 2018;127(1):1–5.

18. Offersen BV, Boersma LJ, Kirkove C, et al. ESTRO consensus guideline on target volume delineation for elective radiation therapy of early stage breast cancer. Radiother Oncol 2015;114(1):3–10.

19. Gregoire V, Evans M, Le QT, et al. Delineation of the primary tumour clinical target volumes (CTV-P) in laryngeal, hypopharyngeal, oropharyngeal and oral cavity squamous cell carcinoma: AIRO, CACA, DAHANCA, EORTC, GEORCC, GORTEC, HKNPCSG, HNCIG, IAG-KHT, LPRHHT, NCIC CTG, NCRI, NRG Oncology, PHNS, SBRT, SOMERA, SRO, SSHNO, TROG consensus guidelines. Radiother Oncol 2018;126(1):3–24.

20. Salembier C, Villeirs G, De Bari B, et al. ESTRO ACROP consensus guideline on CT- and MRI-based target volume delineation for primary radiation therapy of localized prostate cancer. Radiother Oncol 2018;127(1):49–61.

21. Onal C, Cengiz M, Guler OC, et al. The role of delineation education programs for improving interobserver variability in target volume delineation in gastric cancer. Br J Radiol 2017;90(1073):20160826.

22. Cardenas CE, Mohamed ASR, Tao R, et al. Prospective qualitative and quantitative analysis of real-time peer review quality assurance rounds incorporating direct physical examination for head and neck cancer radiation therapy. Int J Radiat Oncol Biol Phys 2017;98(3):532–40.

23. Li G, Citrin D, Camphausen K, et al. Advances in 4D medical imaging and 4D radiation therapy. Technol Cancer Res Treat 2008;7(1):67–81.

24. Giraud P, Garcia R. Respiratory gating for radiotherapy: main technical aspects and clinical benefits. Bull Cancer 2010;97(7):847–56 [in French].

25. Evans PM. Anatomical imaging for radiotherapy. Phys Med Biol 2008;53(12):R151–91.

26. Ahmed N, Venkataraman S, Johnson K, et al. Does motion assessment with 4-dimensional computed tomographic imaging for non-small cell lung cancer radiotherapy improve target volume coverage? Clin Med Insights Oncol 2017;11. 1179554917698461.

27. Wang L, Hayes S, Paskalev K, et al. Dosimetric comparison of stereotactic body radiotherapy using 4D CT and multiphase CT images for treatment planning of

lung cancer: evaluation of the impact on daily dose coverage. Radiother Oncol 2009;91(3):314–24.

28. Beddar AS, Briere TM, Balter P, et al. 4D-CT imaging with synchronized intravenous contrast injection to improve delineation of liver tumors for treatment planning. Radiother Oncol 2008;87(3):445–8.

29. O'Connor JP, Tofts PS, Miles KA, et al. Dynamic contrast-enhanced imaging techniques: CT and MRI. Br J Radiol 2011;(84 Spec No 2):S112–20.

30. Jensen NK, Mulder D, Lock M, et al. Dynamic contrast enhanced CT aiding gross tumor volume delineation of liver tumors: an interobserver variability study. Radiother Oncol 2014;111(1):153–7.

31. Wang JZ, Li JB, Qi HP, et al. Effect of contrast enhancement in delineating GTV and constructing IGTV of thoracic oesophageal cancer based on 4D-CT scans. Radiother Oncol 2016;119(1):172–8.

32. Coursey CA, Nelson RC, Boll DT, et al. Dual-energy multidetector CT: how does it work, what can it tell us, and when can we use it in abdominopelvic imaging? Radiographics 2010;30(4):1037–55.

33. van Elmpt W, Landry G, Das M, et al. Dual energy CT in radiotherapy: current applications and future outlook. Radiother Oncol 2016;119(1):137–44.

34. Ginat DT, Mayich M, Daftari-Besheli L, et al. Clinical applications of dual-energy CT in head and neck imaging. Eur Arch Otorhinolaryngol 2016;273(3):547–53.

35. Pessis E, Sverzut JM, Campagna R, et al. Reduction of metal artifact with dual-energy CT: virtual monospectral imaging with fast kilovoltage switching and metal artifact reduction software. Semin Musculoskelet Radiol 2015;19(5):446–55.

36. Remy C, Lalonde A, Beliveau-Nadeau D, et al. Dosimetric impact of dual-energy CT tissue segmentation for low-energy prostate brachytherapy: a Monte Carlo study. Phys Med Biol 2018;63(2):025013.

37. Zhu J, Penfold SN. Dosimetric comparison of stopping power calibration with dual-energy CT and single-energy CT in proton therapy treatment planning. Med Phys 2016;43(6):2845–54.

38. Kovacs DG, Rechner LA, Appelt AL, et al. Metal artefact reduction for accurate tumour delineation in radiotherapy. Radiother Oncol 2018;126(3):479–86.

39. Noid G, Currey AD, Bergom C, et al. Improvement of breast tumor delineation for preoperative radiation therapy using dual-energy CT. Int J Radiat Oncol Biol Phys 2017;99(2):E704.

40. Weltens C, Menten J, Feron M, et al. Interobserver variations in gross tumor volume delineation of brain tumors on computed tomography and impact of magnetic resonance imaging. Radiother Oncol 2001;60(1):49–59.

41. Barkati M, Simard D, Taussky D, et al. Magnetic resonance imaging for prostate bed radiotherapy planning: an inter- and intra-observer variability study. J Med Imaging Radiat Oncol 2016;60(2):255–9.

42. Geets X, Daisne JF, Arcangeli S, et al. Inter-observer variability in the delineation of pharyngo-laryngeal tumor, parotid glands and cervical spinal cord: comparison between CT-scan and MRI. Radiother Oncol 2005;77(1):25–31.

43. Wee CW, An HJ, Kang HC, et al. Variability of gross tumor volume delineation for stereotactic body radiotherapy of the lung with Tri-(60)Co magnetic resonance image-guided radiotherapy system (ViewRay): a comparative study with magnetic resonance- and computed tomography-based target delineation. Technol Cancer Res Treat 2018;17. 1533033818787383.

44. Al-Hammadi N, Caparrotti P, Divakar S, et al. MRI reduces variation of contouring for boost clinical target volume in breast cancer patients without surgical clips in the tumour bed. Radiol Oncol 2017;51(2):160–8.

45. Anderson CM, Sun W, Buatti JM, et al. Interobserver and intermodality variability in GTV delineation on simulation CT, FDG-PET, and MR images of head and neck cancer. Jacobs J Radiat Oncol 2014;1(1):006.

46. Boon IS, Au Yong TPT, Boon CS. Assessing the role of artificial intelligence (AI) in clinical oncology: utility of machine learning in radiotherapy target volume delineation. Medicines (Basel) 2018;5(4) [pii:E131].

47. Ligtenberg H, Schakel T, Dankbaar JW, et al. Target volume delineation using diffusion-weighted imaging for mr-guided radiotherapy: a case series of laryngeal cancer validated by pathology. Cureus 2018;10(4):e2465.

48. Schernberg A, Balleyguier C, Dumas I, et al. Diffusion-weighted MRI in image-guided adaptive brachytherapy: tumor delineation feasibility study and comparison with GEC-ESTRO guidelines. Brachytherapy 2017;16(5):956–63.

49. Cardoso M, Min M, Jameson M, et al. Evaluating diffusion-weighted magnetic resonance imaging for target volume delineation in head and neck radiotherapy. J Med Imaging Radiat Oncol 2019;63(3):399–407.

50. Vamvakas A, Williams SC, Theodorou K, et al. Imaging biomarker analysis of advanced multiparametric MRI for glioma grading. Phys Med 2019;60:188–98.

51. Wu J, Liu A, Cui J, et al. Radiomics-based classification of hepatocellular carcinoma and hepatic haemangioma on precontrast magnetic resonance images. BMC Med Imaging 2019;19(1):23.

52. Chaddad A, Niazi T, Probst S, et al. Predicting gleason score of prostate cancer patients using radiomic analysis. Front Oncol 2018;8:630.

53. Xu M, Fang M, Zou J, et al. Using biparametric MRI radiomics signature to differentiate between benign and malignant prostate lesions. Eur J Radiol 2019;114: 38–44.

54. Wang H, Hu D, Yao H, et al. Radiomics analysis of multiparametric MRI for the preoperative evaluation of pathological grade in bladder cancer tumors. Eur Radiol 2019. [Epub ahead of print].

55. Fruehwald-Pallamar J, Czerny C, Holzer-Fruehwald L, et al. Texture-based and diffusion-weighted discrimination of parotid gland lesions on MR images at 3.0 Tesla. NMR Biomed 2013;26(11):1372–9.

56. Zhang H, Mao Y, Chen X, et al. Magnetic resonance imaging radiomics in categorizing ovarian masses and predicting clinical outcome: a preliminary study. Eur Radiol 2019;29(7):3358–71.

57. Lardinois D, Weder W, Hany TF, et al. Staging of non-small-cell lung cancer with integrated positron-emission tomography and computed tomography. N Engl J Med 2003;348(25):2500–7.

58. De Wever W, Ceyssens S, Mortelmans L, et al. Additional value of PET-CT in the staging of lung cancer: comparison with CT alone, PET alone and visual correlation of PET and CT. Eur Radiol 2007;17(1):23–32.

59. Bural GG, Muthukrishnan A, Oborski MJ, et al. Improved benefit of SPECT/CT compared to SPECT alone for the accurate localization of endocrine and neuroendocrine tumors. Mol Imaging Radionucl Ther 2012;21(3):91–6.

60. Satoh Y, Ichikawa T, Motosugi U, et al. Diagnosis of peritoneal dissemination: comparison of 18F-FDG PET/CT, diffusion-weighted MRI, and contrast-enhanced MDCT. AJR Am J Roentgenol 2011;196(2):447–53.

61. McKay MJ, Taubman KL, Foroudi F, et al. Molecular imaging using PET/CT for radiation therapy planning for adult cancers: current status and expanding applications. Int J Radiat Oncol Biol Phys 2018;102(4):783–91.

62. Prathipati A, Manthri RG, Subramanian BV, et al. A prospective study comparing functional imaging ((18)F-FDG PET) versus anatomical imaging (contrast

enhanced CT) in dosimetric planning for non-small cell lung cancer. Asia Ocean J Nucl Med Biol 2017;5(2):75–84.

63. Flavell RR, Naeger DM, Aparici CM, et al. Malignancies with low fluorodeoxyglucose uptake at PET/CT: pitfalls and prognostic importance: resident and fellow education feature. Radiographics 2016;36(1):293–4.

64. Strauss LG. Fluorine-18 deoxyglucose and false-positive results: a major problem in the diagnostics of oncological patients. Eur J Nucl Med 1996;23(10):1409–15.

65. Reske SN, Blumstein NM, Glatting G. [11C]choline PET/CT imaging in occult local relapse of prostate cancer after radical prostatectomy. Eur J Nucl Med Mol Imaging 2008;35(1):9–17.

66. Vees H, Buchegger F, Albrecht S, et al. 18F-choline and/or 11C-acetate positron emission tomography: detection of residual or progressive subclinical disease at very low prostate-specific antigen values (<1 ng/mL) after radical prostatectomy. BJU Int 2007;99(6):1415–20.

67. Souvatzoglou M, Krause BJ, Purschel A, et al. Influence of (11)C-choline PET/CT on the treatment planning for salvage radiation therapy in patients with biochemical recurrence of prostate cancer. Radiother Oncol 2011;99(2):193–200.

68. Alongi F, Comito T, Villa E, et al. What is the role of [11C]choline PET/CT in decision making strategy before post-operative salvage radiation therapy in prostate cancer patients? Acta Oncol 2014;53(7):990–2.

69. Banerjee SR, Pomper MG. Clinical applications of Gallium-68. Appl Radiat Isot 2013;76:2–13.

70. Wong TZ, van der Westhuizen GJ, Coleman RE. Positron emission tomography imaging of brain tumors. Neuroimaging Clin N Am 2002;12(4):615–26.

71. Dunet V, Pomoni A, Hottinger A, et al. Performance of 18F-FET versus 18F-FDG-PET for the diagnosis and grading of brain tumors: systematic review and meta-analysis. Neuro Oncol 2016;18(3):426–34.

72. Thie JA. Understanding the standardized uptake value, its methods, and implications for usage. J Nucl Med 2004;45(9):1431–4.

73. Kwee TC, Cheng G, Lam MG, et al. SUVmax of 2.5 should not be embraced as a magic threshold for separating benign from malignant lesions. Eur J Nucl Med Mol Imaging 2013;40(10):1475–7.

74. Suzuki O, Nishiyama K, Morimoto M, et al. Defining PET standardized uptake value threshold for tumor delineation with metastatic lymph nodes in head and neck cancer. Jpn J Clin Oncol 2012;42(6):491–7.

75. Hong R, Halama J, Bova D, et al. Correlation of PET standard uptake value and CT window-level thresholds for target delineation in CT-based radiation treatment planning. Int J Radiat Oncol Biol Phys 2007;67(3):720–6.

76. Walker AJ, Chirindel A, Hobbs RF, et al. Use of standardized uptake value thresholding for target volume delineation in pediatric Hodgkin lymphoma. Pract Radiat Oncol 2015;5(4):219–27.

77. Daisne JF, Sibomana M, Bol A, et al. Tri-dimensional automatic segmentation of PET volumes based on measured source-to-background ratios: influence of reconstruction algorithms. Radiother Oncol 2003;69(3):247–50.

78. Schinagl DA, Vogel WV, Hoffmann AL, et al. Comparison of five segmentation tools for 18F-fluoro-deoxy-glucose-positron emission tomography-based target volume definition in head and neck cancer. Int J Radiat Oncol Biol Phys 2007;69(4):1282–9.

79. Khan N, Oriuchi N, Zhang H, et al. A comparative study of 11C-choline PET and [18F]fluorodeoxyglucose PET in the evaluation of lung cancer. Nucl Med Commun 2003;24(4):359–66.

80. Minamimoto R, Jamali M, Barkhodari A, et al. Biodistribution of the (1)(8)F-FPPRGD(2) PET radiopharmaceutical in cancer patients: an atlas of SUV measurements. Eur J Nucl Med Mol Imaging 2015;42(12):1850–8.
81. Dirix P, Vandecaveye V, De Keyzer F, et al. Dose painting in radiotherapy for head and neck squamous cell carcinoma: value of repeated functional imaging with (18)F-FDG PET, (18)F-fluoromisonidazole PET, diffusion-weighted MRI, and dynamic contrast-enhanced MRI. J Nucl Med 2009;50(7):1020–7.
82. Houweling AC, Wolf AL, Vogel WV, et al. FDG-PET and diffusion-weighted MRI in head-and-neck cancer patients: implications for dose painting. Radiother Oncol 2013;106(2):250–4.
83. Mohamed ASR, Cardenas CE, Garden AS, et al. Patterns-of-failure guided biological target volume definition for head and neck cancer patients: FDG-PET and dosimetric analysis of dose escalation candidate subregions. Radiother Oncol 2017;124(2):248–55.

Principles and Applications of Stereotactic Radiosurgery and Stereotactic Body Radiation Therapy

Stephen Abel, DO[a], Soyoung Lee, PhD[a], Ethan B. Ludmir, MD[b],
Vivek Verma, MD[a],*

KEYWORDS

- Stereotactic radiosurgery • Stereotactic body radiation therapy
- Stereotactic ablative radiotherapy

KEY POINTS

- Stereotactic radiation therapy (RT) involves the delivery of high dose-per-fraction treatments to small intracranial (stereotactic radiosurgery or SRS) and extracranial (stereotactic body radiotherapy or SBRT) sites.
- SRS and SBRT share several overarching principles that differentiate stereotactic RT from conventionally fractionated radiation techniques.
- SRS and SBRT represent advanced RT technologies to further the goal of radiation oncology and deliver highly conformal radiation therapy in a safe and efficacious way.
- Hallmarks of SRS/SBRT include superior tumor localization and patient immobilization, smaller treatment margins, image guidance, careful treatment planning, high fractional doses, and distinct radiobiology compared with conventionally fractionated regimens.

INTRODUCTION

At its core, the goal of radiation oncology is to balance the beneficial, antitumoral effects of radiation therapy (RT) with radiation-induced toxicities. To this end, radiation oncology maintains its commitment to patients by continually seeking to deliver RT with the utmost technological precision possible; these advances afford the opportunity to optimize the therapeutic ratio, improving disease control while limiting toxicity. The development of stereotactic RT represents an important step toward this goal.

Disclosures: None. This article has never been presented or published before in any form. There was no research funding for this study. All authors declare that conflicts of interest do not exist.
[a] Division of Radiation Oncology, Allegheny Health Network Cancer Institute, 320 East North Avenue, Pittsburgh, PA 15212, USA; [b] Department of Radiation Oncology, University of Texas M.D. Anderson Cancer Center, Unit 097, 1515 Holcombe Boulevard, Houston, TX 77030, USA
* Corresponding author.
E-mail address: vivek333@gmail.com

Stereotactic RT involves the delivery of high dose-per-fraction treatments to a relatively small volumetric target(s). To safely deliver such high doses, a high degree of target conformality is essential and dose constraints of adjacent organs at risk must be respected. Although stereotactic RT is not applicable to every clinical scenario (ie, large tumors and nearby critical structures), the ablative potential of stereotactic RT has shown increasing preclinical and clinical interest for numerous neoplasms.

Both stereotactic radiosurgery (SRS) and stereotactic body radiation therapy (SBRT, also known as stereotactic ablative body radiotherapy or SABR) refer to the highly conformal, targeted delivery of conformal radiation made possible by advanced technological capabilities (**Fig. 1**). These sophisticated capabilities include aspects of the radiation delivery system (via either teletherapy or linear accelerator [LINAC] for the purposes of this review) as well as developments in patient positioning and image guidance of RT. These advancements have allowed practitioners to use smaller target margins when better accounting for patient setup and motion uncertainties. Similarly, the use of multiple static beams and arcs has facilitated increasingly conformal treatment plans, whereby the target volume is tightly fitted by the desired radiation dose, and surrounding structures are well spared from high radiation doses. Additionally, in comparison with conventional fractionation (fractional doses of 1.8–2.0 Gy; definitive treatment of many malignancies involves 20–45 fractions), stereotactic techniques involve fewer treatment fractions and are nearly always hypofractionated (an umbrella term referring to fractional doses >2.0 Gy). SRS is most used in a single fraction to an intracranial area (ie, a brain metastasis), whereas SBRT largely refers to extracranial locations and administers 5 or fewer fractions. The reader is advised that these are generalized definitions, noting that the most contemporary era has blurred these "classical" definitions as will be further discussed later.

The goal of this review is to discuss the historical, technical, and clinical aspects of stereotactic radiotherapy (both SRS and SBRT) in an effort to introduce the audience to a RT modality that has expanded, and will continue to expand, the reach of RT for a variety of applications.

BRIEF HISTORY

The initial concept of SRS began in the 1950s by Lars Leksell, a Swedish neurosurgeon, who later introduced the first clinical SRS device in the late 1960s.[1] The purpose of SRS was to provide a noninvasive treatment system capable of targeting lesions

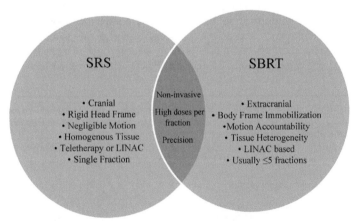

Fig. 1. Venn diagram comparing and contrasting classical definitions of SRS and SBRT.

located in the skull base or eloquent regions of the brain; these sites represent surgical challenges, where the risks of morbidity from invasive surgical interventions could be substantial. To overcome this, Leksell designed and implemented his SRS device; the treatment system consisted of multiple, hemispherically arranged cobalt-60 sources responsible for the production of multiple γ-radiation beams that converged in the desired target area. Interestingly, SRS was first used for nonmalignant intracranial conditions[2–4] before the more widespread modern application of SRS for the treatment of neoplasms.

The success of SRS, or "performing surgery by means of radiation," for intracranial targets led to a desire in applying this technology to other areas of the body. Whereas the machine developed by Leksell was uniquely tailored for treatment of intracranial lesions, LINAC-based SRS platforms were introduced in the 1980s,[5,6] thus paving the way for adaption of the technique to treat extracranial targets, which was termed SBRT (used interchangeably with the term SABR).[7,8] Over the subsequent decades, advances in treatment delivery and radiologic technologies helped to further refine SRS and SBRT techniques, leading to increased use globally.

MODERN SEMANTICS

Both intracranial SRS and extracranial SBRT were initially developed for single- or ≤3-fraction treatments; however, multiple experiences have shown that targets in close proximity to organs at risk (OARs) may be suboptimal for these regimens.[9,10] As a result, more fractionated approaches are often used for these conditions, and/or large treatment volumes more at risk of developing toxicities. As time has brought a better understanding of OAR dosimetry with stereotactic techniques, semantic definitions of SRS/SBRT have blurred, resulting in discontinuities between historical versus modern functional definitions of SRS/SBRT.

Although SRS has historically referred to single-fraction delivery, particularly for medical billing purposes, the term "fractionated SRS" or "fractionated stereotactic RT" can be used in the context of treating brain metastases that may not meet OAR dose constraints with single-fraction regimens. For these cases, RT is most commonly delivered in 2 to 5 fractions.[11] However, the literature also recognizes a subtype of "fractionated SRS" or "fractionated stereotactic RT" whereby RT is delivered using conventional fractionation (1.8–2.0 Gy per fraction).[11] This may be applied for unique cases with close abutment or invasion of an OAR (eg, brainstem or optic apparatus) where ≤5-fraction schedules (or potentially even 10- to 20-fraction schedules) may not meet OAR dose constraints. As a functional definition, conventionally fractionated SRS or stereotactic RT may not require the "stereotactic" moniker therein, but this is often still included owing to the more precise "stereotactic" patient setup with smaller target margins, neither of which are commonly used with conventionally fractionated RT in other body areas (eg, pelvis).

Similarly, the definition of SBRT with regard to medical billing has referred to ≤5 fractions. Although this remains an appropriate option for lung tumors that are larger and/or close to central mediastinal structures,[12,13] other proposed schemes have used 8 to 10 fractions.[14,15] The latter are often referred to as either "SBRT" or "hypo-fractionated SBRT," recognizing that patient setup, target margins, and daily image guidance are virtually identical to ≤5-fraction schedules.

HALLMARKS AND PRINCIPLES

Despite the semantic complexities already noted, there are several overarching common characteristics of modern SRS and SBRT. However, the reader is cautioned that the following factors may be neither specific to SRS/SBRT nor necessarily representative of all possible clinical scenarios.

First, stereotactic RT places extra emphasis on precisely localizing the target. This point is particularly important because the treatment course includes usually not more than a few fractions, meaning that suboptimal tumor localization for even one fraction of the treatment course may result in marked underdosing of the lesion and/or overdosing of an OAR. To achieve superior tumor localization, patients are immobilized to a greater extent than with conventional RT. Examples include rigid head frames for intracranial SRS and custom body-fixation molds for thoracoabdominal SBRT. Moreover, optimal target delineation requires advanced techniques. In the setting of intracranial SRS, this includes the use of MRI obtained with the rigid head frame in place; this allows for excellent soft tissue detail to delineate specific intracranial target volumes and avoidance structures with the patient in the treatment position. For thoracic and abdominal lesions to be treated with SBRT, for instance, respiratory tracking and motion management methods are used. This approach encompasses a number of techniques, such as 4-dimensional computed tomography (CT) simulation (whereby the patient is scanned with CT imaging during the simulation/treatment planning process in all respiratory phases), which captures the complete cycle of tumor movement associated with respiration. Breath-hold techniques may similarly be used, whereby patients are coached (often with biofeedback systems) in holding their breath at a specific point in the respiratory cycle (generally end-inhalation and end-expiration for thoracic and gastrointestinal malignancies, respectively). Breath-hold is especially useful when motion of a thoracic or abdominal tumor during the course of the respiratory cycle is substantial, and designing a treatment plan to target the tumor over the full range of respiratory motion would lead to larger fields than desired. Isolating the position of the tumor at one point in the respiratory cycle allows for smaller treatment fields and less dose delivered to uninvolved structures. Respiratory management, including breath-hold techniques, are further discussed later in this article.

Second, the result of these more precise immobilization and tracking techniques is the use of smaller treatment margins. Following radiologic delineation of clinical/subclinical disease involvement, additional margins are placed to account for uncertainties in patient setup and/or motion, termed planning target volume (PTV) margins. In the setting of conventional RT, PTV margins usually range from 0.5 to 1.0 cm depending on the clinical and anatomic context, in addition to additional expansion for microscopic disease. However, for stereotactic treatment these margins are largely $\leq$0.5 cm, sometimes with no PTV margin at all (for instance, in the context of teletherapy-based SRS for intracranial lesions). The use of smaller PTV margins enables dose intensification and results in a smaller volume of normal tissue treated to full dose, and hence the potential for reduced toxicities without compromise of disease control (**Fig. 2**).

Third, another factor allowing use of smaller PTV margins with SRS/SBRT is the increased reliance on high-quality image-guided RT (IGRT). IGRT is an umbrella term referring to obtaining imaging before (or, in some cases, during) each RT fraction, in efforts to ensure adequate patient positioning/setup. This imaging, by definition, is performed with the patient in the treatment position, and therefore IGRT is generally incorporated into the treatment delivery system. Imaging systems built into the LINAC allow radiation therapists to obtain images with the patient in the treatment position immediately before RT delivery. Whereas conventional RT may use simpler IGRT techniques (eg, kilovoltage or megavoltage radiographs), SRS/SBRT nearly always involves high-quality IGRT with advanced modes of image registration. Broadly, this

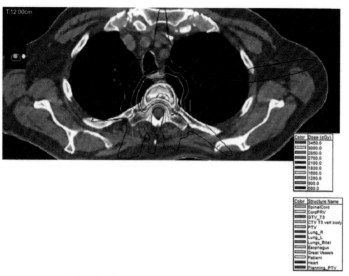

Fig. 2. Retreatment of T3 spinal metastasis using SBRT. Note the relatively narrow (ie, 0.2 cm) PTV margin (*orange line*).

can refer to repeated plain radiographs (ie, fluoroscopy on the LINAC and CyberKnife platform) or volumetric imaging with superior soft tissue detail such as kilovoltage fan-beam or cone-beam CT (CBCT) (discussed subsequently). These allow for 3-dimensional or 4-dimensional volumetric imaging in the treatment position immediately before RT delivery. Moreover, a rapidly emerging area of interest has been the use of MRI-based IGRT, which affords MRI-quality soft-tissue contrast as part of axial imaging for IGRT; in the appropriate clinical contexts, MRI-based IGRT has the potential to substantially further adaptive therapy with enhanced precision.[16]

Fourth, the ability of SRS/SBRT to offer a sharp radiation dose gradient between the target and surrounding OARs speaks to advanced treatment planning capabilities. Although not always the case, SRS/SBRT treatment planning is generally conducted in a more specialized manner than many conventional RT techniques. This approach may involve the use of inverse RT planning (using iterative computational algorithms to modulate fluence patterns of each radiation beam to meet prespecified OAR constraints), respiratory-gated RT administration, and/or delivering continuous arcs of RT instead of fixed beams. Although these nuances are not specific for SRS/SBRT, they are often liberally applied to this setting to allow for precise RT delivery.

Fifth, SRS/SBRT are by definition hypofractionated (>2.0 Gy per fraction), and very often categorized as ablative. Although the term "ablative" does not have a specific predefined cutoff, it has historically referred to ≥10 Gy per fraction. More recently, the definition of ablative RT doses has been roughly broadened to refer to fractional doses of ≥6 Gy. Not only do large fractional doses allow for faster completion of a prescribed RT course and increased patient convenience, they also offer certain radiobiological benefits compared with conventional RT. Based on the linear-quadratic radiobiological model (the most commonly used model for understanding the cell-killing properties of fractionated RT), the biologically effective dose (BED) of x Gy delivered in y fractions is not equivalent to the same x Gy dose delivered in z fractions; the greater BED corresponds to the regimen delivering the same total dose over fewer treatment fractions. Mathematically, the BED of a radiotherapeutic regimen equals $nd\left(1+\frac{d}{\alpha/\beta}\right)$, where n is the number of RT fractions, d is the fractional dose, and α/β is a constant (assumed to be 10 for most tumors of malignant behavior). Hence, administering high fractional doses with SRS/SBRT delivers BEDs that are difficult to replicate by conventionally fractionated RT. As an example, one can compare a common SBRT regimen for early-stage lung cancer (50 Gy in 4 fractions) with a common conventional RT regimen for locally advanced lung cancers (60 Gy in 30 fractions). Comparing these 2 regimens, the BED for SBRT regimen (112.5 Gy_{10}) is substantially higher than that of conventional regimen (72.0 Gy_{10}); this highlights the impact of SBRT fractionation on BED even for regimens with lower total doses than conventionally fractionated regimens. Most tumors show an RT dose response, indicating that escalating BED values are associated with a greater chance of tumor control.[17] Hence, SRS/SBRT may indirectly affect tumor control by means of allowing safer BED escalation.

Lastly, hypofractionated—and especially ablative—RT may act in a radiobiologically distinct manner from conventional RT. Whereas the latter is predicated on tumor cell killing by means of lethal DNA damage from double-stranded DNA breaks, ablatively dosed RT may offer an additional, indirect mode of cell death. This involves causing profound alterations in the tumor microenvironment by means of substantial local oncovascular damage. This hypothesis may account for why ablative RT is theorized to more often produce an antitumoral inflammatory response and augment the effects of immunotherapies than nonablative RT doses.[18–21]

TECHNIQUES AND TECHNOLOGY

Intracranial SRS uses a stereotactic technique,[1] which was first performed using the Gamma Knife (GK) platform. The GK platform involves use of a rigid head frame, which immobilizes the patient's skull; the frame is placed via a surgical procedure (generally involving a 4-pin placement of the frame around the largest axially circumferential portion of the skull), and subsequently localized onto a stereotactic coordinate system. However, given that LINAC-based radiosurgery offers acceptable accuracy, precision, and stability, frameless SRS is a reasonable alternative option. Hybridizing both approaches, the most contemporary GK machine is the GK Icon (Elekta, Stockholm, Sweden), which does not use a head frame, and is equipped with C-arm CBCT and high-definition motion management systems (**Fig. 3**). Patients are fixed with a patient-specific thermoplastic mask and a customized head rest, and are rigidly aligned based on coregistration of CBCT images with MRI and/or CT images. Intrafractional motion during irradiation is monitored by an infrared stereoscopic camera that tracks a marker attached to the patient's nasal tip relative to the reference markers on the GK head-support system.

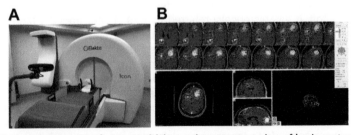

Fig. 3. (*A*) Elekta Gamma Knife Icon and (*B*) sample treatment plan of brain metastases. ([*A*] Elekta, Atlanta, GA.)

Thoracoabdominal SBRT, regardless of platform or equipment, must involve a strategy to address respiratory motion. Methods include abdominal compression, breath-hold treatment, gated delivery, and tumor tracking. Abdominal compression, coupled with a stereotactic body frame, is aimed at restricting target and organ motion. Shallow breathing is forced until diaphragmatic excursion is within a predefined acceptable limit. The breath-hold technique (**Fig. 4**) uses a spirometer to set a prespecified air volume in the lung and freezes the target for a predetermined amount of time, permitting improved target positional reproducibility and consistency. Once the predetermined volume of air is reached, the spirometer valve closes, preventing further exhalation or inhalation. Gated SBRT delivery allows the administration of radiation within a few phases of the respiratory cycle; the respiratory signal can be traced either by surgically implanted fiducials or external markers as a surrogate. For instance, the Varian RPM system (Varian, Palo Alto, CA) uses infrared markers placed on the patient's abdomen. The gating technique can reduce the treated lung volume, but may prolong the treatment time owing to the limited gating window. Lastly, tumor-tracking methods detect implanted fiducials (or the tumor directly) to administer real-time RT. For example, the Cyber Knife (Accuray, Sunnyvale, CA) system tracks implanted fiducials in or near the tumor by a stereotactic x-ray system, allowing for real-time dose delivery.

IGRT for SRS/SBRT is diverse, and any one modality is not necessarily superior to another; rather, knowing limitations of each is crucial in the overall treatment process. The most common modern IGRT method is kilovoltage CBCT mounted to the LINAC apparatus; this provides 3-dimensional volumetric images, resulting in high soft-tissue visibility. Megavoltage CBCT is sometimes used, but generally does not provide higher-quality soft tissue detail owing to the abundance of Compton scattering at megavoltage energies (in contrast to the predominant photoelectric effect observed

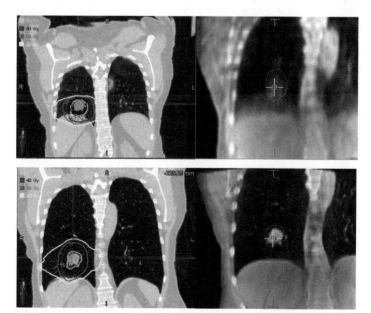

Fig. 4. Comparison between free-breathing (top) and breath-hold treatment (bottom) for lung SBRT. The SBRT plans are shown in the left panels, and representative CBCT images in the right panels. Internal target volume on free-breathing CBCT and gross target volume on breath-hold CBCT are indicated.

at kilovolt energies, which results in higher soft-tissue contrast). Fan-beam CT systems, although associated with a higher radiation dosage to patients than CBCT, offer even further improved soft tissue resolution than CBCT. This is especially true for kilovoltage fan-beam CT, although the TomoTherapy HiArt System (TomoTherapy, Madison, WI) (MV fan-beam CT) is also in extensive use.

Intrafractional tumor motion management is not mandatory for SRS/SBRT, but can be checked intermittently by obtaining images during treatment or continuously monitored by an optical tracking system. The BrainLAB ExacTrac system (BrainLAB, Feldkirchen, Germany) uses 2-dimensional orthogonal kilovoltage images, with 2 x-ray sources on the room's floor and 2 detectors mounted on the room's ceiling. In addition, implanted fiducials in orthogonal radiograph images or/and external markers through optical imaging systems (eg, Cyber Knife as already mentioned) can be used to track, trigger, and terminate the treatment beam based on tumor motion. Another example of intrafractional tumor management technology is the Elekta XVI Symmetry, in which 4-dimensional image guidance is used. Once the patient has reached the required threshold, pinch valves in the spirometer remotely close, preventing the patient from exhaling or inhaling outside the required threshold, to assess respiratory-associated target motion before treatment. Similarly, the Varian TrueBeam IGRT package allows kilovolt imaging during treatment delivery to monitor the target in real time. Other platforms using nonionizing surface image guidance include the Align[RT] (Vision RT, London, UK), in which target motion is correlated with the surface.

CLINICAL APPLICATIONS

The clinical data on SRS/SBRT for a wide variety of neoplasms and clinical scenarios is beyond the scope of this article. However, broad summaries are provided based on nationally recognized indications as put forth by the National Comprehensive Cancer Network and other consensus guidelines. The readership is advised that this is not a complete list encompassing currently investigative approaches but rather an array of conditions for which SRS/SBRT is routinely accepted.

SRS was initially described for benign intracranial lesions such as meningioma, vestibular schwannoma, pituitary adenoma, arteriovenous malformation, and functional disorders (eg, trigeminal neuralgia).[22,23] However, the most frequent use of SRS in clinical practice is for brain metastases, which will likely continue to increase worldwide owing to the increasing emphasis on preventing radiation-induced neurocognitive decline of whole brain radiation.[24]

SBRT in extracranial sites has been best studied in the setting of early-stage non–small cell lung cancer (NSCLC).[17] However, it has since expanded to (and shows promise for) early-stage small cell lung cancer,[25–27] hepatocellular carcinoma,[28] pancreatic cancer,[29] prostate cancer,[30] spinal disease,[31] oligometastatic disease,[32] and clinical scenarios involving reirradiation of previously treated regions.[33] Of note, the aforementioned sites (with the exception of NSCLC[34]) do not have phase 3 data supporting the use of SBRT over conventional fractionation at the time of writing. However, SBRT's conformality, convenience, and cost-effectiveness, yielding similar efficacy and equivalent or lower toxicities compared with conventional fractionation, has led to rapid adoption despite the lack of phase 3 data. This parallels its trajectory in early-stage NSCLC, for which SBRT was used worldwide for nearly 3 decades[7] before the eventual publication of phase 3 data.[34]

Despite these shortcomings regarding available evidence, SBRT continues to be actively investigated prospectively for numerous clinical settings. These active areas of investigation include: assessing the effects of SBRT and immunotherapy in the treatment of early-stage NSCLC (NCT03110978); defining the oncologic role of SBRT in the treatment of oligometastatic (NCT03137771, NCT02364557) and potentially polymetastatic disease (NCT03721341); and treatment of refractory ventricular tachycardia (NCT03349892). In each investigation, SBRT use continues to be synonymous with aiming to achieve high rates of disease control while minimizing treatment-related toxicities.

SUMMARY

Stereotactic RT describes a specialized highly conformal radiation technique whereby high doses of radiation are focally delivered using multiple collimated beams to small 3-dimensionally defined intracranial (SRS) or extracranial (SBRT) targets. Whereas SRS and SBRT have many principal commonalities, technical challenges vary based on structural and functional anatomic differences. As such, a multidisciplinary team approach is essential considering the increased complexities associated with stereotactic RT. The use of stereotactic RT has increased drastically over the past decade and is an active area of multiple ongoing clinical trials.

REFERENCES

1. Leksell L. The stereotaxic method and radiosurgery of the brain. Acta Chir Scand 1951;102(4):316–9.
2. Leksell L. Cerebral radiosurgery. I. Gammathalanotomy in two cases of intractable pain. Acta Chir Scand 1968;134(8):585–95.
3. Leksell L. Sterotaxic radiosurgery in trigeminal neuralgia. Acta Chir Scand 1971; 137(4):311–4.
4. Steiner L, Leksell L, Greitz T, et al. Stereotaxic radiosurgery for cerebral arteriovenous malformations. Report of a case. Acta Chir Scand 1972;138(5):459–64.
5. Betti OO, Derechinsky VE. Hyperselective encephalic irradiation with linear accelerator. In: Advances in stereotactic and functional neurosurgery6. Vienna (Austria): Springer Vienna; 1984. p. 385–90.
6. Lutz W, Winston KR, Maleki N. A system for stereotactic radiosurgery with a linear accelerator. Int J Radiat Oncol 1988;14(2):373–81.
7. Blomgren H, Lax I, Näslund I, et al. Stereotactic high dose fraction radiation therapy of extracranial tumors using an accelerator. Clinical experience of the first thirty-one patients. Acta Oncol 1995;34(6):861–70.
8. Uematsu M, Shioda A, Tahara K, et al. Focal, high dose, and fractionated modified stereotactic radiation therapy for lung carcinoma patients: a preliminary experience. Cancer 1998;82(6):1062–70.
9. Timmerman R, McGarry R, Yiannoutsos C, et al. Excessive toxicity when treating central tumors in a phase II study of stereotactic body radiation therapy for medically inoperable early-stage lung cancer. J Clin Oncol 2006;24(30):4833–9.
10. Schellenberg D, Goodman KA, Lee F, et al. Gemcitabine chemotherapy and single-fraction stereotactic body radiotherapy for locally advanced pancreatic cancer. Int J Radiat Oncol Biol Phys 2008;72(3):678–86.
11. Kirkpatrick JP, Soltys SG, Lo SS, et al. The radiosurgery fractionation quandary: single fraction or hypofractionation? Neuro Oncol 2017;19(suppl2):ii38–49.
12. Verma V, Shostrom VK, Kumar SS, et al. Multi-institutional experience of stereotactic body radiotherapy for large (≥5 centimeters) non-small cell lung tumors. Cancer 2017;123(4):688–96.
13. Verma V, Shostrom VK, Zhen W, et al. Influence of fractionation scheme and tumor location on toxicities after stereotactic body radiation therapy for large (≥5 cm)

non-small cell lung cancer: a multi-institutional analysis. Int J Radiat Oncol Biol Phys 2017;97(4):778–85.

14. Haasbeek CJA, Lagerwaard FJ, Slotman BJ, et al. Outcomes of stereotactic ablative radiotherapy for centrally located early-stage lung cancer. J Thorac Oncol 2011;6(12):2036–43.

15. Li Q, Swanick CW, Allen PK, et al. Stereotactic ablative radiotherapy (SABR) using 70 Gy in 10 fractions for non-small cell lung cancer: exploration of clinical indications. Radiother Oncol 2014;112(2):256–61.

16. Raaymakers BW, Jürgenliemk-Schulz IM, Bol GH, et al. First patients treated with a 1.5 T MRI-Linac: clinical proof of concept of a high-precision, high-field MRI guided radiotherapy treatment. Phys Med Biol 2017;62(23):L41–50.

17. Onishi H, Araki T, Shirato H, et al. Stereotactic hypofractionated high-dose irradiation for 285 stage I nonsmall cell lung carcinoma: clinical outcomes in 245 subjects in a Japanese multi-institutional study. Cancer 2004;101(7):1623–31.

18. Song CW, Cho LC, Yuan J, et al. Radiobiology of stereotactic body radiation therapy/stereotactic radiosurgery and the linear-quadratic mode. Int J Radiat Oncol Biol Phys 2013;87(1):18–9.

19. Song CW, Park I, Cho LC, et al. Is there indirect cell death involved in response of tumor to SRS and SBRT? Int J Radiat Oncol Biol Phys 2014;89(4):924–5.

20. Song CW, Lee YJ, Griffin RJ, et al. Indirect tumor cell death after high-dose hypofractionated irradiation: implications for stereotactic body radiation therapy and stereotactic radiation surgery. Int J Radiat Oncol Biol Phys 2015;93(1):166–72.

21. Menon H, Ramapriyan R, Cushman TR, et al. Role of radiation therapy in modulation of the tumor stroma and microenvironment. Front Immunol 2019;10:193.

22. Tsao MN, Wara WM, Larson DA. Radiation therapy for benign central nervous system disease. Semin Radiat Oncol 1999;9(2):120–33.

23. Gilbo P, Zhang I, Knisely J. Stereotactic radiosurgery of the brain: a review of common indications. Chin Clin Oncol 2017;6(Suppl2):S14.

24. Saad S, Wang TJ. Neurocognitive deficits after radiation therapy for brain malignancies. Am J Clin Oncol 2015;38(6):634–40.

25. Verma V, Simone CB 2nd, Allen PK, et al. Multi-institutional experience of stereotactic ablative radiation therapy for stage I small cell lung cancer. Int J Radiat Oncol Biol Phys 2017;97(2):362–71.

26. Verma V, Simone CB 2nd, Allen PK, et al. Outcomes of stereotactic body radiotherapy for T1-T2N0 small cell carcinoma according to addition of chemotherapy and prophylactic cranial irradiation: a multicenter analysis. Clin Lung Cancer 2017;18(6):675–81.e1.

27. Verma V, Hasan S, Wegner RE, et al. Stereotactic ablative radiation therapy versus conventionally fractionated radiation therapy for stage I small cell lung cancer. Radiother Oncol 2019;131:145–9.

28. Rim CH, Kim HJ, Seong J. Clinical feasibility and efficacy of stereotactic body radiotherapy for hepatocellular carcinoma: a systematic review and meta-analysis of observational studies. Radiother Oncol 2019;131:135–44.

29. Myrehaug S, Sahgal A, Russo SM, et al. Stereotactic body radiotherapy for pancreatic cancer: recent progress and future directions. Expert Rev Anticancer Ther 2016;16(5):523–30.

30. Haque W, Butler EB, Teh BS. Stereotactic body radiation therapy for prostate cancer-a review. Chin Clin Oncol 2017;6(Suppl2):S10.

31. Sprave T, Verma V, Förster R, et al. Randomized phase II trial evaluating pain response in patients with spinal metastases following stereotactic body

radiotherapy versus three-dimensional conformal radiotherapy. Radiother Oncol 2018;128(2):274–82.

32. Ning MS, Gomez DR, Heymach JV, et al. Stereotactic ablative body radiation for oligometastatic and oligoprogressive disease. Transl Lung Cancer Res 2019; 8(1):97–106.

33. Høyer M. Re-irradiation with stereotactic body radiation therapy (SBRT). Chin Clin Oncol 2017;6(Suppl2):S15.

34. Ball D, Mai GT, Vinod S, et al. Stereotactic ablative radiotherapy versus standard radiotherapy in stage 1 non-small-cell lung cancer (TROG 09.02 CHISEL): a phase 3, open-label, randomised controlled trial. Lancet Oncol 2019. https://doi.org/10.1016/S1470-2045(18)30896-9.

Proton Therapy

Michael J. LaRiviere, MD[a], Patricia Mae G. Santos, MD, MS[b],
Christine E. Hill-Kayser, MD[a], James M. Metz, MD[a],*

KEYWORDS

- Protons • Proton therapy • Ion therapy • Charged ion therapy • Particle therapy
- Charged particle therapy • Single-room proton unit • Bragg peak

KEY POINTS

- Proton therapy is a form of external beam radiotherapy that has several key advantages over conventional photon (x-ray) radiotherapy.
- Unlike x-rays, protons deposit their maximum dose at a specific depth, with no exit dose to normal tissues, exploiting a phenomenon known as the Bragg peak.
- Lack of exit dose allows for delivery of a therapeutic radiation dose to tumors in challenging anatomic locations.
- Reduction in integral dose (low-dose bath) to normal tissues may reduce the risk of late toxicities and secondary cancers.
- The emergence of smaller, more economically viable single-room proton units has led to the expansion in use of this technology across the world.

INTRODUCTION

The concept of harnessing protons as an anticancer therapy was first proposed in 1946 by Robert R. Wilson, physicist at the Harvard cyclotron, who posited that protons' unique physical characteristics would be advantageous in the treatment of deep-seated cancers.[1] Less than a decade later, the first patients were treated with protons at the Lawrence Berkeley National Laboratory in 1954.[2] Today, proton therapy is emerging as a promising improvement on conventional, x-ray–based external beam radiotherapy.

Both x-rays and protons are forms of ionizing radiation, which produce free radicals and reactive oxygen species within cells. The overarching goal of radiotherapy is to maximize the therapeutic ratio: delivering lethal doses of ionizing radiation to the tumor

Disclosure Statement: M.J. LaRiviere, P.M.G. Santos, C.E. Hill-Kayser: nothing to disclose. J.M. Metz: advisory boards for Varian, IBA, and Provision.
[a] Department of Radiation Oncology, University of Pennsylvania, 3400 Civic Center Boulevard, Philadelphia, PA 19104, USA; [b] Department of Medicine, Memorial Sloan Kettering Cancer Center, 1275 York Avenue, New York, NY 10065, USA
* Corresponding author.
E-mail address: James.Metz@pennmedicine.upenn.edu
twitter: @mjlariviere (M.J.L.)

Hematol Oncol Clin N Am 33 (2019) 989–1009
https://doi.org/10.1016/j.hoc.2019.08.006
0889-8588/19/© 2019 Elsevier Inc. All rights reserved.

while delivering the lowest possible dose to normal tissues (**Fig. 1**). Although conventional x-ray radiotherapy relies on a linear accelerator to deliver a therapeutic dose of ionizing radiation to the tumor (**Fig. 2**), x-rays also deliver substantial dose to normal tissues distal to the tumor, because the physics of massless, chargeless x-rays dictate that they can pass through material even if they are attenuated to some extent. Improvements in x-ray–based conventional radiotherapy have greatly improved the therapeutic ratio. Two-dimensional (2-D) radiotherapy (**Fig. 3**) was supplanted by 3-dimensional (3-D) conformal radiotherapy (CRT) with the advent of computed tomography (CT) in the 1970s to 1980s (**Fig. 4** and **Fig. 5**), followed by intensity-modulated radiotherapy (IMRT) beginning in the late 1990s and early 2000s (**Fig. 6**). IMRT with image-guided radiotherapy, or the use of regular imaging to verify both target and patient position, represents the current standard of care for x-ray radiotherapy.

X-ray–based treatment, however, still suffers from the physically insurmountable radiation exit dose. Because complex beam arrangements often produce exit dose in 360°, nearby tissues may receive significant integral dose—a larger volume of lower-dose radiation—the long-term consequences of which are not yet fully understood (**Fig. 7**). Late radiation toxicity is known to depend on both dose and volume irradiated, and risk increases with time. Particularly for younger patients, integral dose has the potential to increase some risks compared with the 2-D era, including second cancers and pathologic fractures. X-ray exit dose also presents challenges for tumors requiring high doses in anatomically sensitive regions, such as skull base tumors near the brainstem, cranial nerves, and/or optic structures; hepatocellular carcinomas requiring preservation of normal liver parenchyma; mediastinal lymphomas; and a variety of other scenarios.

Proton therapy overcomes these limitations, because they have no exit dose. Protons are heavy, charged particles that can be stripped from hydrogen gas and accelerated toward the speed of light using an accelerator, such as a cyclotron or synchrotron. The resultant proton beam is delivered to the tumor in a manner that is conceptually similar to conventional x-ray radiotherapy: tumor and normal organs are delineated, beam arrangements, and modulation patterns are planned with the

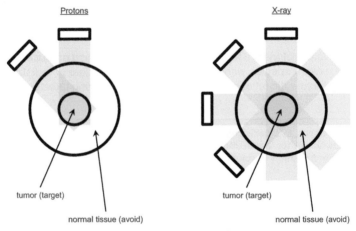

Fig. 1. The therapeutic ratio—delivering lethal doses of ionizing radiation to tumor, while sparing dose to normal tissues—for proton versus x-ray therapy. Left: Proton therapy. Right: X-ray therapy.

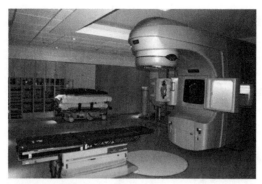

Fig. 2. A linear accelerator, which produces therapeutic (rather than diagnostic) x-rays. (*Courtesy of* Penn Medicine, Philadelphia, PA; and Varian Medical Systems, Inc. All rights reserved.)

intent of maximizing the therapeutic ratio; image guidance is used to ensure the patient is set up to within millimeters of the computer simulation; and the patient is treated daily over several weeks. In contrast to x-ray radiotherapy, however, proton therapy exploits the Bragg peak to deliver its maximum dose at a specific depth, with no exit dose to tissues beyond this point (**Fig. 8**). Although protons and x-rays are theorized to have similar biologic effectiveness, research into the question of whether the regions surrounding the proton Bragg peak see a higher biologic effect is ongoing.[3] By contrast, charged ions that are heavier than protons have a greater

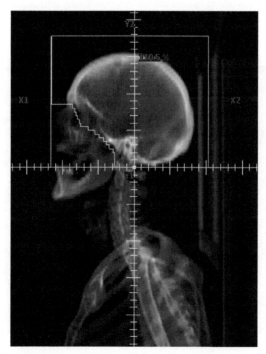

Fig. 3. An x-ray 2-D radiotherapy plan for whole-brain radiation.

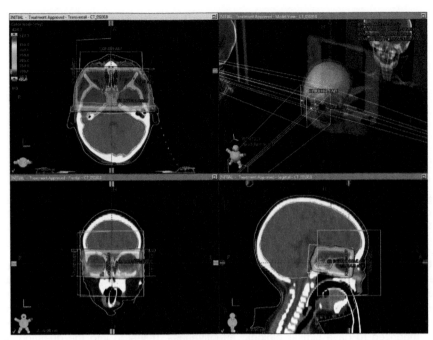

Fig. 4. An x-ray 3-D–CRT for focal radiation to the optic nerves. Top left: axial view. Lower left: coronal view. Lower right: sagittal view. Top right: 3D reconstruction.

biologic effectiveness in addition to the ability to stop at a specific depth. Carbon ion therapy, for instance, is being tested primarily in Germany and Japan. First-generation passive scattering or double-scattering proton technology uses devices placed along

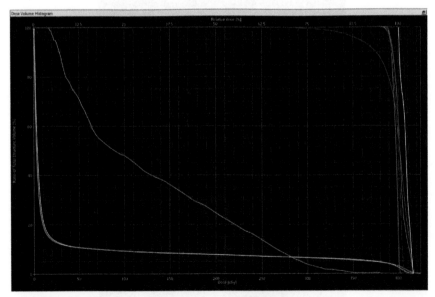

Fig. 5. The dose-volume histogram is evaluated to determine the radiation dose coverage of the target structures (*upper right*) and organs at risk (*lower left*).

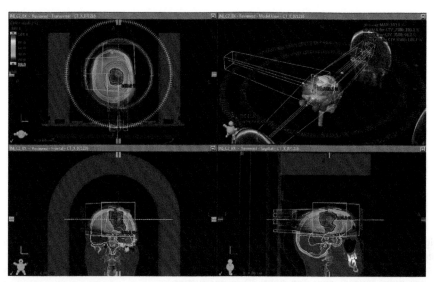

Fig. 6. An x-ray IMRT plan depicting beams directed in arcs to achieve a highly conformal, high-dose region (*red*) that covers the target. Top left: axial view. Lower left: coronal view. Lower right: sagittal view. Top right: 3D reconstruction.

the path of the proton beam to modify its width and depth (**Fig. 9**). In contrast, current state-of-the-art pencil beam scanning directs small proton beamlets, or pencil beams, to deposit doses at specified x, y, and z coordinates that correspond to the 3-D tumor volume (**Fig. 10**).

Proton therapy's lack of exit dose offers 2 key clinical advantages:

1. The avoidance of normal tissues distal to the Bragg peak
2. The marked reduction in integral dose.

For younger patients who are still growing—especially children, adolescents, and young adults—as well as in some cases involving nonelderly adults, avoiding normal

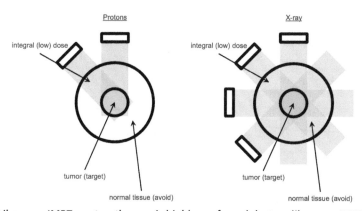

Fig. 7. Like x-ray IMRT, proton therapy is highly conformal, but, unlike x-ray IMRT, proton therapy yields a much smaller integral dose (low-dose bath). Left: Proton therapy. Right: X-ray therapy.

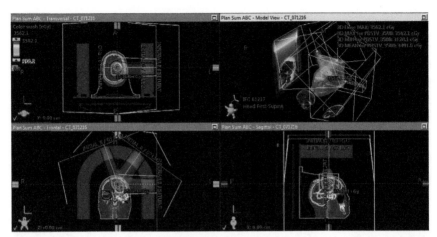

Fig. 8. A proton therapy plan comprising 3 beams achieves a highly conformal, high-dose region (*red*) that covers the target. Compared with x-ray IMRT, protons produce less integral dose (*blue*)—the contralateral brain is spared. Top left: axial view. Lower left: coronal view. Lower right: sagittal view. Top right: 3D reconstruction.

tissues and minimizing the integral dose with proton therapy is advantageous. Proton therapy has been associated with decreased incidence of secondary cancers after craniospinal irradiation for medulloblastoma and other clinical scenarios,[4–6] mediastinal irradiation for lymphomas,[7–9] nodal irradiation for germ cell tumors,[10] and others pediatric cancers. For pediatric patients in particular, radiation oncologists aim to minimize or eliminate exposure to developing normal tissues that otherwise would be permanently damaged by even small doses of radiation.[11,12] Protons also allow older adults with anatomically challenging tumors—such as hepatocellular carcinoma, for example—to receive tumoricidal doses of radiation that otherwise may not be safe to deliver with conventional x-ray–based radiotherapy (**Fig. 11**).[13] With conventional x-ray radiotherapy, delivering the full dose would potentially cure the tumor but at the risk of lethal hepatic decompensation[14,15]; on the other hand, delivering a lower dose to the tumor may be safer for the normal liver but may not control the cancer.[14–17]

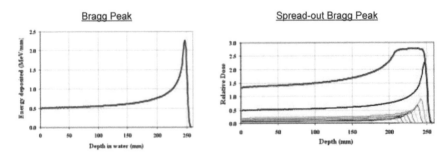

Fig. 9. A proton beam deposits most of its energy at the Bragg peak. Because a tumor is not a point in space, a spread-out Bragg peak comprises protons with a spectrum of energies—and, therefore, stops at different distances—to deliver a homogeneous dose over the entire tumor. Left: Bragg peak. Right: Spread-out Bragg peak. (*Courtesy of* Penn Medicine, Philadelphia, PA.)

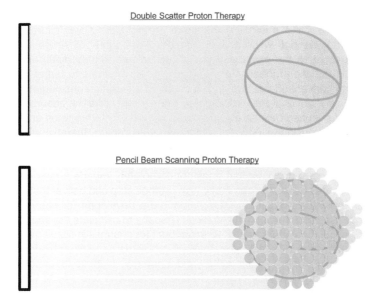

Fig. 10. A double-scattering proton beam has a higher entrance dose and is less conformal than pencil beam scanning, which delivers beamlets across the tumor, varying energies to achieve different depths. Pencil beam scanning may better avoid normal tissues but is more sensitive to setup error, anatomic changes, and radiation oncologist experience. Upper: Double scattering proton therapy. Lower: Pencil beam scanning proton therapy.

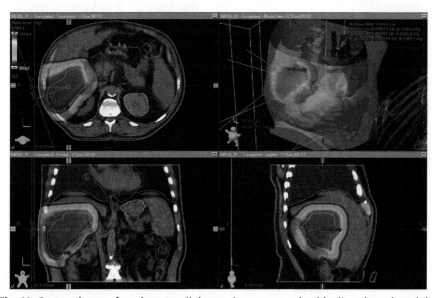

Fig. 11. Proton therapy for a hepatocellular carcinoma spares healthy liver, bowel, and the contralateral kidney. Top left: axial view. Lower left: coronal view. Lower right: sagittal view. Top right: 3D reconstruction.

Proton therapy, by contrast, has the potential to safely deliver the full dose while sparing normal liver, thus controlling the tumor without risking liver failure.[16,17]

Proton therapy is not without its limitations. A degree of range uncertainty exists with respect to the exact position of the proton beam's distal edge, which may make this radiation modality less forgiving when it comes to target delineation compared with conventional x-rays. Like a surgeon, a radiation oncologist, therefore, must rely heavily on anatomic expertise, taking great care to accurately define the target of interest and delineate nearby organs at risk, with precision and attention to detail. Not surprisingly, patient outcomes after proton therapy with respect to local control, survival, and associated toxicities may, to some degree, be dependent on provider skill and experience with this technique. Additionally, while dense tissue—such as bone—attenuates but does not completely impede x-rays, differences in tissue density do change the depth at which protons stop and deliver their maximum dose. Thus, individualized proton therapy plans are developed for each patient via software that uses their respective planning CT scans to calculate the specific proton energy and modulation pattern required to account for changes in tissue density along the proton beam path (**Fig. 12**). Nonetheless, problems can still arise due to unexpected changes in daily patient setup and anatomy, leading to underdosing of tumor or overdosing of nearby organs. Image guidance is one way to mitigate this problem. For instance, image guidance can detect new ascites in a hepatocellular carcinoma patient and, with a repeat simulation CT scan, subsequent computer models can account for this abrupt change in anatomy. Another strategy, robust multifield optimization with uncertainty analysis, models setup and beam range errors, to help select multiple beam angles that can minimize differences in delivered dose

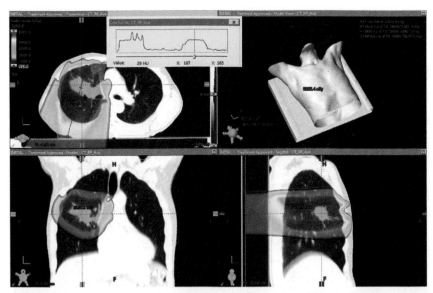

Fig. 12. The patient undergoes a simulation CT scan, set up exactly as will be set up for daily proton therapy treatment. Each voxel of the simulation CT scan encodes tissue density information that is used to model the proton dose distribution; the yellow-boxed inset shows an example of the various tissue densities traversed by the proton beam before it deposits dose at the target. Modern radiotherapy plans, including proton therapy, are patient-specific and demand that the daily setup is within millimeters of the simulation setup. Top left: axial view. Lower left: coronal view. Lower right: sagittal view. Top right: dose-volume histogram.

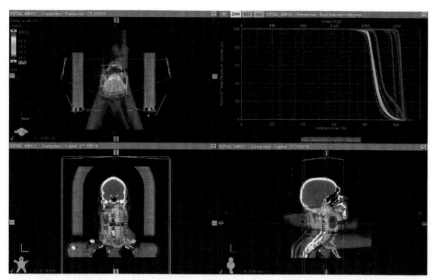

Fig. 13. Proton therapy robust multifield optimization with uncertainty analysis for the treatment of the supraglottic larynx and cervical lymph nodes. The dose-volume histogram (*upper right*) shows the radiation dose coverage of the targets (*solid lines*), with scenarios modeling setup errors (*dotted lines*) used to help select beam arrangements that ensure the targets receive sufficient dose even in the face of setup uncertainty. Top left: axial view. Lower left: coronal view. Lower right: sagittal view. Top right: dose-volume histogram.

(**Fig. 13**). Organ motion represents another challenge in proton therapy planning. Changes in density with moving tissues can have an impact on proton path length, resulting in changes in dose distribution. There also is a risk of missing the target prescribed due to motion. Many motion management techniques are utilized, including breath hold, gating, and abdominal compression but need to be personalized for each patient's tolerance of these techniques. In certain clinical situations, such as significant organ motion, an x-ray–based plan is more appropriate than proton therapy; in other situations, a mixed photon-proton plan can leverage the advantages of both x-ray IMRT and proton therapy. Ultimately, proton therapy's unique considerations underscore the need for experience and volume among the radiation oncologist, the radiation physicist, and the proton center as a whole to best capitalize on proton therapy's potential benefits.

EXPANSION AND USE OF SINGLE-ROOM CENTERS

Until recently, the costs associated with developing and operating a proton center have been a key drawback. Traditional multiroom centers—typically housing 4 to 5 proton treatment rooms—have cost between $100 million and 300 million to build, with estimated annual operating costs of $15 million to $25 million.[18] These centers typically have required bread-and-butter cases—breast cancer and prostate cancer—to economically sustain the center and subsidize the rare, complex cancers most likely to benefit from proton therapy.[19] Complicating matters is the need to service the debt and achieve profitability for the for-profit equity backers that many centers have relied on for construction. Even debt-free, philanthropically funded centers may have difficulty breaking even depending on their case mix and volume, which often depend on the coverage policies of local health insurers.[20] Proton therapy thus has required costlier billing rates than x-ray radiotherapy, increasing costs to the health care system and leading some insurers to deny coverage for protons.[20] Other limitations relate to the relative scarcity of proton centers. Whereas for x-ray radiotherapy, a second or nearby linear accelerator can accommodate maintenance downtime or unavailability of treatment slots for new patients, there generally is no backup proton center for either scenario, potentially resulting in delays to start new patients' treatments.

The development of single-room proton centers has offered a more cost-effective option that addresses these drawbacks. Current start-up costs for single-room proton centers are estimated at $40 million. Hitachi (Tokyo, Japan), IBA (Louvain-La-Neuve, Belgium), Mevion Medical Systems (Littleton, Massachusetts, United States), and Varian Medical Systems (Palo Alto, California, United States) are the largest manufacturers currently marketing single-room proton centers that rely on smaller cyclotrons. Of the 25 proton centers in the United States currently treating patients, 11 are single-room centers. Four more are currently under development (**Fig. 14**). Although substantially more expensive than the sub–$5 million cost for a new conventional x-ray linear accelerator, single-room proton centers require considerably less financial engineering to achieve their initial build-out: such a project may still require debt financing, although less reliant on for-profit equity partners, thus obviating optimizing disease site mix for profit. Washington University School of Medicine contracted with Mevion Medical Systems to build the first integrated single-room proton system, opening for treatment in late 2013. Treating 24 patients daily—of whom under 5% had prostate

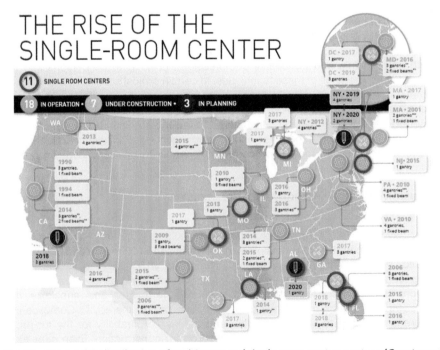

Fig. 14. Geographic distribution of multiroom and single-room proton centers. (*Courtesy of Proton International, Louisville, Kentucky.*)

Table 1
Proton Therapy Phase III Randomized Controlled Trials

Disease	Primary Endpoint	Start Date	Estimated Primary Completion Date	Estimated Study Completion Date	Registry Number
Esophageal Cancer	Progression-free Survival, Total Toxicity Burden	4/2012	4/2020	4/2021	NCT01512589
Lung Cancer	Overall Survival	2/2014	12/2020	12/2025	NCT01993810
Glioblastoma	Overall Survival	10/2014	5/2021	5/2026	NCT02179086
Prostate Cancer	Patient-reported Bowel Symptom Score	7/2012	12/2021	12/2026	NCT01617161
Hepatocellular Carcinoma	Overall Survival	6/2017	8/2022	8/2027	NCT03186898
Low Grade Glioma	Neurocognition	8/2017	1/2025	1/2030	NCT03180502
Breast Cancer	Major Cardiovascular Events	2/2016	8/2022	11/2032	NCT02603341

cancer—achieved financial sustainability.[21] A 75% debt-financed $40 million center would require only $10 million in equity, closer in up-front outlay to a new x-ray linear accelerator, and would require a smaller proportion of bread-and-butter cases to break even.[22] This is certainly within reach of many hospitals and radiation oncology departments without the need of a for-profit equity partner. Newer single-room systems use pencil beam scanning, and those using cyclotrons are capable of delivering high dose rates. Thus, trends toward single-room proton centers will likely drive uptake of proton therapy for clinical scenarios most likely to benefit from this treatment modality.

KEY CLINICAL AREAS OF USE

The National Comprehensive Cancer Network guidelines currently support the use of proton therapy in various scenarios across more than 40 distinct cancer types,[23] and several clinical trials are currently randomizing patients to proton therapy versus x-ray radiotherapy (**Table 1**).[20] The following sections highlight selected key disease sites in which proton therapy may offer key advantages over conventional radiotherapy.

Pediatrics

Proton therapy is a particularly appealing treatment modality for children who require radiotherapy. Despite numerous advances in pediatric oncology and the intention of many recent and ongoing pediatric trials to reduce or eliminate the use of radiotherapy altogether, many children with central nervous system tumors, solid tumors (eg, Ewing sarcoma, rhabdomyosarcoma, and neuroblastoma), and Hodgkin lymphoma still require radiotherapy. The pediatric population is particularly vulnerable to late effects from radiation: not only are children's developing tissues more sensitive to radiation toxicity but also the time from cancer cure until expected death can be many decades long. In essence, survivors of childhood cancer may have a very long time to live and, as such, have greater potential to develop late radiation toxicities. Childhood cancer survivors are at risk for myriad late effects involving nearly every organ system.[24,25]

Survivors of pediatric brain tumors who received brain radiation are at risk for significant neurocognitive sequelae, the degree to which seems to be based on 3 major factors:

1. Age at the time of radiotherapy
2. The volume of brain exposed to radiation
3. The radiation dose received[26]

Data published in the 1980s demonstrated profound neurocognitive damage resulting from conventional x-ray radiotherapy delivered to the brains of very young children.[27] The damage was so severe that treatment paradigms shifted away from offering radiation to this population, often at the cost of cure.[28] In contrast, early data suggest that proton therapy may offer normal tissue brain sparing due to its stopping power, allowing curative treatment to be delivered even to young patients undergoing continued neurodevelopment.[29,30]

The benefits of proton therapy have been demonstrated in other pediatric disease sites as well. For patients requiring radiation to the spine, proton therapy may eliminate exposure of breast tissue, heart, lungs, bowel, and organs of fertility. For patients with pelvic and abdominal tumors, again, proton therapy can reduce exposure to the ovaries, uterus, bladder, liver, kidneys, and bowel. Numerous publications have documented that proton therapy offers excellent rates of local control in experienced hands, and data regarding late and long-term effects are being published, with more forthcoming. In some tumor types, cost effectiveness of proton therapy has been documented due mostly to reduction in late effects. Cooperative groups, notably the Children's Oncology Group and the Pediatric Proton Consortium Registry, will be essential bodies in supporting the collaborative work necessary to examine longitudinal outcomes in a relatively small population worldwide.

Children's cancers remain rare compared with many other types of malignancy, and children requiring radiotherapy are a unique population. Pediatric radiotherapy should be delivered at a center of excellence, with expertise in pediatric radiotherapy and oncology, and with resources, such as pediatric anesthesia, pediatric nursing, and child life support. The selection of patients likely to benefit from proton therapy should be performed at a multidisciplinary level, with consideration of multiple factors. For example, most patients treated palliatively do not benefit from proton therapy. Some patients treated curatively do not benefit dosimetrically from this technology. For others, delays due to insurance approval and/or travel to a proton center may offset the benefit of proton therapy. When patients are selected appropriately, insurance companies in the United States seem likely to approve proton therapy for children, emphasizing the unique and well-established benefits in this population.[31] These benefits support consideration of proton therapy for any pediatric patient receiving curative radiotherapy.

Lymphoma

The rationale for proton therapy in lymphomas parallels its rationale for use in pediatric cancers. Many lymphomas can be cured with relatively low-dose radiotherapy, yet even low-dose exposure of large volumes of normal tissues carries significant risk. Secondary malignancy is a well-documented late effect of radiotherapy among lymphoma survivors, in particular those with Hodgkin lymphoma (who have historically been treated with very large radiation fields).[32] To reduce these risks, decades of clinical trials have sought to reduce not only radiation dose but also the volume irradiated. Proton therapy can significantly spare normal tissues that are at risk for a radiation-induced cancer, such as the thyroid, esophagus, lung, breast, and other soft tissues. Equally important is proton therapy's ability to spare the heart, which is commonly adjacent to sites of lymphoma. Cardiac disease, stroke, and lung disease are important noncancerous risks of radiotherapy for survivors of lymphoma. Because late effects and second cancers require decades of follow-up, dosimetric studies have been undertaken to compare proton and x-ray radiotherapy. With some exceptions, a majority of these studies have shown clinically important dose reductions to the heart, coronary arteries, lung, and body; data are more mixed with respect to the breast, thyroid, and esophagus.[32]

Breast

For most patients undergoing adjuvant whole-breast radiotherapy, x-ray 3-D–CRT achieves excellent disease control with minimal toxicity. In certain cases, however, protons may better spare healthy cardiac and lung tissue.[33] The importance of minimizing dose to the heart cannot be overstated: in a seminal 2013 report, Darby and colleagues[34] predicted a dose-dependent increase in major coronary events. Modern x-ray techniques using maneuvers, such as prone positioning or deep inspiratory breath-hold, can significantly reduce heart and lung dose in many cases. When radiation to the internal mammary nodes is required, however, conventional radiotherapy may yield unacceptably high heart and lung dose exposure. Similarly, in patients with rarer anatomic features, such as pectus excavatum, there is a clear advantage to the use of proton therapy to spare the heart and lung. The Radiotherapy Comparative

Effectiveness (RADCOMP) phase III trial is randomizing breast cancer patients to proton versus x-ray therapy with a primary outcome of cardiac toxicity.

Prostate

The first patient was treated with protons for prostate cancer in 1976 at the Harvard cyclotron.[35] At the time, x-ray and proton technologies both lacked the sophistication of the modern-day era, and conventional 4-field box 2-D x-ray radiotherapy was still considered standard of care. Since then, both x-ray and proton radiotherapy have rapidly evolved to adopt increasingly more sophisticated modalities: as the 3-D–CRT of the 1990s was replaced with IMRT in the 2000s, today's standard-of-care x-ray treatment achieves conformal high-dose coverage and good normal tissue sparing. Modern x-ray–based treatment is generally well tolerated, although it does cause both acute and late genitourinary and gastrointestinal toxicities. Because the high-dose radiation region—including the prostatic urethra and portions of the bladder and rectum—are similar with either x-ray or proton therapy, it is not clear if reducing the moderate-dose and low-dose bath with protons reduces toxicity. Two of 4 large claims-based studies found decreased risk of acute genitourinary toxicities with proton therapy,[36,37] whereas three-fourths found increased late gastrointestinal toxicities.[36,38,39] Smaller patient-level data sets also have been mixed, with most demonstrating no significant difference between proton therapy and IMRT.[40–42] The potential of proton therapy to reduce toxicity for prostate cancer treatment remains an open question, and the Prostate Advanced Radiation Technologies Investigating Quality of Life (PARTIQoL) trial is currently accruing.

Sarcoma

Sarcomas of the skull base and spine—primarily chordomas and chondrosarcomas—require high radiation doses (typically 70–80 Gy) of radiation, putting critical structures at high risk for severe, irreversible toxicity, namely myelopathy or necrosis resulting in paralysis or death. A recent National Cancer Database analysis reported that for chordoma and chondrosarcoma treated with definitive radiotherapy, proton therapy was associated with greater 5-year overall survival versus x-rays.[43] Sarcomas arising elsewhere in the body, such as retroperitoneal sarcoma, also may benefit from the organ-sparing effects of proton therapy. Early-phase trials have demonstrated the safety and feasibility of dose escalation using proton therapy for retroperitoneal sarcoma,[44] and an additional trial is currently accruing.

Ophthalmologic, Central Nervous System, and Head and Neck

For ocular uveal melanomas whose large size or proximity to the optic disk increases the risks of photon plaque brachytherapy, proton therapy can achieve 5-year local control in more than 90%[45] and keep 15-year enucleation rates under 20%.[46] In a small series of children with optic gliomas, with a median 3 years of follow-up, local control was 100%, visual outcomes were excellent, and substantial dose reductions were achieved for the contralateral visual optic nerve, optic chiasm, pituitary gland, brainstem, and frontal and temporal lobes compared with conventional photon radiotherapy.[47] In adults with benign meningioma—an intracranial tumor with high rates of cure and thus a need to minimize late toxicity—3-year toxicity-free survival of 76%, with local control of 91%, has been reported.[48] Retrospective comparisons in several head and neck cancers have reported reduced toxicities using proton therapy versus x-ray IMRT in unilateral salivary gland carcinomas; nasopharyngeal, nasal cavity, and paranasal sinus cancers; and oropharyngeal cancer.[49]

Lung

Locally advanced lung cancer requires thoracic radiation to the primary tumor and involved mediastinal lymph nodes—targets that are surrounded by key sensitive structures, such as the lung, heart, and esophagus. Although higher doses to these structures can produce severe toxicities or adversely affect overall survival,[50] an adequate dose to the target is needed to maximize tumor control and survival.[51] Proton therapy has the potential to reduce doses to the lung, heart, and esophagus, while delivering a sufficient dose to the target. Protons' distal beam uncertainty, however, presents unique risks in the thorax, an anatomic region with tissues of widely varying densities (from bone to aerated lung) and a target that moves with respiration: issues that demand accurate heterogeneity correction and motion management. Thus, the clinical treatment planning and delivery team's proton expertise is of particular importance in this disease site, as was suggested by a 2018 randomized trial comparing passive scattering proton therapy versus conventional x-ray IMRT for locally advanced non–small cell lung cancer patients undergoing definitive chemoradiation. Although the primary endpoints were not met, a post hoc analysis found significantly lower rates of radiation pneumonitis among patients receiving passive scattering proton therapy when comparing patients enrolled after versus prior to the trial midpoint, with zero reports of grade 3 or higher radiation pneumonitis among patients enrolled in the second half of the trial. This difference was not seen among patients receiving conventional x-ray IMRT. This likely reflects a learning curve associated with implementing proton therapy, emphasizing the need for experience in treatment with protons before embarking on comparative trials.

Gastrointestinal

Proton therapy has shown a clear benefit over conventional photon radiotherapy in hepatocellular carcinoma. With prior data showing that survival depends on higher doses of radiation delivered to the tumor,[17] a subsequent phase II trial found that that proton therapy could achieve a tumoricidal dose that was nonetheless safe for nearby tissues.[16] With few grade 3 toxicities and no grade 4 or higher toxicities, 2-year local control was nearly 95%, supporting the safety and utility of protons for hepatocellular carcinoma. For esophageal cancer, a provocative retrospective study reported improved overall and progression-free survival with proton therapy versus x-ray IMRT; although this remained the case after controlling for other factors on

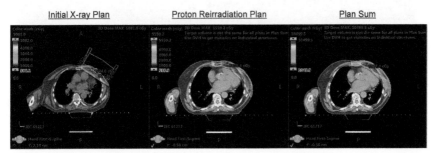

Fig. 15. The dose distribution from a prior, completed x-ray radiotherapy treatment is added to the dose distribution for a planned proton reirradiation course. The resulting plan sum allows the radiation oncologist to evaluate the lifetime dose to normal tissues and organs-at-risk both visually and using the dose-volume histogram (not shown). Left: Initial x-ray plan. Center: Proton reirradiation plan. Right: Plan sum.

multivariable analysis, the investigators concede that socioeconomic factors related to insurance coverage of proton therapy may have confounded their results.[52] Although these data are intriguing, the randomized phase III NRG-GI006 trial may definitively show whether proton therapy is superior to photon IMRT for esophageal cancer, although the study is not anticipated to complete until 2032.

Reirradiation

Several prospective single-arm trials evaluating proton therapy for patients with locally recurrent cancers who have previously undergone radiotherapy have reported results,

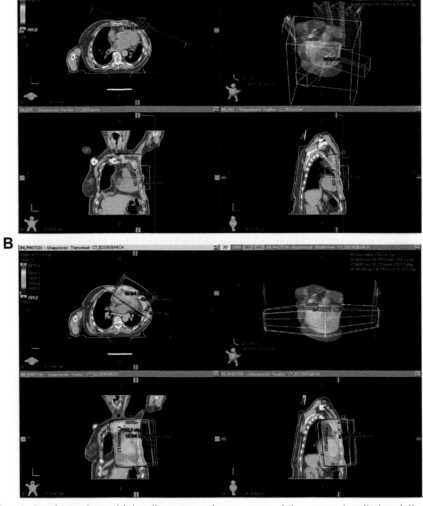

Fig. 16. For this patient with locally recurrent breast cancer, (*A*) proton reirradiation delivers a much lower dose to surrounding tissues, such as the heart and lung, than (*B*) x-ray reirradiation. (A) Top left: axial view. Lower left: coronal view. Lower right: sagittal view. Top right: 3D reconstruction. (B) Top left: axial view. Lower left: coronal view. Lower right: sagittal view. Top right: 3D reconstruction.

and still more are currently in progress. Historically, patients typically have undergone only a single course of radiation to a given site, because high-dose reirradiation could place nearby normal tissues at unacceptable risk—essentially exceeding their lifetime radiation tolerance—with the potential for significant morbidity and mortality. With the advent of software-based radiation treatment planning and dose modeling, a reirradiation plan could be superimposed on and added to the prior radiation treatment plan—creating a plan sum—allowing the radiation oncologist to determine the exact lifetime dose a given tissue would receive (**Fig. 15**). Because proton therapy's key advantage is normal tissue avoidance, reirradiation plans could be created that would yield a plan sum with an acceptable risk of toxicity. Emerging prospective and retrospective data are finding that proton reirradiation can achieve a favorable disease control and toxicity profile in central nervous system,[53] head and neck,[54] breast (**Fig. 16**),[55] esophageal,[56] pancreatic,[57] and rectal cancers.[56]

FUTURE DIRECTIONS FOR RESEARCH AND USE

Future directions for in silico and in vivo research aim to improve the understanding of the physics and biology of proton therapy and how these differ versus those of conventional photon radiation. Specifically, learning exactly where the Bragg peak occurs has key clinical implications, because proton depth dose uncertainty currently requires strategies that involve either treating a margin of normal tissue to ensure tumor coverage or avoiding a margin of tissue to avoid a key organ at risk. Prompt gamma imaging, which detects secondary gamma rays produced by protons' interaction with tissue at the Bragg peak, and triangulating its location, is one strategy to address this issue.[58] As discussed previously, another active area of research aims to determine whether the relative biologic effectiveness of protons versus photons is different at regions surrounding the Bragg peak, where a majority of proton-tissue interactions take place.[3] Currently, it is assumed that protons are 1.1 times more biologically effective than photons, and clinical dose adjustments are made accordingly; however, there is emerging laboratory and clinical evidence that there is a gradient of biologic effectiveness along the proton beam path and at the distal edge where the beam stops.[3] Perhaps the most intriguing—but least certain—area of research surrounds ultrahigh dose rate FLASH radiotherapy, which very preliminary preclinical work suggests may achieve tumor control with markedly reduced toxicity.[59] Unlike conventional x-ray linear accelerators, proton therapy units have the unique ability to deliver this ultrahigh dose rate. Although FLASH represents a potential paradigm shift in radiation oncology, time will tell whether this approach is safe and feasible.

In the near term, future directions for the clinical use of proton therapy will hinge on the results of the randomized phase III trials currently accruing (see **Table 1**).[20] RADCOMP and PARTIQoL, once reported in peer-reviewed literature, may lead to expanded indications for proton therapy to reduce the toxicity of breast and prostate radiotherapy. More broadly, 2 key advances in oncology may lead to new indications for proton therapy in the longer term: first, improvements in radiotherapy, surgical techniques, and systemic therapies—including targeted therapies and immunotherapy—are already yielding remarkable improvements in survival and frank cures; and second, the development and widespread adoption of photon IMRT is exposing patients to a much higher integral dose than ever before, and longer-term follow-up of cured younger patients has the potential to show unexpected late toxicities. With cancer patients living longer and seeing cures at greater rates—particularly in light of emerging data reporting prolonged survival after aggressively treating oligometastatic cancers—the long-term toxicities of treatment are becoming a primary concern, just as they have in pediatric oncology. Proton therapy's lack of integral dose and its reduced volume of normal tissue exposure may thus come to be increasingly important as more long-term follow-up data emerge. The increasing adoption of economical single-room centers, in turn, may make proton therapy a less scarce resource, potentially eliminating delays in treatment starts, reducing treatment costs to payers, driving improved insurance coverage, and ultimately bringing proton therapy to more patients.

REFERENCES

1. Wilson RR. Radiological use of fast protons. Radiology 1946;47(5):487–91.
2. Lawrence JH, Tobias CA, Born JL, et al. Pituitary irradiation with high-energy proton beams: a preliminary report. Cancer Res 1958;18(2):121–34.
3. Jones B, McMahon SJ, Prise KM. The radiobiology of proton therapy: challenges and opportunities around relative biological effectiveness. Clin Oncol (R Coll Radiol) 2018;30(5):285–92.
4. Miralbell R, Lomax A, Cella L, et al. Potential reduction of the incidence of radiation-induced second cancers by using proton beams in the treatment of pediatric tumors. Int J Radiat Oncol Biol Phys 2002;54(3):824–9.
5. St Clair WH, Adams JA, Bues M, et al. Advantage of protons compared to conventional X-ray or IMRT in the treatment of a pediatric patient with medulloblastoma. Int J Radiat Oncol Biol Phys 2004;58(3):727–34.
6. Eaton BR, Esiashvili N, Kim S, et al. Clinical outcomes among children with standard-risk medulloblastoma treated with proton and photon radiation therapy: a comparison of disease control and overall survival. Int J Radiat Oncol Biol Phys 2016;94(1):133–8.
7. Dabaja BS, Hoppe BS, Plastaras JP, et al. Proton therapy for adults with mediastinal lymphomas: the International Lymphoma Radiation Oncology Group guidelines. Blood 2018;132(16):1635–46.
8. Yahalom J, Illidge T, Specht L, et al. Modern radiation therapy for extranodal lymphomas: field and dose guidelines from the International Lymphoma Radiation Oncology Group. Int J Radiat Oncol Biol Phys 2015;92(1):11–31.
9. Hodgson DC, Dieckmann K, Terezakis S, et al. Implementation of contemporary radiation therapy planning concepts for pediatric Hodgkin lymphoma: Guidelines from the International Lymphoma Radiation Oncology Group. Pract Radiat Oncol 2015;5(2):85–92.
10. MacDonald SM, Trofimov A, Safai S, et al. Proton radiotherapy for pediatric central nervous system germ cell tumors: early clinical outcomes. Int J Radiat Oncol Biol Phys 2011;79(1):121–9.
11. Krasin MJ, Constine LS, Friedman DL, et al. Radiation-related treatment effects across the age spectrum: differences and similarities or what the old and young can learn from each other. Semin Radiat Oncol 2010;20(1):21–9.
12. Eaton BR, MacDonald SM, Yock TI, et al. Secondary malignancy risk following proton radiation therapy. Front Oncol 2015;5:261.
13. Qi W-X, Fu S, Zhang Q, et al. Charged particle therapy versus photon therapy for patients with hepatocellular carcinoma: a systematic review and meta-analysis. Radiother Oncol 2015;114(3):289–95.
14. Kalogeridi M-A, Zygogianni A, Kyrgias G, et al. Role of radiotherapy in the management of hepatocellular carcinoma: a systematic review. World J Hepatol 2015; 7(1):101–12.
15. Klein J, Dawson LA. Hepatocellular carcinoma radiation therapy: review of evidence and future opportunities. Int J Radiat Oncol Biol Phys 2013;87(1):22–32.

16. Hong TS, Wo JY, Yeap BY, et al. Multi-institutional phase II study of high-dose hypofractionated proton beam therapy in patients with localized, unresectable hepatocellular carcinoma and intrahepatic cholangiocarcinoma. J Clin Oncol 2016;34(5):460–8.

17. Ben-Josef E, Normolle D, Ensminger WD, et al. Phase II trial of high-dose conformal radiation therapy with concurrent hepatic artery floxuridine for unresectable intrahepatic malignancies. J Clin Oncol 2005;23(34):8739–47.

18. Huff C. Catching the proton wave; hospitals weigh the promise of a breakthrough cancer treatment against the enormous costs. Hosp Health Netw 2007;81(3):62, 64, 66, 2.

19. Johnstone PAS, Kerstiens J, Richard H. Proton facility economics: the importance of "simple" treatments. J Am Coll Radiol 2012;9(8):560–3.

20. Bekelman JE, Denicoff A, Buchsbaum J. Randomized trials of proton therapy: why they are at risk, proposed solutions, and implications for evaluating advanced technologies to diagnose and treat cancer. J Clin Oncol 2018; 36(24):2461–4.

21. Klein EE, Bradley J. Single-room proton radiation therapy systems: no small change. Int J Radiat Oncol Biol Phys 2016;95(1):147–8.

22. Kerstiens J, Johnstone GP, Johnstone PAS. Proton facility economics: single-room centers. J Am Coll Radiol 2018;15(12):1704–8.

23. National Comprehensive Cancer Network. NCCN Clinical Practice Guideline in Oncology–Prostate Cancer Version 2.2017. Available at: https://www.nccn.org/professionals/physician_gls/pdf/prostate.pdf. Accessed April 16, 2017.

24. Effinger KE, Stratton KL, Fisher PG, et al. Long-term health and social function in adult survivors of paediatric astrocytoma: a report from the Childhood Cancer Survivor Study. Eur J Cancer 2019;106:171–80.

25. Friend AJ, Feltbower RG, Newton HL, et al. Late effects of childhood cancer. Lancet 2018;391(10132):1772.

26. Willard VW, Berlin KS, Conklin HM, et al. Trajectories of psychosocial and cognitive functioning in pediatric patients with brain tumors treated with radiation therapy. Neuro Oncol 2019. https://doi.org/10.1093/neuonc/noz010.

27. Duffner PK, Cohen ME, Thomas P. Late effects of treatment on the intelligence of children with posterior fossa tumors. Cancer 1983;51(2):233–7.

28. Duffner PK, Horowitz ME, Krischer JP, et al. Postoperative chemotherapy and delayed radiation in children less than three years of age with malignant brain tumors. N Engl J Med 1993;328(24):1725–31.

29. Pulsifer MB, Duncanson H, Grieco J, et al. Cognitive and adaptive outcomes after proton radiation for pediatric patients with brain tumors. Int J Radiat Oncol Biol Phys 2018;102(2):391–8.

30. Ventura LM, Grieco JA, Evans CL, et al. Executive functioning, academic skills, and quality of life in pediatric patients with brain tumors post-proton radiation therapy. J Neurooncol 2018;137(1):119–26.

31. Ojerholm E, Hill-Kayser CE. Insurance coverage decisions for pediatric proton therapy. Pediatr Blood Cancer 2018;65(1). https://doi.org/10.1002/pbc.26729.

32. Tseng YD, Cutter DJ, Plastaras JP, et al. Evidence-based review on the use of proton therapy in lymphoma from the particle therapy cooperative group (PTCOG) lymphoma subcommittee. Int J Radiat Oncol Biol Phys 2017;99(4):825–42.

33. Kammerer E, Guevelou JL, Chaikh A, et al. Proton therapy for locally advanced breast cancer: a systematic review of the literature. Cancer Treat Rev 2018;63:19–27.

34. Darby SC, Ewertz M, McGale P, et al. Risk of ischemic heart disease in women after radiotherapy for breast cancer. N Engl J Med 2013;368(11):987–98.

35. Shipley WU, Tepper JE, Prout GR, et al. Proton radiation as boost therapy for localized prostatic carcinoma. JAMA 1979;241(18):1912–5.

36. Pan HY, Jiang J, Hoffman KE, et al. Comparative toxicities and cost of intensity-modulated radiotherapy, proton radiation, and stereotactic body radiotherapy among younger men with prostate cancer. J Clin Oncol 2018;36(18):1823–30.

37. Yu JB, Soulos PR, Herrin J, et al. Proton versus intensity-modulated radiotherapy for prostate cancer: patterns of care and early toxicity. J Natl Cancer Inst 2013; 105(1):25–32.

38. Sheets NC, Goldin GH, Meyer A-M, et al. Intensity-modulated radiation therapy, proton therapy, or conformal radiation therapy and morbidity and disease control in localized prostate cancer. JAMA 2012;307(15):1611–20.

39. Kim S, Shen S, Moore DF, et al. Late gastrointestinal toxicities following radiation therapy for prostate cancer. Eur Urol 2011;60(5):908–16.

40. Fang P, Mick R, Deville C, et al. A case-matched study of toxicity outcomes after proton therapy and intensity-modulated radiation therapy for prostate cancer. Cancer 2015;121(7):1118–27.

41. Gray PJ, Paly JJ, Yeap BY, et al. Patient-reported outcomes after 3-dimensional conformal, intensity-modulated, or proton beam radiotherapy for localized prostate cancer. Cancer 2013;119(9):1729–35.

42. Hoppe BS, Michalski JM, Mendenhall NP, et al. Comparative effectiveness study of patient-reported outcomes after proton therapy or intensity-modulated radiotherapy for prostate cancer. Cancer 2014;120(7):1076–82.

43. Palm RF, Oliver DE, Yang GQ, et al. The role of dose escalation and proton therapy in perioperative or definitive treatment of chondrosarcoma and chordoma: An analysis of the National Cancer Data Base. Cancer 2019;125(4):642–51.

44. DeLaney TF, Chen Y-L, Baldini EH, et al. Phase 1 trial of preoperative image guided intensity modulated proton radiation therapy with simultaneously integrated boost to the high risk margin for retroperitoneal sarcomas. Adv Radiat Oncol 2017;2(1):85–93.

45. Gragoudas ES, Lane AM, Regan S, et al. A randomized controlled trial of varying radiation doses in the treatment of choroidal melanoma. Arch Ophthalmol 2000; 118(6):773–8.

46. Egger E, Zografos L, Schalenbourg A, et al. Eye retention after proton beam radiotherapy for uveal melanoma. Int J Radiat Oncol Biol Phys 2003;55(4): 867–80.

47. Fuss M, Hug EB, Schaefer RA, et al. Proton radiation therapy (PRT) for pediatric optic pathway gliomas: comparison with 3D planned conventional photons and a standard photon technique. Int J Radiat Oncol Biol Phys 1999;45(5):1117–26.

48. Weber DC, Lomax AJ, Rutz HP, et al. Spot-scanning proton radiation therapy for recurrent, residual or untreated intracranial meningiomas. Radiother Oncol 2004; 71(3):251–8.

49. Kim JK, Leeman JE, Riaz N, et al. Proton therapy for head and neck cancer. Curr Treat Options Oncol 2018;19(6):28.

50. Bradley JD, Paulus R, Komaki R, et al. Standard-dose versus high-dose conformal radiotherapy with concurrent and consolidation carboplatin plus paclitaxel with or without cetuximab for patients with stage IIIA or IIIB non-small-cell lung cancer (RTOG 0617): a randomised, two-by-two factorial phase 3 study. Lancet Oncol 2015;16(2):187–99.

51. Hong JC, Salama JK. Dose escalation for unresectable locally advanced non-small cell lung cancer: end of the line? Transl Lung Cancer Res 2016;5(1): 126–33.
52. Xi M, Xu C, Liao Z, et al. Comparative outcomes after definitive chemoradiotherapy using proton beam therapy versus intensity modulated radiation therapy for esophageal cancer: a retrospective, single-institutional analysis. Int J Radiat Oncol Biol Phys 2017;99(3):667–76.
53. Galle JO, McDonald MW, Simoneaux V, et al. Reirradiation with proton therapy for recurrent gliomas. Int J Part Ther 2015;2(1):11–8.
54. Romesser PB, Cahlon O, Scher ED, et al. Proton beam reirradiation for recurrent head and neck cancer: multi-institutional report on feasibility and early outcomes. Int J Radiat Oncol Biol Phys 2016;95(1):386–95.
55. LaRiviere MJ, Dreyfuss A, Taunk NK, et al. Acute and late toxicity of hyperfractionated reirradiation for locoregionally recurrent breast cancer. Int J Radiat Oncol Biol Phys 2019;103(5):E25–6.
56. Berman AT, Both S, Sharkoski T, et al. Proton reirradiation of recurrent rectal cancer: dosimetric comparison, toxicities, and preliminary outcomes. Int J Part Ther 2014;1(1):2–13.
57. Boimel PJ, Berman AT, Li J, et al. Proton beam reirradiation for locally recurrent pancreatic adenocarcinoma. J Gastrointest Oncol 2017;8(4):665–74.
58. Richter C, Pausch G, Barczyk S, et al. First clinical application of a prompt gamma based in vivo proton range verification system. Radiother Oncol 2016; 118(2):232–7.
59. Durante M, Bräuer-Krisch E, Hill M. Faster and safer? FLASH ultra-high dose rate in radiotherapy. Br J Radiol 2018;91(1082):20170628.

Modern Brachytherapy

Sophie J. Otter, MBBChir, MRCP, FRCR[a],*,
Alexandra J. Stewart, MD, MRCP, FRCR[a], Phillip M. Devlin, MD, FFRCSI[b]

KEYWORDS

- Brachytherapy • Radionuclide • Normal tissue sparing • Prostate cancer
- Cervix cancer • Breast cancer • Rectal cancer • Skin cancer

KEY POINTS

- Brachytherapy can be used in a wide variety of situations to treat multiple tumor sites, such as gynecological, urologic, rectal, skin, and breast cancers.
- Brachytherapy enables the delivery of a high dose of radiation to the tumor while sparing the surrounding normal tissue, therefore often allowing dose escalation that would not be possible with other forms of radiotherapy.
- Modern brachytherapy involves sophisticated image guidance for the accurate placement of catheters/sources and real-time adaptive planning to facilitate highly conformal dose distribution.

INTRODUCTION

Brachytherapy is the placement of radioactive sources within or very close to target tissue. The target tissue may be a tumor or a postoperative tumor bed. The dosimetric benefit of brachytherapy is that a high dose of radiation can be delivered to the tumor while keeping within normal tissue tolerance limits.

Radium was first discovered in 1889 and was initially used for the brachytherapy treatment of skin cancers. Radium has been superseded by other radioisotopes that have more favorable safety profiles. Radioisotopes decay and emit radiation in the form of alpha particles, beta particles, or gamma rays as they do so **(Table 1)**. These particles or rays interact with living cells and damage DNA, leading to cell death.

The physical properties of a radioisotope determine whether it delivers high dose rate (HDR, >12 Gy/h), low dose rate (LDR, 0.4–2 Gy/h), or very low dose rate (vLDR, <0.4 Gy/h) brachytherapy. In many instances, HDR brachytherapy is more convenient for the patient because of shorter treatment times, which can potentially lead to fewer complications, such as venous thromboembolism. For example, cervical

Disclosures: There are no conflicts of interest to disclose.
[a] Royal Surrey County Hospital, Egerton Road, Guildford GU2 7XX, UK; [b] Dana Farber Cancer Institute, Harvard Medical School, 75 Francis Street, Boston, MA 02115, USA
* Corresponding author.
E-mail address: sophie.otter1@nhs.net

Hematol Oncol Clin N Am 33 (2019) 1011–1025
https://doi.org/10.1016/j.hoc.2019.08.011
0889-8588/19/© 2019 Elsevier Inc. All rights reserved.

hemonc.theclinics.com

Table 1
Radioisotopes in common clinical use with their relevant physical properties and radium-226 for comparison

Isotope	Half-life	Emission Type	Mean Therapeutic Energy	Half Value Layer of Lead (mm)	Dose Rate	Uses
Radium-226	1626 y	Alpha, beta, and gamma	830 keV	16	LDR	No longer used clinically
Cobalt-60	5.26 y	Gamma	1.17, 1.33 MeV	11	HDR	Intracavitary
Cesium-131	9.7 d	Gamma	30.4 keV	Not known	vLDR	Permanent interstitial implants; eg, prostate, breast, head and neck, lung
Cesium-137	30 y	Gamma	662 keV	3.28	LDR	LDR intracavitary brachytherapy; eg, cervical Rarely used now
Iodine-125	59.6 d	Gamma	28 keV	0.025	vLDR	Permanent interstitial implants; eg, prostate
Iridium-192	74.2 d	Gamma	380 keV	6	HDR/PDR	HDR/PDR interstitial and intracavitary
Strontium-90/ yttrium-90	28.8 y/2.7 d	Beta	2.27 MeV	<1	HDR	Plaques used for treatment of superficial ocular lesions
Ruthenium-106	1.02 y	Beta	3.54 MeV	3.28	HDR	Plaques

Abbreviations: HDR, high dose rate; LDR, low dose rate; PDR, pulsed dose rate; vLDR, very low dose rate.

brachytherapy took approximately 24 hours to deliver when cesium-137 was routinely used, whereas, with iridium-192, treatments often last less than 10 minutes. However, when changing dose rate from LDR to HDR, the total dose must be reduced to account for the increased biological effect of HDR. Pulsed dose rate (PDR) mimics LDR delivery by delivering small pulses of HDR intermittently; for example, hourly.

Brachytherapy is most commonly used to treat cancers of the uterus, cervix, prostate, skin, breast, and rectum (because of accessibility). Brachytherapy can be used as a monotherapy in these tumor types or as a means to deliver a high-dose boost to the primary tumor after external beam radiotherapy (EBRT) (eg, in high-risk prostate cancer) or after surgery (eg, in breast cancer). Therefore, this article focuses on the clinical indications of brachytherapy in the treatment of these tumor sites and the practicalities of delivering brachytherapy.

CLINICAL APPLICATIONS OF BRACHYTHERAPY
Gynecological Brachytherapy

Cervical cancer
Brachytherapy is an essential part of the treatment of locally advanced cervical cancers (LACCs) in combination with EBRT and concomitant chemotherapy.[1] There was a decline in the use of brachytherapy in the United States from 83% in 1988 to 58% in 2009 because of the introduction of other radiotherapy techniques, such as intensity-modulated radiotherapy (IMRT) and stereotactic radiotherapy (SBRT).[2] However, brachytherapy is independently associated with an improved cancer-specific survival and overall survival (OS) and therefore cannot be replaced by alternative methods such as IMRT.[3] Planning studies have also shown that IMRT is not able to achieve doses as high as image-guided brachytherapy (IGBT) when dose constraints (D1cc and D2cc) to the bladder, sigmoid, and rectum are adhered to.[4]

Patients with LACC should ideally receive pelvic IMRT with concomitant cisplatin-based chemotherapy.[1] Brachytherapy in the modern era is usually delivered using PDR or HDR brachytherapy using an iridium-192 source. Many HDR patients can therefore be treated as day cases. Depending on tumor size, brachytherapy usually starts after at least 20 fractions of IMRT and can be interdigitated with the EBRT so that the overall treatment time is kept as short as possible because improved local control is associated with a shorter overall treatment time of less than 56 days (**Fig. 1** shows an example treatment schema).[5,6]

An MRI scan before the procedure is helpful to assess the tumor response to chemoradiotherapy and to plan the brachytherapy.[7] The insertional procedure is typically performed under a general or spinal anesthetic. The cervix is dilated and a tandem is

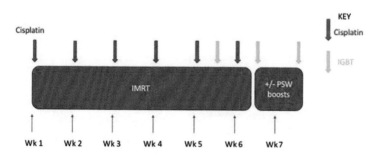

Fig. 1. An example treatment schema for chemoradiotherapy and brachytherapy. Cisplatin is given weekly at 40 mg/m². PSW, pelvic side wall boosts.

inserted through the cervix into the uterine cavity (**Fig. 2**). The use of intraoperative ul-trasonography can minimize the rate of perforation because it allows direct visualiza-tion of the position of the tandem (**Fig. 3**A).[8,9] Two ovoids or a ring then sit against the cervix. A variety of applicators can be used based on patient anatomy, tumor geom-etry, and availability at a particular center. In addition, interstitial needles can be used to ensure adequate tumor coverage in larger tumors or if there is parametrial invasion. A rectal retractor or packing is used to move the rectum away from the source, thereby reducing the dose that the rectum receives. The patient then has a computed tomog-raphy (CT) or MRI scan with the applicators in situ[10].

Cervical brachytherapy has evolved significantly over the past 100 years. Initially, the brachytherapy dose was prescribed to point A on a plain radiograph, which is 2 cm lateral to the midline and 2 cm superior to the surface of the ovoid. This method was the Manchester system, which was developed in the 1930s.[11] However, bulky tumors larger than 4 cm probably did not receive an adequate dose with this method. Interna-tional Commission on Radiation Units and Measurements (ICRU 38)[12] was published in 1985 and encouraged the use of target volume for dose prescription rather than point A (dose specification to the 60-Gy volume). It also specified the bladder and rectal refer-ence points, therefore taking the organs at risk and risk of toxicity into consideration.

GEC-ESTRO (The Groupe Européen de Curiethérapie [GEC] and the European SocieTy for Radiotherapy & Oncology [ESTRO]) guidelines were published in 2005 to aid with the implementation of IGBT.[13,14] IGBT uses CT or MRI scans to define an at-risk volume (predominantly the high-risk clinical target volume [HR-CTV]; see **Fig. 3**B, C). The evaluation of dose to organs at risk has also shifted away from the ICRU 38 reference points to a dose-volume histogram–based approach. This approach allows more accurate definition of where the dose will be rather than predicting where it may be (**Fig. 4**). Retrospective single-institutional studies have shown that IGBT leads to a reduction in local recurrence and an improvement in survival compared with conventional brachytherapy (CBT).[15,16] The Retro-EMBRACE and EMBRACE studies have shown excellent pel-vic control rates with limited major morbidity with IGBT but have also shown that clinical outcome is related to dose prescription and technique.[17,18] IGBT should therefore ideally be the standard of care at every institution, but it requires appro-priate skills and training. The planning aim for the HR-CTV should be to deliver at

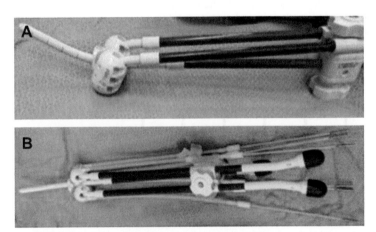

Fig. 2. The MRI/CT-compatible intracavitary equipment used for cervical cancer brachyther-apy. (*A*) A tandem and ovoids. (*B*) Interstitial needles attached to the ovoids.

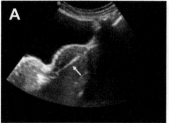
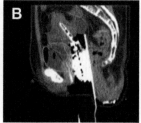
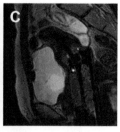

Fig. 3. IGBT. (*A*) Sagittal view of ultrasonography-guided insertion of the tandem (*arrow*). (*B*) Sagittal CT view of the tandem and ovoids in situ. HR-CTV is outlined in red. (*C*) Sagittal MRI of the tandem and ovoids in situ.

least 80 to 85 Gy (including both the external beam and brachytherapy components).

For patients with early-stage cervical cancer (stage IB1–IIA), radical surgery is the typical management. However, if they are subsequently found to have involved pelvic lymph nodes, parametrial invasion, a positive surgical margin, or modified Sedlis criteria,[19,20] then postoperative chemoradiotherapy and/or vaginal cylinder brachytherapy may be indicated. Vaginal cylinder brachytherapy is discussed in more detail later.

Endometrial cancer

Endometrial cancer is predominantly treated surgically. Postoperative brachytherapy with or without radiotherapy is indicated for stage I cancers if there are certain high-risk features, such as grade 3, lymphovascular space invasion or invasion into the outer half of the muscle.[21–23] Stage II and III cancers routinely receive postoperative radiotherapy and brachytherapy, with stage III endometrial cancers also being offered chemotherapy with radiotherapy.[24]

A single-channel cylinder is often used for vaginal brachytherapy (**Fig. 5**). It comes in a variety of widths, chosen according to patient anatomy and comfort. The target for vaginal vault brachytherapy is the vaginal mucosa and the vaginal cuff. The most common site of recurrence of endometrial cancer following a radical hysterectomy is the vaginal cuff.[25] Therefore, in most cases, the upper third to half of the vagina is treated. This technique decreases the morbidity associated with treating the whole vagina, such as vaginal dryness or shortening. However, in

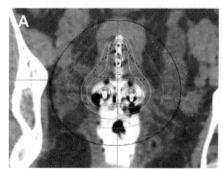
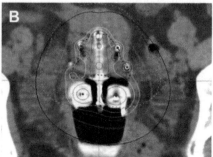

Fig. 4. Brachytherapy plans for cervical IGBT. (*A*) The classic pear-shaped distribution of dose with a tandem and ovoids. (*B*) The use of interstitial needles allows the dose to be pushed laterally to enable coverage of more bulky tumors.

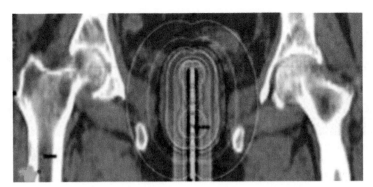

Fig. 5. A coronal CT of the vaginal cylinder in situ and the dose distribution it delivers.

higher-risk cases (eg, papillary serous or clear cell histology), the whole vaginal length may be treated. Brachytherapy can be prescribed at the cylinder surface or at 5 mm into the tissue, a depth that approximates the vaginal lymphatics. The most common endometrial cancer HDR postoperative vaginal vault brachytherapy fractionation schedule in the United States in 2014 was 15 Gy in 3 fractions when given with EBRT and 21 Gy in 3 fractions when brachytherapy alone was used, both prescribed at 0.5 cm from the cylinder surface.[26]

Prostate Brachytherapy

Prostate brachytherapy can be used as monotherapy in patients with low or intermediate risk with T1 or T2 disease or as a boost after EBRT for intermediate-risk to high-risk disease (**Table 2** shows risk stratification). Prostate brachytherapy can be delivered at a vLDR over several months, usually using permanently implanted iodine-125 seeds. Other isotopes used in LDR brachytherapy are palladium-103 (^{103}Pd) and cesium-131 (^{131}Cs). There is no published difference in clinical outcomes between ^{125}I or ^{103}Pd seeds.[27] Alternatively, prostate brachytherapy can be delivered using HDR brachytherapy with a temporary iridium-192 source. The benefits of HDR compared with LDR are that much larger prostate glands can be treated with HDR. Also, patients with extracapsular spread or seminal vesicle invasion (T3a or T3b disease) can be treated adequately with HDR brachytherapy.

Before prostate brachytherapy, patients need to be assessed for suitability. Relative contraindications for vLDR brachytherapy include high International Prostate Symptom Score (>15), prior pelvic radiotherapy, large transurethral resection defects, large median lobe, gland size greater than 60 cm^3, and inflammatory bowel disease.[28]

Table 2
Risk stratification for prostate cancer from the European Association of Urology guidelines

Level of Risk	Clinical Stage	Gleason Score	PSA
Low	T1-T2a	≤6	<10
Intermediate	T2b	7	10–20
High	≥T2c	8–10	>20

Abbreviation: PSA, prostate-specific antigen.
Adapted from Mottet N, Bellmunt J, Bolla M, et al. EAU-ESTRO-SIOG Guidelines on Prostate Cancer. Part 1: Screening, Diagnosis, and Local Treatment with Curative Intent. Eur Urol 2017;71(4):619; with permission.

The implantation procedure for LDR brachytherapy should ideally be done in a single stage with real-time planning during the procedure. However, some centers still use a 2-stage procedure whereby a volume study is performed in a separate step before implantation under anesthesia. Single-stage brachytherapy involves the measurements being taken in clinic using transrectal ultrasonography with the patient awake. This method allows an initial plan to be created detailing the number and position of seeds. At implantation, the transrectal ultrasonography probe is used to delineate the clinical target volume (CTV), rectum, and urethra (**Fig. 6**) and to allow accurate positioning of the seeds (**Figs. 7** and **8**). The seeds are implanted either in strands or individual seeds or as a combination of both. The plan can be adapted during the implantation procedure depending on the position of the implanted seeds. A postimplant CT scan at 30 days is recommended to ensure an adequate dose is delivered to the prostate. If necessary, the patient can be recalled for additional seeds if the dosimetry is suboptimal on the postimplant CT scan. MRI is an alternative imaging modality for postimplant dosimetry.

Prostate brachytherapy as monotherapy

Large single-institution series have shown very good outcomes from vLDR prostate brachytherapy monotherapy in low-risk and low-intermediate–risk patients.[29–33] Fifteen-year biochemical relapse-free survival from the Seattle group was 85.9%, 79.9%, and 62.2% for low-risk, intermediate-risk, and high-risk patients respectively.[29] One of the benefits of brachytherapy compared with surgery and EBRT is the reduction in long-term toxicity such as incontinence, erectile dysfunction, and proctitis. The standard dose for vLDR prostate brachytherapy as monotherapy is 145 Gy.

HDR monotherapy in favorable/intermediate-risk prostate cancers has been shown to be safe and effective in large single-institution cohorts. The 10-year biochemical relapse-free survival following HDR prostate brachytherapy (43.5 Gy in 6 fractions) for low-risk or intermediate-risk prostate cancer is 97.8% and the OS is 76.7%.[34]

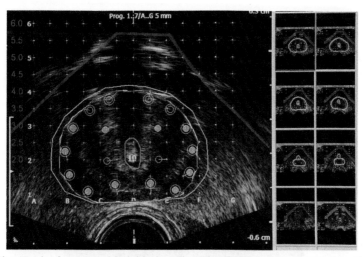

Fig. 6. The CTV (*red*), rectum (*dark blue*), and urethra (*green*) are contoured on the transverse ultrasonography image. The filled circles indicate the position of seeds and the unfilled circles indicate the needle path. The purple line shows the pubic arch. (*Courtesy of* S. Langley, MS, FRCS, Urol, Guildford, UK.)

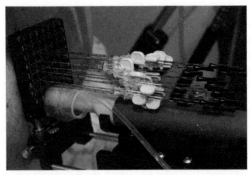

Fig. 7. The needles are inserted using transrectal ultrasonography and a grid to ensure accurate replication of the needle positions from the original plan. (*Courtesy of* S. Langley, MS, FRCS, Urol, Guildford, UK.)

HDR brachytherapy has also been used as monotherapy for high-risk disease (45.5–54 Gy in 7–9 fractions over 4–5 days).[35–39] Most high-risk patients also received neoadjuvant androgen deprivation therapy. The 8-year cancer-specific survival was 93%, metastasis-free survival was 74%, and the biochemical failure–free survival was 77%. Further investigation, ideally with a randomized controlled trial, is required to determine whether it is safe to omit EBRT in these high-risk patients.

Prostate brachytherapy as a boost

For higher-risk patients, brachytherapy can be used as a boost for dose escalation purposes. The ASCENDE-RT trial randomized men with intermediate-risk and high-risk disease to 12 months of androgen deprivation therapy, plus pelvic irradiation including lymph nodes to 46 Gy and either a dose-escalated EBRT boost to 78 Gy or an LDR prostate brachytherapy boost.[40–44] Men randomized to the EBRT boost arm were twice as likely to experience biochemical failure (hazard ratio, 2.04; $P = .004$);

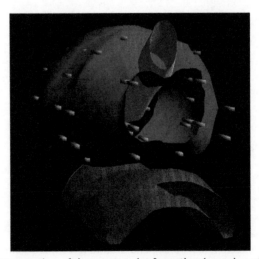

Fig. 8. A digital reconstruction of the prostate (*red*), urethra (*green*), and the rectum (*blue*), with the position of the seeds shown in orange. (*Courtesy of* S. Langley, MS, FRCS, Urol, Guildford, UK.)

however, there was no significant difference in OS. The LDR prostate brachytherapy boost benefitted both intermediate-risk and high-risk patients. Therefore, dose escalation with a brachytherapy boost can lead to an improvement in biochemical relapse–free survival and can be delivered in various ways either as a vLDR permanent implant or an HDR boost.

Breast Brachytherapy

Breast-conserving surgery followed by whole-breast irradiation (WBI) is a standard of care for most early breast cancers. However, there is increasing interest in accelerated partial breast irradiation. Multiple options exist for partial breast irradiation delivery, such as catheters, seeds, balloon, EBRT, and intraoperative radiotherapy (IORT). Some studies have shown similar ipsilateral breast tumor recurrence and survival rates to WBI but lower acute and late toxicities and potentially better cosmetic outcomes.[45–48] However, there are other studies using IORT that have reported increased IBTR,[49–51] and therefore more data are required before this becomes standard practice.

Rectal Brachytherapy

Brachytherapy can also be used in rectal cancer either palliatively or radically. The use of rectal brachytherapy in the radical setting is being evaluated in trials as a technique to increase the rates of organ preservation. It is not yet standard practice in the United States, although it is being used more frequently in Europe. There are 2 methods that can be used for rectal brachytherapy: contact brachytherapy (using the Papillon technique), which delivers superficial 50-kV photons directly to the tumor (**Fig. 9**), and HDR brachytherapy using a flexible silicone applicator. HDR brachytherapy can treat larger or deeper fields with deeper penetration than contact brachytherapy.

Rectal brachytherapy can be used in low rectal cancers to allow anal sphincter preservation and therefore enable patients to avoid having a colostomy. It can also be used for higher tumors in elderly patients who may have other medical comorbidities and therefore may avoid the morbidity and mortality associated with surgery. For T1 tumors, contact brachytherapy alone can be delivered. A dose of 110 Gy in 4 fractions delivered at 2-weekly intervals is used and, for greater than or equal to T2 tumors, 85 to 90 Gy in 3 fractions is used in addition to EBRT 45 to 50 Gy in 25 fractions.

In a randomized trial, patients assigned to 39 Gy in 13 fractions with EBRT alone had a 63% rate of colostomy at 10 years compared with 29% in the group receiving 85 Gy in 3 fractions of contact brachytherapy in addition to the EBRT.[52] Contact brachytherapy does have a higher recurrence rate than surgery, therefore patients who are eligible for surgery must be counseled accordingly and accept the requirement for increased sigmoidoscopic and MRI screening for the first 2 years.

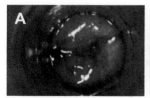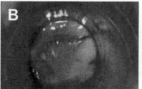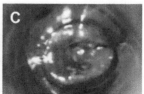

Fig. 9. A rectal tumor being treated with the Papillon technique at (A) fraction 1, (B) fraction 2, and (C) fraction 3. There is clear regression of the tumor from fraction 1 to fraction 3.

However, most patients remain colostomy free and OS is unchanged.[53] A further randomized trial, the OPERA trial, is examining this technique in combination with chemoradiotherapy.

For HDR brachytherapy, the superior and inferior extents of the tumor are marked with clips. The applicator is then inserted and the treatment field defined, preferably using CT or MRI. HDR brachytherapy can also be used radically or palliatively. In the radical setting, it can be used as monotherapy (eg, 36 Gy in 6 fractions 2–3 times per week[54]) or as a boost after EBRT in patients who are medically unfit or refuse to have surgery (eg, 30 Gy in 3 fractions weekly[55]). The Herbert trial was a dose-finding trial using an HDR brachytherapy boost after EBRT (39 Gy in 13 fractions) in elderly patients with rectal cancer.[56] The recommended dose from this trial was 21 Gy in 3 fractions. There was a 60% complete response rate. OS was 63% at 2 years; however, a significant proportion of patients experienced acute and late toxicity. Acute grade 2 and 3 toxicity occurred in 68% and 13% respectively, and late grade 2 and grade 3 proctitis occurred in 48% and 40%.[57] However, a wide range of doses and fractionations are used at other centers.

In addition, there is interest in the use of HDR brachytherapy as a neoadjuvant treatment instead of external beam after results were published from a single institution.[58] In this setting, HDR brachytherapy has comparable complete response rates and leads to improved tumor downstaging (but not nodal downstaging) compared with EBRT.

Skin Brachytherapy

Brachytherapy can be used to treat nonmelanoma skin cancers, such as basal cell carcinomas and squamous cell carcinomas, and may preferential to surgery in elderly or frail patients. Brachytherapy has advantages compared with the other radiation treatments (eg, superficial photons or electrons) in areas of the body with complex superficial targets because it allows higher conformality and shorter treatment courses (**Fig. 10**). Either interstitial or surface techniques can be used. Superficial techniques can use either custom molds or surface applicators (Freiberg flap and so forth) or commercial contact applicators such as the Leipzig applicator (Nucletron, an Elekta company, Veenendaal, The Netherlands). A single-institution study of 200 patients has shown that 36 Gy in 12 fractions delivered using the Leipzig applicator had a local control rate of 98% with good to excellent cosmesis in 85% of patients.[59]

Interstitial brachytherapy is usually used for tumors thicker than 5 mm or on curved surfaces such as the face. Insertion of the catheters involves a general or local anesthetic. A CT scan can be used to define the CTV. In addition, electronic brachytherapy is an increasingly popular technique that uses a 50-kV electronic source with a skin applicator.[60] This technique reduces treatment time and dependency on HDR equipment and can be used to treat small-volume lesions on regular surfaces.[61] In a retrospective study of 127 patients treated with 40 Gy in 8 fractions, the recurrence rate was 1.3% after a median follow-up of 16 months and the cosmetic results were excellent in 94%[62].

Other Tumor Sites

It is not possible to cover all of the possible applications of brachytherapy in this article. Brachytherapy can essentially be used at any tumor site where access can be gained to the tumor. For example, endocavitary brachytherapy can be used for bronchial or esophageal tumors, whereby the brachytherapy catheter is placed over a guidewire sited using bronchoscopy or endoscopy respectively. This method can provide palliation or could be used in combination with EBRT as a boost.

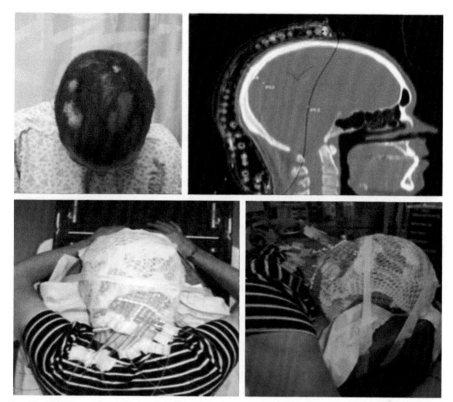

Fig. 10. Whole-scalp surface applicator HDR brachytherapy (8 Gy in 2 fractions) for stage IB follicular cutaneous T-cell lymphoma with refractory patch/plaque disease of the scalp and prominent partial alopecia. There was resolution of plaques and the disease is still controlled at 5 years with full resolution of alopecia.

SUMMARY

Brachytherapy is integral in the treatment of cervical, endometrial, and prostate cancers and shows significant benefit in the treatment of many other malignancies. It can be used either as monotherapy or to deliver a highly conformal boost to the tumor as part of multimodal therapy, whether that be EBRT or surgery.

REFERENCES

1. Green J, Kirwan J, Tierney J, et al. Concomitant chemotherapy and radiation therapy for cancer of the uterine cervix. Cochrane Database Syst Rev 2005;(3):CD002225.
2. Han K, Milosevic M, Fyles A, et al. Trends in the utilization of brachytherapy in cervical cancer in the United States. Int J Radiat Oncol Biol Phys 2013;87(1):111–9.
3. Gill BS, Lin JF, Krivak TC, et al. National Cancer Data Base analysis of radiation therapy consolidation modality for cervical cancer: the impact of new technological advancements. Int J Radiat Oncol Biol Phys 2014;90(5):1083–90.
4. Georg D, Kirisits C, Hillbrand M, et al. Image-guided radiotherapy for cervix cancer: high-tech external beam therapy versus high-tech brachytherapy. Int J Radiat Oncol Biol Phys 2008;71(4):1272–8.

5. Nag S, Erickson B, Thomadsen B, et al. The American Brachytherapy Society recommendations for high-dose-rate brachytherapy for carcinoma of the cervix. Int J Radiat Oncol Biol Phys 2000;48(1):201–11.

6. Stewart AJ, Viswanathan AN. Current controversies in high-dose-rate versus low-dose-rate brachytherapy for cervical cancer. Cancer 2006;107(5):908–15.

7. Otter S, Franklin A, Ajaz M, et al. Improving the efficiency of image guided brachytherapy in cervical cancer. J Contemp Brachytherapy 2016;8(6):557–65.

8. Schaner PE, Caudell JJ, De Los Santos JF, et al. Intraoperative ultrasound guidance during intracavitary brachytherapy applicator placement in cervical cancer: the University of Alabama at Birmingham experience. Int J Gynecol Cancer 2013; 23(3):559–66.

9. Small W Jr, Strauss JB, Hwang CS, et al. Should uterine tandem applicators ever be placed without ultrasound guidance? No: a brief report and review of the literature. Int J Gynecol Cancer 2011;21(5):941–4.

10. Viswanathan AN, Dimopoulos J, Kirisits C, et al. Computed tomography versus magnetic resonance imaging-based contouring in cervical cancer brachytherapy: results of a prospective trial and preliminary guidelines for standardized contours. Int J Radiat Oncol Biol Phys 2007;68(2):491–8.

11. Meredith W. Radium dosage: the Manchester system. Edinburgh (Scotland): Livingstone; 1967.

12. ICRU ICoRUaMDavsfritigIR. Dose and volume specification for reporting intracavitary therapy in gynaecology. 1985. Available at: https://academic.oup.com/jicru/article-abstract/os20/1/NP/2923724?redirectedFrom=PDF.

13. Haie-Meder C, Potter R, Van Limbergen E, et al. Recommendations from Gynaecological (GYN) GEC-ESTRO Working Group (I): concepts and terms in 3D image based 3D treatment planning in cervix cancer brachytherapy with emphasis on MRI assessment of GTV and CTV. Radiother Oncol 2005;74(3):235–45.

14. Potter R, Haie-Meder C, Van Limbergen E, et al. Recommendations from gynaecological (GYN) GEC ESTRO working group (II): concepts and terms in 3D image-based treatment planning in cervix cancer brachytherapy-3D dose volume parameters and aspects of 3D image-based anatomy, radiation physics, radiobiology. Radiother Oncol 2006;78(1):67–77.

15. Potter R, Georg P, Dimopoulos JC, et al. Clinical outcome of protocol based image (MRI) guided adaptive brachytherapy combined with 3D conformal radiotherapy with or without chemotherapy in patients with locally advanced cervical cancer. Radiother Oncol 2011;100(1):116–23.

16. Rijkmans EC, Nout RA, Rutten IH, et al. Improved survival of patients with cervical cancer treated with image-guided brachytherapy compared with conventional brachytherapy. Gynecol Oncol 2014;135(2):231–8.

17. Sturdza A, Potter R, Fokdal LU, et al. Image guided brachytherapy in locally advanced cervical cancer: improved pelvic control and survival in RetroEMBRACE, a multicenter cohort study. Radiother Oncol 2016;120(3):428–33.

18. Potter R, Tanderup K, Kirisits C, et al. The EMBRACE II study: the outcome and prospect of two decades of evolution within the GEC-ESTRO GYN working group and the EMBRACE studies. Clin Transl Radiat Oncol 2018;9:48–60.

19. Sedlis A, Bundy BN, Rotman MZ, et al. A randomized trial of pelvic radiation therapy versus no further therapy in selected patients with stage IB carcinoma of the cervix after radical hysterectomy and pelvic lymphadenectomy: a Gynecologic Oncology Group Study. Gynecol Oncol 1999;73(2):177–83.

20. NCCN. NCCN guidelines Version 1.2017 cervical cancer 2017. Available at: https://www.tri-kobe.org/nccn/guideline/gynecological/english/cervical.pdf. Accessed June 14, 2018.

21. Creutzberg CL, Nout RA, Lybeert ML, et al. Fifteen-year radiotherapy outcomes of the randomized PORTEC-1 trial for endometrial carcinoma. Int J Radiat Oncol Biol Phys 2011;81(4):e631–8.

22. Wortman BG, Creutzberg CL, Putter H, et al. Ten-year results of the PORTEC-2 trial for high-intermediate risk endometrial carcinoma: improving patient selection for adjuvant therapy. Br J Cancer 2018;119(9):1067–74.

23. Keys HM, Roberts JA, Brunetto VL, et al. A phase III trial of surgery with or without adjunctive external pelvic radiation therapy in intermediate risk endometrial adenocarcinoma: a Gynecologic Oncology Group study. Gynecol Oncol 2004; 92(3):744–51.

24. de Boer SM, Powell ME, Mileshkin L, et al. Adjuvant chemoradiotherapy versus radiotherapy alone for women with high-risk endometrial cancer (PORTEC-3): final results of an international, open-label, multicentre, randomised, phase 3 trial. Lancet Oncol 2018;19(3):295–309.

25. Creutzberg CL, van Putten WL, Koper PC, et al. Survival after relapse in patients with endometrial cancer: results from a randomized trial. Gynecol Oncol 2003; 89(2):201–9.

26. Harkenrider MM, Grover S, Erickson BA, et al. Vaginal brachytherapy for postoperative endometrial cancer: 2014 Survey of the American Brachytherapy Society. Brachytherapy 2016;15(1):23–9.

27. Peschel RE, Colberg JW, Chen Z, et al. Iodine 125 versus palladium 103 implants for prostate cancer: clinical outcomes and complications. Cancer J 2004;10(3): 170–4.

28. Davis BJ, Horwitz EM, Lee WR, et al. American Brachytherapy Society consensus guidelines for transrectal ultrasound-guided permanent prostate brachytherapy. Brachytherapy 2012;11(1):6–19.

29. Sylvester JE, Grimm PD, Wong J, et al. Fifteen-year biochemical relapse-free survival, cause-specific survival, and overall survival following I(125) prostate brachytherapy in clinically localized prostate cancer: Seattle experience. Int J Radiat Oncol Biol Phys 2011;81(2):376–81.

30. Henry AM, Al-Qaisieh B, Gould K, et al. Outcomes following iodine-125 monotherapy for localized prostate cancer: the results of leeds 10-year single-center brachytherapy experience. Int J Radiat Oncol Biol Phys 2010;76(1):50–6.

31. Bowes D, Crook J. A critical analysis of the long-term impact of brachytherapy for prostate cancer: a review of the recent literature. Curr Opin Urol 2011;21(3): 219–24.

32. Prestidge BR, Winter K, Sanda MG, et al. Initial Report of NRG Oncology/RTOG 0232: a phase 3 study comparing combined external beam radiation with transperineal interstitial permanent brachytherapy alone for selected patients with intermediate-risk prostatic carcinoma. Int J Radiat Oncol Biol Phys 2016; 96(2):S4.

33. Schlussel Markovic E, Buckstein M, Stone NN, et al. Outcomes and toxicities in patients with intermediate-risk prostate cancer treated with brachytherapy alone or brachytherapy and supplemental external beam radiation therapy. BJU Int 2018;121(5):774–80.

34. Hauswald H, Kamrava MR, Fallon JM, et al. High-dose-rate monotherapy for localized prostate cancer: 10-year results. Int J Radiat Oncol Biol Phys 2016; 94(4):667–74.

35. Yoshioka Y, Suzuki O, Isohashi F, et al. High-dose-rate brachytherapy as monotherapy for intermediate- and high-risk prostate cancer: clinical results for a median 8-year follow-up. Int J Radiat Oncol Biol Phys 2016;94(4):675–82.

36. Hoskin P, Rojas A, Ostler P, et al. Single-dose high-dose-rate brachytherapy compared to two and three fractions for locally advanced prostate cancer. Radiother Oncol 2017;124(1):56–60.

37. Krauss DJ, Ye H, Martinez AA, et al. Favorable preliminary outcomes for men with low- and intermediate-risk prostate cancer treated with 19-gy single-fraction high-dose-rate brachytherapy. Int J Radiat Oncol Biol Phys 2017;97(1):98–106.

38. Prada PJ, Cardenal J, Blanco AG, et al. High-dose-rate interstitial brachytherapy as monotherapy in one fraction for the treatment of favorable stage prostate cancer: toxicity and long-term biochemical results. Radiother Oncol 2016;119(3):411–6.

39. Morton G, Chung HT, McGuffin M, et al. Prostate high dose-rate brachytherapy as monotherapy for low and intermediate risk prostate cancer: early toxicity and quality-of life results from a randomized phase II clinical trial of one fraction of 19Gy or two fractions of 13.5Gy. Radiother Oncol 2017;122(1):87–92.

40. Morris WJ, Tyldesley S, Rodda S, et al. Androgen suppression combined with elective nodal and dose escalated radiation therapy (the ASCENDE-RT trial): an analysis of survival endpoints for a randomized trial comparing a low-dose-rate brachytherapy boost to a dose-escalated external beam boost for high- and intermediate-risk prostate cancer. Int J Radiat Oncol Biol Phys 2017;98(2):275–85.

41. Kishan AU, Cook RR, Ciezki JP, et al. Radical prostatectomy, external beam radiotherapy, or external beam radiotherapy with brachytherapy boost and disease progression and mortality in patients with gleason score 9-10 prostate cancer. JAMA 2018;319(9):896–905.

42. Sathya JR, Davis IR, Julian JA, et al. Randomized trial comparing iridium implant plus external-beam radiation therapy with external-beam radiation therapy alone in node-negative locally advanced cancer of the prostate. J Clin Oncol 2005;23(6):1192–9.

43. Hoskin PJ, Rojas AM, Bownes PJ, et al. Randomised trial of external beam radiotherapy alone or combined with high-dose-rate brachytherapy boost for localised prostate cancer. Radiother Oncol 2012;103(2):217–22.

44. Zumsteg ZS, Spratt DE, Pei I, et al. A new risk classification system for therapeutic decision making with intermediate-risk prostate cancer patients undergoing dose-escalated external-beam radiation therapy. Eur Urol 2013;64(6):895–902.

45. Livi L, Meattini I, Marrazzo L, et al. Accelerated partial breast irradiation using intensity-modulated radiotherapy versus whole breast irradiation: 5-year survival analysis of a phase 3 randomised controlled trial. Eur J Cancer 2015;51(4):451–63.

46. Ott OJ, Strnad V, Hildebrandt G, et al. GEC-ESTRO multicenter phase 3-trial: accelerated partial breast irradiation with interstitial multicatheter brachytherapy versus external beam whole breast irradiation: early toxicity and patient compliance. Radiother Oncol 2016;120(1):119–23.

47. Strnad V, Ott OJ, Hildebrandt G, et al. 5-year results of accelerated partial breast irradiation using sole interstitial multicatheter brachytherapy versus whole-breast irradiation with boost after breast-conserving surgery for low-risk invasive and in-situ carcinoma of the female breast: a randomised, phase 3, non-inferiority trial. Lancet 2016;387(10015):229–38.

48. Polgar C, Ott OJ, Hildebrandt G, et al. Late side-effects and cosmetic results of accelerated partial breast irradiation with interstitial brachytherapy versus whole-breast irradiation after breast-conserving surgery for low-risk invasive and in-situ carcinoma of the female breast: 5-year results of a randomised, controlled, phase 3 trial. Lancet Oncol 2017;18(2):259–68.

49. Veronesi U, Orecchia R, Maisonneuve P, et al. Intraoperative radiotherapy versus external radiotherapy for early breast cancer (ELIOT): a randomised controlled equivalence trial. Lancet Oncol 2013;14(13):1269–77.

50. Leonardi MC, Maisonneuve P, Mastropasqua MG, et al. How do the ASTRO consensus statement guidelines for the application of accelerated partial breast irradiation fit intraoperative radiotherapy? A retrospective analysis of patients treated at the European Institute of Oncology. Int J Radiat Oncol Biol Phys 2012;83(3):806–13.

51. Vaidya JS, Wenz F, Bulsara M, et al. An international randomised controlled trial to compare TARGeted Intraoperative radioTherapy (TARGIT) with conventional postoperative radiotherapy after breast-conserving surgery for women with early-stage breast cancer (the TARGIT-A trial). Health Technol Assess 2016; 20(73):1–188.

52. Ortholan C, Romestaing P, Chapet O, et al. Correlation in rectal cancer between clinical tumor response after neoadjuvant radiotherapy and sphincter or organ preservation: 10-year results of the Lyon R 96-02 randomized trial. Int J Radiat Oncol Biol Phys 2012;83(2):e165–71.

53. Sun Myint A, Grieve RJ, McDonald AC, et al. Combined modality treatment of early rectal cancer: the UK experience. Clin Oncol (R Coll Radiol) 2007;19(9): 674–81.

54. Corner C, Bryant L, Chapman C, et al. High-dose-rate afterloading intraluminal brachytherapy for advanced inoperable rectal carcinoma. Brachytherapy 2010; 9(1):66–70.

55. Devic S, Bekerat H, Garant A, et al. Optimization of HDRBT boost dose delivery for patients with rectal cancer. Brachytherapy 2019;18(4):559–63.

56. Rijkmans EC, Cats A, Nout RA, et al. Endorectal brachytherapy boost after external beam radiation therapy in elderly or medically inoperable patients with rectal cancer: primary outcomes of the phase 1 HERBERT study. Int J Radiat Oncol Biol Phys 2017;98(4):908–17.

57. Rijkmans EC, van Triest B, Nout RA, et al. Evaluation of clinical and endoscopic toxicity after external beam radiotherapy and endorectal brachytherapy in elderly patients with rectal cancer treated in the HERBERT study. Radiother Oncol 2018; 126(3):417–23.

58. Garfinkle R, Lachance S, Vuong T, et al. Is the pathologic response of T3 rectal cancer to high-dose-rate endorectal brachytherapy comparable to external beam radiotherapy? Dis Colon Rectum 2019;62(3):294–301.

59. Gauden R, Pracy M, Avery AM, et al. HDR brachytherapy for superficial non-melanoma skin cancers. J Med Imaging Radiat Oncol 2013;57(2):212–7.

60. Devlin PM, Gaspar LE, Buzurovic I, et al. American College of Radiology-American Brachytherapy Society practice parameter for electronically generated low-energy radiation sources. Brachytherapy 2017;16(6):1083–90.

61. Guinot JL, Rembielak A, Perez-Calatayud J, et al. GEC-ESTRO ACROP recommendations in skin brachytherapy. Radiother Oncol 2018;126(3):377–85.

62. Paravati AJ, Hawkins PG, Martin AN, et al. Clinical and cosmetic outcomes in patients treated with high-dose-rate electronic brachytherapy for nonmelanoma skin cancer. Pract Radiat Oncol 2015;5(6):e659–64.

Treatment Toxicity: Radiation

Thomas J. FitzGerald, MD[a,b,]*, Maryann Bishop-Jodoin, MEd[c],
Fran Laurie, BS[c], Alexander Lukez, BS[d], Lauren O'Loughlin, BS[d],
Allison Sacher, MD[a]

KEYWORDS

- Radiation exposure dose volume • Cell damage • Treatment effects
- Normal tissue tolerance

KEY POINTS

- Intentional and unintentional radiation exposures have a powerful impact on normal tissue function and can induce short-term and long-term injury to all cell systems.
- A broad understanding of the effects of intentional and unintentional radiation exposures is essential for health care providers.
- During evaluation of acute-phase management, assessing radiation dose and exposure is essential.

INTRODUCTION

More than 60% of patients with cancer have radiation therapy (RT) as part of primary treatment. Although tissue effects may not be clinically apparent during evaluation, exposure is important to patient medical history because it leaves an invisible footprint that may be relevant decades after exposure. Intentional exposure is well documented with dose/volume precision in the radiation oncology treatment record. The RT record, however, often is not directly linked to hospital informatics system. Information valuable to the health care team may be cursory, incomplete, or even inaccurate if obtained from a service unfamiliar with RT.[1–5] Therefore, information relevant to the patient may be unavailable to practitioners involved in patient care.

Exposure from nontherapeutic sources, including imaging, is more challenging to document and often limited to mathematical models of duration and distance from the primary incident. Although helpful, the models can be less accurate.[1,6,7]

Disclosure Statement: The authors have nothing to disclose.
[a] Department of Radiation Oncology, University of Massachusetts Medical School/UMass Memorial Health Care, 55 Lake Avenue North, Worcester, MA 01655, USA; [b] Imaging and Radiation Oncology Core (IROC), 640 George Washington Highway, Building B, Suite 201, Lincoln, RI 02865, USA; [c] Department of Radiation Oncology, University of Massachusetts Medical School, 55 Lake Avenue North, Worcester, MA 01655, USA; [d] University of Massachusetts Medical School, 55 Lake Avenue North, Worcester, MA 01655, USA
* Corresponding author.
E-mail addresses: TJ.Fitzgerald@umassmemorial.org; Thomas.FitzGerald@umassmed.edu

Hematol Oncol Clin N Am 33 (2019) 1027–1039
https://doi.org/10.1016/j.hoc.2019.08.010
0889-8588/19/© 2019 Elsevier Inc. All rights reserved.
hemonc.theclinics.com

Fluoroscopy, during interventional radiology/cardiology procedures, can lead to a surprisingly high-radiation dose to underlying structures that is often not or poorly documented, again a relatively hidden risk in patient care.[2–4]

There exists a knowledge gap among providers concerning the effects of radiation exposure and the interrelation to health care. With increasing number of cancer survivors, closing this gap is essential to mission moving forward.

ACUTE RADIATION EFFECTS
Management of Acute Effects of Radiation Therapy

Acute effects from therapeutic RT are typically associated with organ systems with rapid self-renewal potential. Acute effects generally occur during RT. Clinical manifestations can be influenced by chemotherapy and/or molecularly targeted small molecule agents delivered before/during RT and the mucosal tissue volume in the RT treatment field. Multiple organ systems with mucosal surfaces (skin, head/neck, gastrointestinal [GI] tract, and bone marrow) can be affected during therapy. Although not well validated through mechanism, patients can experience visible acute effects from low-dose RT to skin and mucosa if they have received prior sensitizing medications as low-dose chemotherapy for autoimmune disease (methotrexate for rheumatoid arthritis) and selected antibiotics (tetracycline).

Skin

The epidermis is site of visible acute reactions to radiation exposure. Dermal stem cells abut the basement membrane and are the active proliferating cell component underneath layers of keratinized cells. Stem cells are the primary target for injury. The time for dermal cell division and migration is between 14 days and 21 days depending on the area of the body. Single doses of 5 Gy generate early erythema followed by vasodilation, fluid exudation, cellular migration, and loss of proteins/other plasma product constituents.[8–10] Investigators have shown this process can be identified on hyperspectral imaging within 12 h of exposure with evidence that imaging evaluation can be dose-specific despite that clinical expression of change may not become apparent for 2 weeks to 3 weeks.[11,12] Fluoroscopy procedures use orthovoltage (low-energy) x-rays, which deliver higher percentages of radiation dose to the skin surface.[2,3] Complicated interventional radiology procedures requiring significant fluoroscopy time can create acute dermal injury because acute injuries are influenced by fractionation (daily dose) and total dose, which can be substantial in complex procedures.[13] Radiation beams resonate on skin surfaces within dermal folds; these intertriginous areas are more vulnerable to injury during treatment. There are reported soft tissue injuries to skin during stereotactic body radiosurgery (SRS) when immobilization devices unintentionally functioned as bolus devices augmenting dose to skin surfaces.[13] As information matures on molecularly targeted therapies, increasing evidence of skin toxicity to multiple new agents: epidermal growth factor receptor inhibitors (rash 2–4 weeks into therapy), BRAF inhibitors (rash/photosensitivity), BCR-ABL inhibitors (keratosis pilaris/maculopapular rash), and mammalian target of rapamycin (m-TOR) inhibitors (rash/pruritus) is seen.[14] Treatment with fragrance-free skin creams and topical skin care generally ameliorates sequelae with near-complete healing 1 month posttherapy. The degree of skin reaction is associated with both the total radiation dose and daily treatment dose. Efforts are made through treatment planning to limit areas of radiation dose asymmetry to skin with skin sparing technology. This has permitted investigators to increase daily dose to breast cancer patients with hypofractionation techniques. These seem successful because the skin is not the intended target; therefore, dose gradients can be placed through dermal surfaces to achieve goal of skin sparing.

Hematopoietic System

Effects on the hematopoietic system are driven by bone marrow volume and lymphoid system treated, previous chemotherapy and RT, and radiation total dose. Total body exposure results in a near-immediate decrease in circulating B lymphocytes and T lymphocytes. A total body dose of 3.0 Gy to 4.0 Gy likely inhibits the ability to respond to new antigen stimuli. Most patients receiving RT for malignancy are treated to a partial organ volume that has a limited effect on immune response unless a patient is neutropenic from concurrent chemotherapy.[15] Recovery occurs post-therapy through self-renewal. In modern radiation oncology, radiation dose has been

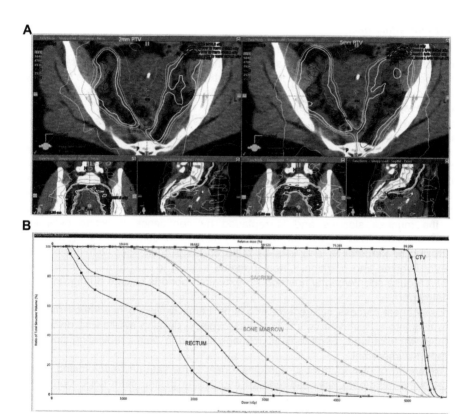

Fig. 1. (*A*) Comparing the difference between a 2-mm expanded target and a 5-mm expanded target in the pelvis on a treatment plan and (*B*) dose volume histogram. Panel A left: Isodose distribution with 2mm PTV in orthogonal views (axial on top and coronal and sagittal at the bottom). Panel A right: Isodose distribution with 2mm PTV in orthogonal views (axial on top and coronal and sagittal at the bottom) Note increased coverage of sacrum by prescription isodose line. Panel B: Dose volume histogram with DVH lines on the sacrum, bone marrow in iliac crest, rectum and CTV. (The squares represent distribution with 2 mm PTV and the triangles represent the distribution with the 5 mm PTV.) (*Courtesy of* the University of Massachusetts Medical School, Department of Radiation Oncology, Worcester, MA.)

prescribed through volumes. As daily RT image guidance has improved through the past decade, radiation oncologists are more comfortable limiting the planning target volume, which was designed to accommodate for daily patient set-up variability. **Fig. 1** shows the difference between a 2-mm expanded target and a 5-mm expanded target in the pelvis. As can be seen, a shaper dose gradient can be placed through the bone marrow in the sacrum with a smaller planning target volume. This has been accomplished with the routine use of cone-beam computer tomography for daily patient set-up. Lukez and colleagues[16] have evaluated exercise before and during therapy to improve patient set-up.

Patient set-up with the clinical trial developed by Moni and Baima permitted appropriate treatment of the target with less variability and limiting dose to bone marrow. Other investigators have evaluated magnetic resonance as a vehicle to define red marrow volumes and fuse these images into planning computer tomography for conformal avoidance of bone marrow as best as possible.[17]

Gastrointestinal Tract

The GI tract mucosa has similar organization to skin tissues as stem cells reside at the basal layer and migrate to the surface at varied time points during their life cycle. In general, cells that line segments of the GI tract possess a shorter life span than their counterparts in skin. The mucosa of the head/neck and large bowel self-renew every 2 weeks, the gastric region mucosa renews nearly every day, and the small intestine renews every 3 days. This explains why symptoms can be apparent early postexposure.

Because the mucosal systems have rapid self-renewal potential, acute sequela from management can be substantial and is driven by radiation dose, fractionation, and volume of mucosa in the treatment field. By week 2 of treatment, the mucosa of the head/neck becomes denuded with increasing pain. Secondary tissues, including salivary glands and taste buds also display limited function. By week 4, the mucosa sloughs and is replaced by confluence of white cells and fibrin exudate. The impact on secondary tissues becomes more pronounced with severe xerostomia and loss of taste creating challenges with maintaining dental hygiene and nutrition. Often, patients treated to substantial mucosal volumes require supplemental nutrition for extended periods of time during and after treatment.[15]

Esophageal mucosa self-renews in a time frame similar to head/neck mucosa; 2 weeks into a treatment course, patients begin to develop swallowing discomfort related to treatment. Symptomatic management with pain medication and fluid support is important.

Treatment of gastric mucosa can cause near-immediate nausea/vomiting largely due to the rapid/near daily self-renewal capacity of gastric stem cells. During RT, delayed gastric emptying can be observed as a result of edema in bowel wall and development of ulcerations due to limited stem cell renewal capacity.

Early complications of small/large bowel are similarly driven by total dose, fractionation, bowel volumes in the treatment field, and previous abdominal surgery. Upper abdominal injury often is manifest by nausea and vomiting whereas injury to both small and large bowel can lead to bowel frequency and limited absorption of nutrients. Previous abdominal surgery can result in adhesions that fix bowel segments into a specific location, potentially exacerbating acute injury due to blood supply limitation and repeated high-dose treatment to fixed segments.[18,19] From a clinical perspective, patients treated for recurrent disease often have more acute and potentially more serious sequelae than patients treated in a neoadjuvant or adjuvant manner. The root cause for this is multifactorial, likely driven in part by tumor compromise of normal tissue function and vasculature prior to initiation of therapy.[15]

SUBACUTE AND LATE (DELAYED) EFFECTS OF TREATMENT

For health care providers, late effects of cancer management can become a highly visible component to patient care decades after primary cancer care is completed. Possible late effects are specific to a patient's cancer treatment, although some late effects, as psychosocial effects, may occur with any cancer survivor. Patients experiencing acute effects of treatment do not always indicate the potential for late effects and patients without acute effects during primary management remain at risk for late effects.

The relationship of chemotherapy to delayed effects from RT to normal tissue is less well described.[20] Although recognized in a qualitative manner that chemotherapy exacerbates acute effects of RT to tissues of rapid self-renewal potential, chemotherapeutic impact on late effects of treatment is not understood. The Quantitative Analysis of Normal Tissue Effects in the Clinic (QUANTEC) is a significant effort by radiation oncologists to define dose volumetrics for thresholds of normal tissue injury. This effort reviewed most of the available, recent, and relevant published data and provides injury prevention guidelines for physicians.[18] Building on this experience provides a quantitative infrastructure to optimize dose-volume tolerance metrics with/without systemic therapy.

In this section, the late effects of radiotherapy are described. Improved knowledge of late effects influence and improve evaluation and care in the acute care setting.

Skin

Acute effects (described previously) of radiation injury to skin resolve within 1 month of therapy completion. The effects are associated with the volume of tissue treated, technique of therapy, total radiation dose, and daily radiation dose. As a consequence, there can be epidermal thinning with prominence of the vascular pattern (telangiectasia) in the dermis. The degree of vascularity decreases over time; epidermal thinning can make the vessels in the dermis appear more prominent.[8] Hyperspectral imaging demonstrates oxygenation is decreased, providing explanation to wound healing limitations when there is secondary injury and infection to these tissues.[11,14] Local immunity and moisture glands significantly diminish; therefore, injury to irradiated tissue can result in delay of healing.[8] The current standard of care is to follow optimal wound care strategies. On rare occasion, reactions to the skin can reappear years after therapy when certain chemotherapy and related antibiotics are given to the patient. Adriamycin, methotrexate, and tetracyclines are common causes of this phenomenon, however innumerable agents are now associated with what is called *recall*. Delayed and late fibrosis can be seen in patients with scleroderma.

Skin tissue can also demonstrate the recall phenomenon, which can occur years after primary RT.

Patients with autoimmune disorders, including lupus and scleroderma, may be vulnerable to accelerated fibrosis from traditional RT.[8]

Bone Marrow

Although the primary focus is acute effects, bone marrow can remain fragile years after therapy and vulnerable to medications and external agents after RT. This is especially true for white cell elements and platelets. Pancytopenia, bone marrow aplasia, and secondary malignancies are becoming more common consequences of cancer therapy and often are first identified in a primary care environment.[15,21]

Gastrointestinal Tract

Residual compromise of the oral cavity is long-standing. The floor of the mouth is taut and lacks mucosal redundancy; it is susceptible to injury and heals less well than other oral cavity structures. If ulceration occurs, debris and particles can sequester in the open space and cause necrosis of underlying structures including the mandible. This requires careful management, including in extreme situations, hyperbaric therapy, and surgery. Patients have dry mouth resulting from radiation to the parotid/submandibular/submucosal glands that provide moisture to the mucosal surface, creating secondary issues for dentition. RT affects the growth and development of teeth in children and the oral cavity for adults. Saliva becomes more acidic and prone to fungal overgrowth. The mucosa of gingival tissues becomes thin and denuded. These changes can lead to chronic decay and demineralization of teeth. Fluoride mouthwash periodically used with baking soda/water rinses helps deacidify the oral cavity and promotes more optimal oral hygiene; however, these changes are often unrelenting and difficult to control. Optimal radiation planning strategies with intensity-modulated RT (IMRT) may help mitigate these changes. Building a strong relationship with dental medicine facilitates optimal care.[15,21]

GI tract motility is not a well-described side effect of radiation management and is becoming an important issue in managing head/neck and esophageal cancers.[19] Contractility of the medial constrictor muscles of the hypopharynx seem to mimic swallowing issues often seen in patients with neurodegenerative disorders.[19] At times these changes are related to treatment-associated dermal and interstitial edema and addressing the edema through lymphedema clinics can be helpful. Delayed GI emptying associated with antral fibrosis and denudement of the mucosa of the gastric lining cells can be seen in patients treated to the gastric region, usually at doses of greater than 45 Gy to the gastric region or gastric resection site. In surgical reconstruction sites, including biliary and bowel anastomosis sites, RT can accelerate stricture formation, which needs to be monitored by the entire treatment team.

Late effects to small and large bowel include mucosa atrophy, resulting in limited absorption of protein, carbohydrate, and fat. This contributes to various degrees of malabsorption syndromes and inconsistent bowel function. If there is previous abdominal surgery, bowel may be fixed in position resulting in stenosis and ulceration requiring surgery. Relatively little is known about effects to the exocrine/endocrine pancreas, although pancreas atrophy can be seen on imaging years after upper abdominal malignancy treatment.[15,21] Mucosal thinning of the lower bowel can lead to limited reabsorption of water, which also is exacerbated by bowel resection, especially in the sigmoid colon and upper rectum.

Liver

There is renewed interest in defining radiation dose effects to the liver as stereotactic techniques (SRS) have been effectively treating metastatic disease to the liver and primary hepatocellular carcinoma. Sequela to the liver, known as radiation-induced liver disease, is driven by the liver volume treated and functional status at the time of therapy. Primary and metastatic disease can impose varying degrees of veno-occlusive changes in the parenchyma and treatment can induce scar tissue that can limit the functional status of the remaining liver. Magnetic resonance imaging (MRI) is valuable in validating the degree of veno-occlusive changes and has evolved into a quantitative metric in predicting veno-occlusive liver injury prior to the administration of RT.[21]

Investigators are using metrics identified on dynamic-contrast imaging to establish the appropriate radiation dose to target. The threshold of injury to the liver is significantly decreased when the entire organ volume is treated. Sioshansi and colleagues[22] have demonstrated diaphragmatic injury without changes in the chest wall resulting in chronic pleuritic pain among patients undergoing SRS. The liver is sensitive to interactions with chemotherapy perhaps best demonstrated in the pediatric population when RT is delivered with actinomycin D for Wilms tumor. Sequelae can include a dramatic decrease in blood counts as well as changes consistent with liver failure, including coagulation disorders.[15]

Kidney

The kidney, like the liver, is a relatively late-responding radiosensitive critical organ. Radiation doses of greater than 20 Gy in 2-Gy fractions can result in renal damage with anemia and hypertension. Although not yet validated through clinical trials, the injury threshold is thought to be lower when chemotherapy is used with RT. Using IMRT, radiation oncologists can be creative with partial volume therapy and spare as much renal parenchyma as possible. In comparison with siblings, there is increased risk of renal failure in the cancer survivor, and investigators should attempt to limit renal dose to as little as possible during treatment planning.[15,20,23] The dose for threshold to injury is not well described; therefore, efforts are made to apply as little dose as possible to renal tissues at risk. This is becoming a visible issue as society ages and patients with renal masses and pelvic calyceal lesions are not amenable to surgery due to medical comorbidities.

Lung

As with the liver and kidney, the lung is a sensitive intermediate-to late-responding tissue. Injury to the lung can be life threatening in extreme situations. There are generally 2 periods of damage that can be identified. Pneumonitis (period of active inflammation) can occur 2 months to 6 months after RT completion, and fibrosis can occur years after treatment. During the pneumonitis phase of injury, there is active inflammation often visible on thoracic imaging. If a patient is asymptomatic, observation is reasonable. Symptoms, including cough and shortness of breath, associated with these image changes often are managed by corticosteroids and antibiotics as appropriate.[24] There are reports of radiation injury to the lung tissue outside of the RT field. Investigators have suggested that production of nitric oxide gas as a by-product of radiation-induced injury may play a role in generating injury in other parts of pulmonary parenchyma not directly in the RT treatment region.[25] Fibrosis as a late change can result in parenchymal scar as well as pleural and pericardial effusions, resulting in limitation of pulmonary reserve. Modern radiation techniques, including the use of motion management and IMRT, may constrain the risk of injury by limiting the parenchyma volume receiving both higher and lower doses. Dose-volume histogram analysis also suggests it is likewise important to limit the normal lung parenchyma volume receiving 20 Gy, although data continue to emerge suggesting that lung injury can be driven by the volume receiving high dose, intermediate dose, and low dose. Accordingly, current RT techniques seek to limit the volume of lung receiving high doses and low doses. Optical tracking may help decrease planning tumor volumes and limit parenchyma in the therapy field. Interactions with other pulmonary toxic agents, such as bleomycin, influence the dose-volume effect of RT. Recent studies reveal an increased risk of chronic pulmonary disease in cancer survivors compared with siblings.[20,26–28]

Heart and Peripheral Vessels

With modern cardiology evaluation techniques, including MRI and nuclear medicine studies, previously unforeseen cardiac events can be identified. This is important because studies are suggesting an association between RT and development of cardiovascular disease when the heart is an unintended target of treatment. Tangential irradiation to the left breast as treatment of breast cancer can deliver a measurable mean dose to the heart.[29] These issues are exacerbated by chemotherapy, including adriamycin and herceptin. Modern optical tracking systems, as with breath monitoring systems, serve to limit cardiac dose to patients receiving direct and indirect dose to the heart.

Anterior-posterior treatment were historically used to treat (define) Hodgkin lymphoma (HL) with non–image-guided techniques. This resulted in full-dose RT to multiple critical cardiac structures. Reviewing the anterior-posterior cardiac anatomy using traditional RT treatment fields for HL, multiple critical structures reside in the plane of the vertebral body including the primary cardiac vessels, the electrical conduction nodes, and the aortic valve. These tissues remain at risk for a patient's lifetime. IMRT decreases radiation dose to the heart; however, patients treated with RT in the pre-IMRT era will be at risk for heart disease during the next several decades. Recent studies demonstrate a significant risk of heart disease in the cancer survivor compared with their siblings.[9,22,28–42]

Large peripheral vessels were historically viewed as resistant to RT; however, injuries are being reported to the carotid vessels. Injury pathology includes intimal hyperplasia and weakening of the carotid muscle. There are reports of fistula formation and sudden death due to rupture of the carotid vessels.[9,39] Injury reports to other large vessels (subclavian, femoral, and so forth) were reported when there was overlap with RT treatment fields necessitating large radiation dose to a tubular structure.[39] With modern RT and traditional fractionation strategies, radiation injury to large vessels is uncommon. Higher daily doses to tubular structures can result in late injury and become clinically important. Symptomatic injury to veins is less common, and injury to capillaries can be visible at radiation doses of 50 Gy. Retreatment of patients is now more commonplace and the impact of RT to both large and small vessels remains to be determined.

Central and Peripheral Nervous System

The brain has several categories of cells susceptible to injury, including the glia (support cells), primary neurons, and blood vessels. All tissues generally are considered as late-responding tissues and most sequelae occur as late events. The most important sequela is necrosis, which can occur within 6 months of RT; however, reports of late injury indicate that events can occur several years after treatment, now seen in patients treated with immunotherapy.[43,44] Necrosis is detected more as radiosurgery techniques frequently are used in patient care. Rarely, demyelinating syndromes can occur in the central nervous system. Reversible syndromes can occur in the spinal cord with doses as low as 35 Gy; however, irreversible changes, including myelitis, begin occurring at 45 Gy to 50 Gy, with traditional fractionation and seem to incrementally increase with larger radiation dose and larger volume of the spinal cord in the treatment field. Toxicity may increase with neurotoxic chemotherapy including cisplatinum, vinblastine, Ara-C, gemcitabine, and methotrexate. Peripheral nerves can likely tolerate a higher dose of RT because the cauda equina and larger nerves seem to tolerate radiation doses more than 55 Gy without evidence of injury.[45] Visual field changes are seen in radiation doses higher than 5400 cGy to the optic nerve and chiasm.[46] It is thought that the chiasm is sensitive to RT because it has an end-arterial blood supply. This was first described in patients treated to the pituitary gland for pituitary adenomas using daily treatment fractions of greater than 200 cGy/d.[47] With today's image guidance and partial volume therapy, some investigators think that tolerance of these structures may be higher than described in historical literature. The cochlea can be affected by radiation and can be more pronounced at lower doses with chemotherapy, including cis-platinum. Historically the lens is very sensitive to RT, with cataract formation identified at very low dose (500 cGy). This may be influenced negatively with the use of prednisone.

Brachial plexopathy has been described in patients with breast cancer treated to peripheral lymph nodes. Although the radiation dose threshold for injury is thought to be 6600 cGy in series of patients with breast cancer, this is an uncommon side effect for patients with head/neck cancer treated with higher radiation doses. The prevailing thought is the more sensitive part of the plexus is the region where the nerve bundles coalesce immediately inferior to the lateral third of the clavicle. In RT's early days, this area was calculated using an anterior field to a depth of 5 cm. The nerves can be as superficial, 1 cm below skin surface; therefore, the nerve region received a higher percent dose (>120% of prescribed dose). Posterior axillary boosts were often calculated as separate fields with exit overlap at the egress points of the brachial plexus into the upper extremity. It is entirely possible that the threshold dose for brachial plexus injury may be higher than described in historical literature due to unintentional overlap of radiation fields and increases in daily fraction size to a critical target. Today, using 3-dimensional volumetrics, the axilla is a volume and planning permits more uniform radiation dose distribution through a volume than 2-dimensional treatment planning constructs.[48]

Reproductive Organs, Genitalia, and Endocrine Organs

Spermatogonia are among the few cell systems that can die an intermitotic death; the absolute number of sperm cells markedly decreases with modest radiation doses. Stem cells develop into spermatozoa in 75 days; therefore, radiation exposure can induce damage to mature sperm. Most oncologists offer sperm banking to patients with known direct RT exposure. Leydig cells secrete testosterone and their specific function is regulated by pituitary gonadotropins, prolactin, and luteinizing hormone. Pituitary gland treatment may impose secondary events to gonadal function. Although Leydig cells are more resistant to radiation exposure, there is incremental decrease in testosterone with doses exceeding 20 Gy. Various chemotherapy agents, including vincristine and mechlorethamine (Mustargen), influence sterility. Oocytes are very sensitive to radiation and, like sperm, die an intermitotic death. Because hormonal secretion is associated with follicular maturation, unlike the testicle, treatment of ovaries results in more immediate suppression of hormonal function. Female genitalia can demonstrate mucosal atrophy and loss of moisture.[15,20,49] RT to children for pelvic malignancies, including rhabdomyosarcoma, can result in significant atrophy and maldevelopment of gonadal organs and pelvic anatomy. Cardiovascular health and other medical comorbidities as problems associated with growth can be significantly influenced by diminution of hormonal function at a young age. For patients treated for gynecologic malignancies, the use of vaginal dilators helps maintain vaginal function. Fertility assessment pretherapy is an important aspect to patient care.

Hypothyroidism is a common sequela associated with surgery and RT to low neck. This is prevalent in patients treated for head/neck cancer and HL. For patients with head/neck cancer, neck dissection and primary surgery also influence hypothyroidism incidence. Pituitary therapy creates panhypopituitary syndrome with need for replacement therapies as appropriate. This can have significant health issues in multiple endocrine organs. There are few data for adrenal function; there are reported cases of adrenal malfunction and decreased cortisol with high-dose RT. More often, adrenal malfunction occurs in patients as a secondary bystander effect to pituitary therapy.[15,20,49] Endocrinopathies, including but not limited to thyroiditis and adrenal dysfunction, are now seen with immunotherapy and the impact of RT with immunotherapy on this point remains to be defined.

Bone: Pediatrics and Adults

Treatment of children is unique because every cell system has self-renewal potential; unlike adults, sequelae are visible and identified in all tissues due to growth and development. Bone and cartilage are key areas distinguishing adults from children. With radiation doses of 20 Gy, growth deficits in bone may be irreversible.[15,50] Deficits in bone and cartilage development are more visible with higher radiation doses and younger age. In adults, the threshold dose for bone necrosis may be 55 Gy with traditional fractionation; there are interesting reports using advanced technology imaging, including MRI, demonstrating sacral fractures in gynecologic patients receiving less than 50 Gy to bone.[50] Radiosurgery techniques, particularly to targets close to the chest wall, are reinviting injury to rib and chest wall that is often nonhealing. Treatment techniques, including volume-modulated arc therapy,[51] seem essential in decreasing this risk.

SUMMARY

Intentional and unintentional radiation exposures have a powerful impact on normal tissue function and can induce short-term and long-term injury to all cell systems. During evaluation of acute-phase management, assessing radiation dose and exposure is essential. Appropriate support can be given to those at risk for serious acute injury. Effects of RT and exposure last for a patient's lifetime with implications for all organ systems. A broad understanding of these effects is essential for health care providers.

REFERENCES

1. Hall EJ, Giaccia AJ. Radiobiology for the radiologist. 7th edition. Philadelphia: Lippincott, Williams and Wilkins; 2012.
2. Miller DL, Balter S, Cole PE, et al. Radiation doses in interventional radiology procedures: the RAD-IR study: part II: skin dose. J Vasc Interv Radiol 2003;14(8): 977–90.
3. Miller DL, Balter S, Wagner LK, et al. Quality improvement guidelines for recording patient radiation dose in the medical record. J Vasc Interv Radiol 2004;15(5):423–9.
4. Shope TB. Radiation-induced skin injuries from fluoroscopy. Radiographics 1996; 16(5):1195–9.
5. Donnelly EH, Nemhauser JB, Smith JM, et al. Acute radiation syndrome: assessment and management. South Med J 2010;103(6):541–6.
6. Turai I, Veress K. Radiation accidents: occurrence, types, consequences, medical management, and lessons learned. Central European Journal of Occupational and Environmental Medicine 2001;7(1):3–14.

7. Wikipedia contributors. Acute radiation syndrome wikipedia, the free encyclopedia 2014. Available at: https://en.wikipedia.org/w/index.php?title=Acute_radiation_syndrome&oldid=914494978. Accessed March 22, 2019.

8. Fitzgerald TJ, Jodoin MB, Tillman G, et al. Radiation therapy toxicity to the skin. Dermatol Clin 2008;26(1):161–72, ix.

9. Fajardo L, Berthrong M, Anderson RE. Radiation pathology. 1st edition. New York: Oxford University Press; 2001.

10. Majno G, Joris I. Cells, tissues, and disease: principles of general pathology. 2nd edition. New York: Oxford University Press; 2004.

11. Chin MS, Freniere BB, Bonney CF, et al. Skin perfusion and oxygenation changes in radiation fibrosis. Plast Reconstr Surg 2013;131(4):707–16.

12. Chin MS, Freniere BB, Lo YC, et al. Hyperspectral imaging for early detection of oxygenation and perfusion changes in irradiated skin. J Biomed Opt 2012;17(2): 026010.

13. Hoppe BS, Laser B, Kowalski AV, et al. Acute skin toxicity following stereotactic body radiation therapy for stage I non-small-cell lung cancer: who's at risk? Int J Radiat Oncol Biol Phys 2008;72(5):1283–6.

14. Citrin D, Cotrim AP, Hyodo F, et al. Radioprotectors and mitigators of radiation-induced normal tissue injury. Oncologist 2010;15(4):360–71.

15. FitzGerald TJ, Aronowitz J, Giulia Cicchetti M, et al. The effect of radiation therapy on normal tissue function. Hematol Oncol Clin North Am 2006;20(1):141–63.

16. Lukez A, O'Loughlin L, Bodla M, et al. Positioning of port films for radiation: variability is present. Med Oncol 2018;35(5):77.

17. Mell LK, Tiryaki H, Ahn KH, et al. Dosimetric comparison of bone marrow-sparing intensity-modulated radiotherapy versus conventional techniques for treatment of cervical cancer. Int J Radiat Oncol Biol Phys 2008;71(5):1504–10.

18. Quantitative Analyses of Normal Tissue Effects in the Clinic. Int J Radiat Oncol Biol Phys 2010;76(3, Supplement):S1–160.

19. McCulloch TM, Jaffe D. Head and neck disorders affecting swallowing. GI Motil online 2006. Available at: https://www.nature.com/gimo/contents/pt1/full/gimo36. html. Accessed August 6, 2019.

20. Bentzen SM. Preventing or reducing late side effects of radiation therapy: radiobiology meets molecular pathology. Nat Rev Cancer 2006;6(9):702–13.

21. Guha C, Kavanagh BD. Hepatic radiation toxicity: avoidance and amelioration. Semin Radiat Oncol 2011;21(4):256–63.

22. Sioshansi S, Rava PS, Karam AR, et al. Diaphragm injury after liver stereotactic body radiation therapy. Pract Radiat Oncol 2014;4(6):e227–30.

23. Moulder JE, Cohen EP. Future strategies for mitigation and treatment of chronic radiation-induced normal tissue injury. Semin Radiat Oncol 2007;17(2):141–8.

24. Rosiello RA, Merrill WW. Radiation-induced lung injury. Clin Chest Med 1990; 11(1):65–71.

25. Sugihara T, Hattori Y, Yamamoto Y, et al. Preferential impairment of nitric oxide-mediated endothelium-dependent relaxation in human cervical arteries after irradiation. Circulation 1999;100(6):635–41.

26. Anscher MS, Thrasher B, Rabbani Z, et al. Antitransforming growth factor-beta antibody 1D11 ameliorates normal tissue damage caused by high-dose radiation. Int J Radiat Oncol Biol Phys 2006;65(3):876–81.

27. Anscher MS, Thrasher B, Zgonjanin L, et al. Small molecular inhibitor of transforming growth factor-beta protects against development of radiation-induced lung injury. Int J Radiat Oncol Biol Phys 2008;71(3):829–37.

28. Armstrong GT, Kawashima T, Leisenring W, et al. Aging and risk of severe, disabling, life-threatening, and fatal events in the childhood cancer survivor study. J Clin Oncol 2014;32(12):1218–27.

29. Evans SB, Sioshansi S, Moran MS, et al. Prevalence of poor cardiac anatomy in carcinoma of the breast treated with whole-breast radiotherapy: reconciling modern cardiac dosimetry with cardiac mortality data. Am J Clin Oncol 2012;35(6):587–92.

30. Lenihan DJ, Cardinale DM. Late cardiac effects of cancer treatment. J Clin Oncol 2012;30(30):3657–64.

31. Marks LB, Yu X, Prosnitz RG, et al. The incidence and functional consequences of RT-associated cardiac perfusion defects. Int J Radiat Oncol Biol Phys 2005;63(1):214–23.

32. Yusuf SW, Sami S, Daher IN. Radiation-induced heart disease: a clinical update. Cardiol Res Pract 2011;2011:317659.

33. Ng AK, Bernardo MP, Weller E, et al. Long-term survival and competing causes of death in patients with early-stage Hodgkin's disease treated at age 50 or younger. J Clin Oncol 2002;20(8):2101–8.

34. Swerdlow AJ, Higgins CD, Smith P, et al. Myocardial infarction mortality risk after treatment for Hodgkin disease: a collaborative British cohort study. J Natl Cancer Inst 2007;99(3):206–14.

35. Hooning MJ, Botma A, Aleman BM, et al. Long-term risk of cardiovascular disease in 10-year survivors of breast cancer. J Natl Cancer Inst 2007;99(5):365–75.

36. Weintraub NL, Jones WK, Manka D. Understanding radiation-induced vascular disease. J Am Coll Cardiol 2010;55(12):1237–9.

37. Lipshultz SE, Sallan SE. Cardiovascular abnormalities in long-term survivors of childhood malignancy. J Clin Oncol 1993;11(7):1199–203.

38. Gayed IW, Liu HH, Yusuf SW, et al. The prevalence of myocardial ischemia after concurrent chemoradiation therapy as detected by gated myocardial perfusion imaging in patients with esophageal cancer. J Nucl Med 2006;47(11):1756–62.

39. Lam WW, Leung SF, So NM, et al. Incidence of carotid stenosis in nasopharyngeal carcinoma patients after radiotherapy. Cancer 2001;92(9):2357–63.

40. Adams MJ, Hardenbergh PH, Constine LS, et al. Radiation-associated cardiovascular disease. Crit Rev Oncol Hematol 2003;45(1):55–75.

41. Katz NM, Hall AW, Cerqueira MD. Radiation induced valvulitis with late leaflet rupture. Heart 2001;86(6):E20.

42. Slama MS, Le Guludec D, Sebag C, et al. Complete atrioventricular block following mediastinal irradiation: a report of six cases. Pacing Clin Electrophysiol 1991;14(7):1112–8.

43. Weingarten N, Kruser TJ, Bloch O. Symptomatic radiation necrosis in brain metastasis patients treated with stereotactic radiosurgery and immunotherapy. Clin Neurol Neurosurg 2019;179:14–8.

44. Diao K, Bian SX, Routman DM, et al. Combination ipilimumab and radiosurgery for brain metastases: tumor, edema, and adverse radiation effects. J Neurosurg 2018;129(6):1397–406.

45. Pieters RS, Niemierko A, Fullerton BC, et al. Cauda equina tolerance to high-dose fractionated irradiation. Int J Radiat Oncol Biol Phys 2006;64(1):251–7.

46. Giese WL, Kinsella TJ. Radiation injury to peripheral and cranial nerves. In: Gutin P, Leibel S, Sheline GE, editors. Radiation injury to the nervous system. New York: Raven; 1991. p. 383–403.

47. Harris JR, Levene MB. Visual complications following irradiation for pituitary adenomas and craniopharyngiomas. Radiology 1976;120(1):167–71.

48. Powell S, Cooke J, Parsons C. Radiation-induced brachial plexus injury: follow-up of two different fractionation schedules. Radiother Oncol 1990;18(3):213–20.

49. World Nuclear Association. Nuclear radiation and health effect. London: World Nuclear Association; 2018. Available at: http://www.world-nuclear.org/information-library/safety-and-security/radiation-and-health/nuclear-radiation-and-health-effects.aspx. Accessed March 12, 2019.

50. Hopewell JW. Radiation-therapy effects on bone density. Med Pediatr Oncol 2003;41(3):208–11.

51. Ding L, Lo YC, Kadish S, et al. Volume Modulated Arc Therapy (VMAT) for pulmonary Stereotactic Body Radiotherapy (SBRT) in patients with lesions in close approximation to the chest wall. Front Oncol 2013;3:12.

Radiation Modifiers

Deborah E. Citrin, MD

KEYWORDS

- Radiation modifier • Radiation sensitizer • Radiation protector • Therapeutic ratio

KEY POINTS

- Radiation modifiers are agents that can alter the response of tissues to radiation, such as radiation sensitizers and radiation protectors.
- Radiation sensitizers often target DNA repair, cell cycle checkpoints, or prosurvival signaling in tumor.
- Radiation protectors are often antioxidants that have the capacity to efficiently scavenge damaging-free radicals.
- To be effective radiation modifiers, agents must have selectivity of effect between tumor and normal tissues.

INTRODUCTION

Radiation therapy plays a central role in the management of cancers originating in many organs and tissues. The goal of radiotherapy is often to provide local or regional control of tumors when delivered as the definitive local therapy or in combination with surgical resection and chemotherapy. Because systemic therapeutic options have improved, the importance of local control in the curative treatment of cancers has become more evident. Indeed, the use of local and regional radiotherapy following surgery and/or chemotherapy has been shown to extend survival in several settings.[1–4]

Radiotherapy has undergone a continuous technologic evolution, including enhanced tumor detection and demarcation for planning, enhanced accuracy and precision of treatment delivery, and a proliferation of highly conformal therapies. Although these technological advances have fundamentally altered the practice of radiation oncology, a significant number of patients with cancer experience local or regional failure after definitive therapy. Although some patients with local and regional failure may be salvaged, many patients in this setting have no curative options. Thus, improving the efficacy of radiotherapy remains an important goal.

Disclosure Statement: The authors have nothing to disclose.
This research was supported by the Intramural Research Program of the NIH, NCI, Center for Cancer Research.
Radiation Oncology Branch, Center for Cancer Research, National Cancer Institute, Building 10 CRC, Room B2-3500, 10 Center Drive, Bethesda, MD 20892, USA
E-mail address: citrind@mail.nih.gov

Radiation dose escalation has been one method explored in the attempts to enhance local control after radiotherapy, which has led to enhanced outcomes in certain settings, such as prostate cancer.[5] In contrast, increasing radiation dose beyond the current standard has not led to improvements in local control in the setting of gliomas, despite the preponderance of local failure.[6] Further, in some settings, such as non-small cell lung cancer, there seems to be an increase in normal tissue toxicity as a result of dose escalation that negates any benefit in local control when the overall survival of the cohort is considered.[7] Thus, attempts have been made to identify agents that can modify the effects of radiation to improve the therapeutic ratio.

CONCEPTS OF COOPERATION

Agents that can modify the sensitivity of tumor or normal tissue to radiation are collectively called radiation modifiers. To be useful therapeutically, radiation modifiers should enhance the capacity to cure tumor without increasing normal tissue injury. As a result, these agents should enhance the therapeutic index, either through enhancing tumor cell kill or through protecting normal tissues (**Fig. 1**). Agents that selectively enhance radiation response of tumors are called radiation sensitizers, whereas agents that prevent radiation injury in normal tissues are considered radiation protectors.

For agents present during a radiation exposure, either for sensitization or protection, there are several methods by which these agents may show selectivity for normal tissue or tumor. One method for selectivity can be the pharmacokinetics of the agent, which can result in a selective local concentration of the agent in tumor or normal tissue. For example, a radiation protector may be selectively taken up or retained by normal tissues relative to tumor, thus resulting in selective protection. Similarly, an agent that enhances radiation response may be selectively retained or modified within a tumor cell to an active intermediate, whereas the concentration in normal tissues remains low. These effects in regard to selectivity may also be due to physiology of the tumor (hypoxia, leaky vasculature, expression of specific enzymes that modify the agent, pH, active drug transport) relative to the normal tissues. Aside from enhanced local concentrations due to the pharmacokinetics of the radiation modifier, the presence or absence of target may also dictate selectivity. Thus, if the radiation modifier targets a molecule expressed at a higher level in tumor versus normal (for a sensitizer), or vice versa (for a protector/mitigator), selectivity can also be afforded by this mechanism. Further, even with equal expression of a molecule, tumor and normal tissues may have different dependence on the target in terms of radiation response, such that inhibition affects radiation response selectively (**Fig. 2**). Examples of these interactions will be highlighted with specific examples, which are discussed later.

RADIATION SENSITIZERS

Radiation sensitizers are one class of radiation modifier. A true radiation sensitizer is capable of enhancing tumor cell kill from irradiation with no single-agent toxicity to tumor or normal tissues.[8] In reality, few true radiations sensitizers have been described, as most agents capable of enhancing tumor response also exhibit single-agent activity or some degree of normal tissue sensitization. If the degree of tumor sensitization is greater than that of normal tissue, use of the agent may still provide an opportunity to enhance the therapeutic window. Similarly, although agents that exhibit single-agent activity against tumor may not be a classical radiation sensitizer, the capacity to simultaneously enhance tumor response to radiation and target tumor cells outside of the radiation field is potentially advantageous. Thus, many agents that do not meet

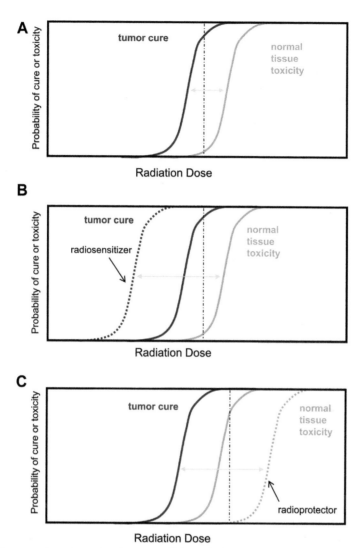

Fig. 1. Therapeutic ratio and radiation modifiers. (*A*) The probability of tumor cure (*red*) and normal tissue toxicity (*blue*) can be plotted as a factor of radiation dose. Note that these are parallel idealized sigmoidal curves that may not be representative of the clinical condition. A therapeutic dose may be selected that delivers a high chance of tumor cure with an acceptable rate of toxicity (*black dashed line*). (*B*) A tumor selective radiation sensitizer increases the probability of tumor cure for a given dose (*red dashed line*), hence the tumor control curve is shifted to the left. This results in a higher chance of cure for the same radiation dose as delivered in (*A*) (*black dashed line*). Alternatively, a lower dose may be delivered to yield the same rate of cure with less normal tissue toxicity. (*C*) A normal tissue radioprotector decreases the probability of normal tissue toxicity for a given dose of radiation, thus pushing the toxicity curve to the right (*blue dashed line*). This allows a higher dose to be given to obtain a higher rate of cure with less or equivalent normal tissue injury. (*From* Citrin DE, Mitchell JB. Altering the response to radiation: sensitizers and protectors. Semin Oncol 2014;41(6):850; with permission.)

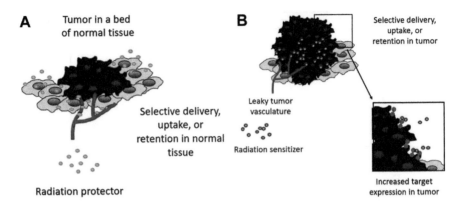

Fig. 2. Methods of selectivity of radiation modifiers. (*A*) Tumor (*dark brown*) arises in a bed of normal tissue (tan). Radiation protectors (*green*) can exhibit selective uptake in normal tissues through enhanced delivery, uptake, or retention in normal tissues compared with tumor. Higher concentrations provide a greater protective effect in normal tissues relative to tumor. (*B*) Radiosensitizing agents (*purple*) may have higher concentrations in tumor relative to normal tissues through similar mechanisms of enhanced delivery due to leaky tumor vasculature, uptake in tumor cells, or retention in tumor relative to normal tissues. Pathways targeted by the radiation sensitizer or receptors affected by the agent (*light blue* in expanded panel) may have higher expression in tumor relative to normal. Thus, even if concentration in tumor and normal tissues are similar, selectivity is afforded by selective expression of a target or selective dependence on that target in tumor.

the classical definition of radiation sensitizer could have the capacity to provide therapeutic benefit.

SENSITIZING CHEMOTHERAPY

In current practice, sensitizing chemotherapy is the most commonly used radiation sensitizer. Several chemotherapies have been described as having sensitizing properties, such as platins, pyrimidine analogues, gemcitabine, taxanes, topoisomerase inhibitors, and alkylating agents. The addition of radiosensitizing chemotherapy has led to clear local control survival benefits compared with radiation alone in a range of tumors, including glioblastoma,[9] cervical cancer,[10,11] non-small cell lung cancer,[12] head and neck cancer,[13] and gastrointestinal malignancies.[14]

Chemotherapeutic agents can augment radiation response through a variety of mechanisms, with some notable agents briefly described later to highlight the diversity of mechanism of enhancement. A common method of radiation sensitization is inducing DNA damage or inhibiting DNA repair. The platins, for example, form DNA adducts. In the case of Cisplatin, repair of these adducts can lead to additional strand breaks at the time of mismatch repair.[15] These single strand breaks can then combine with closely located single-strand breaks from irradiation to result in the more lethal DNA double-strand breaks.

Another frequently used sensitizing chemotherapy is 5-flurouracil, which exerts its radiation sensitizing effects via inhibition of DNA synthesis and repair through inhibition of thymidylate synthase.[16] In contrast, metabolites of gemcitabine can deplete intracellular adenosine triphosphate pools at the same time cells are redistributed into a radiosensitive sensitive phase of the cell cycle.[17,18] Finally, taxanes promote microtubule assembly and inhibit disaggregation, thus arresting cells in the most radiosensitive phase of the cell cycle.[19] Thus, cytotoxic chemotherapies can act via diverse mechanisms to enhance radiation response.

The use of sensitizing chemotherapy has led to enhanced local control and survival for patients with numerous types of cancers but not without a cost in terms of toxicity. In several settings, the use of sensitizing chemotherapy increases the risk of moderate to severe toxicity, such as the risk of severe cytopenias, mucositis, gastrointestinal toxicities, and cutaneous toxicity. Aside from the expected chemotherapy-related side effects, these agents may also sensitize normal tissues to irradiation, exacerbating in-filed toxicity. Despite the benefits afforded by sensitizing chemotherapy, recurrences continue to occur, leading to interest in developing nonchemotherapeutic radiation sensitizers that could be used in concert with chemotherapy or as an alternative in select situations.

RADIATION SENSITIZERS TARGETING PATHWAYS IMPORTANT IN RADIATION RESPONSE

A growing knowledge of the molecular events that occur after radiation and the cellular determinants of radiation sensitivity, coupled with the development of agents capable of targeting aspects of signal transduction, metabolism, cell cycle, and DNA repair have led to interest in developing novel radiosensitizing combinations. The goal of these studies is to develop agents that enhance cure rates with acceptable toxicity. A few examples of classes of agents that have been shown to sensitize to radiation are described later.

DNA Repair Inhibitors

Unrepaired DNA double-strand breaks are a potentially lethal event after irradiation.[20] Agents capable of inhibiting DNA repair or increasing DNA double-strand breaks often enhance the cytotoxicity of radiation.[21] Several small molecules have been developed that target DNA repair pathways, such as Poly (ADP-ribose) polymerase (PARP) inhibitors, Ataxia telangiectasia-mutated/ataxia telangiectasia and Rad3-related inhibitors, and other proteins involved in DNA repair.[22] These agents have demonstrated efficacy as radiation sensitizers in preclinical tumor model systems and are in varying stages of clinical development.[23–25] Because DNA repair inhibitors target a process that is critical for both tumor and normal cell survival after irradiation, demonstrating a selectivity for tumor becomes an important component of the evaluation of the agent.[26–28]

Inhibition of PARP has been known to enhance cellular sensitivity to radiation since the 1980s.[27,29] The availability of newer small molecule inhibitors with favorable pharmacology, selectivity, and tolerability led to the investigation of PARP inhibitors as a therapeutic option in the treatment of diverse tumor types when delivered alone and in combination with other agents, such as chemotherapy and/or radiation. Preclinical studies have demonstrated broad efficacy of PARP inhibitors as radiation sensitizers.[1–4] The mechanism of this radiation sensitization seems to primarily reflect increase in DNA damage in both tumor and tumor stroma, although additional mechanisms have been suggested.[4]

The capacity of PARP inhibition to sensitize tumor cells to radiation has included several recent and ongoing clinical trials, including numerous Phase I and II trials. The only published randomized trial of radiation with or without PARP inhibition evaluated a standard whole brain radiotherapy regimen (30 Gy in 10 fractions) with/without veliparib in patients with brain metastases from non-small cell lung cancer.[30] This trial found no improvement in the primary endpoint of overall survival with the addition of veliparib, as well as no statistically different effect on intracranial response rate, time to progression, or adverse events.

Recent work has attempted to elucidate molecular and genetic phenotypes most sensitive to PARP inhibitor–mediated radiation sensitization, and preclinical studies have demonstrated that p53 status is an important indicator of efficacy of PARP inhibition for radiation sensitization.[1,3] It is possible that a more comprehensive understanding of molecular predictors of radiation sensitization with PARP inhibitors will allow for evaluation of these agents in selected populations that may have a better chance of demonstrating efficacy.

Signal Transduction

Several signaling pathways that contribute to growth and survival are activated in tumors, such as the Ras/MAPK, NFκB, PI3K/AKT/mTOR pathways. These pathways may be activated in tumors due to activating mutations of pathway intermediates, deactivating mutations of pathway inhibitors, overexpression of receptors, or elaboration of ligands. In addition, radiation can activate these pathways and increase elaboration of ligands that stimulate them. These pathways may be important in proliferation, migration, invasion, and stress response. In addition, several pathways activated by tumor cell exposure to ionizing radiation may also enhance DNA repair, activate cell cycle blocks that facilitate DNA repair, and signal through other pathways that contribute to tumor cell survival.

Cell cycle location can alter cellular sensitivity to radiation,[31] with cells in G1 and late S exhibiting relative resistance to radiation compared with cells in G2 and M. The resistance of cells in G2 and M may be due to the capacity of these cells to activate cell cycle checkpoints that allow for DNA repair. An example of agents that can alter cell cycle checkpoints and sensitize to radiation are Chk1 inhibitors. These agents selectively sensitize p53 mutant cells to radiation through abrogation of the G2 checkpoint after irradiation.[32] As with many sensitizers, these agents must have selective uptake, retention, or activity in regard to tumor versus normal tissues in order to enhance the therapeutic ratio.

The epidermal growth factor receptor (EGFR)/Ras/MAPK pathway is an example of a pathway that has been extensively explored as pathway to target for radiation sensitization. The EGFR signaling pathway is known to enhance proliferation, tumor cell survival, and DNA repair.[33] Further, EGFR signaling is activated after irradiation and has been implicated in accelerated repopulation during radiation.[34]

Several methods of inhibiting the EGFR/Ras/MAPK pathway have been explored, including using monoclonal antibodies that bind to EGFR, such as cetuximab and panitumumab, as well as tyrosine kinase inhibitors, such as erlotinib, gefitinib, and lapatinib. In addition to targeting EGFR, several attempts have been made to target inhibitors of downstream signaling intermediates, such as Ras and ERK, as a method to sensitize tumors to radiation.[35,36] It is important to note that intermediates such as Ras and ERK/MAPK are involved in perpetuating signaling from numerous growth factor receptors other than EGFR, and signaling through this pathway is also generally activated by irradiation.

Clinical trials evaluating EGFR inhibition combined with radiotherapy ± chemotherapy have been extensive and will only briefly be highlighted here. The landmark trial by Bonner and colleagues[37,38] demonstrated a survival benefit with the addition of cetuximab to radiation when compared with radiotherapy alone in patients with locoregionally advanced head and neck cancers. Because chemoradiotherapy became the standard of care in this patient subgroup, later trials tested the addition of cetuximab to cisplatin-based chemoradiation regimens. These studies revealed no benefit in survival and an increase in acute toxicities with the addition of cetuximab.[39] Additional approaches have included using cetuximab as an adjuvant after concurrent chemoradiation or concurrently with neoadjuvant chemotherapy in locoregionally advanced head and neck cancers, with varied results. Recently, the results of RTOG 1016 were published, in which patients with human papilloma virus (HPV)-positive oropharyngeal cancer were randomized to radiation with concurrent cisplatin versus cetuximab. Patients treated with cetuximab had significantly worse locoregional control and overall survival with cetuximab compared with cisplatin.[40] Similar results were obtained in the De-ESCALaTE HPV trial of cisplatin versus cetuximab with radiation in the treatment of patients with low-risk HPV-positive oropharyngeal cancer, in which patients treated with cetuximab exhibited higher rates of local recurrence and lower overall survival.[41] Thus, the future of EGFR inhibition combined with radiotherapy in head and neck cancer remains uncertain at the present time.

Additional Targets for Sensitization

Several additional classes of agents that target unique aspects of tumor physiology or molecular characteristics of tumor have been described (summarized in **Table 1**). Many of these agents target unique aspects of tumor biology that allow a selective sensitization of tumor compared with normal tissues.

One common target is abnormal tumor vasculature, which can lead to chronic and intermittent hypoxia, low pH, and altered metabolism.[58] Hypoxic cells are known (<0.5% oxygen) to exhibit resistance to radiation relative to oxygenated tumor cells.[59,60] In addition, the stresses of hypoxia and low nutrient availability can reduce

Table 1
Radiation sensitizers

	Target	Selected Examples
Cell-cell and cell-matrix interactions	Integrins, FAK[42,43]	Cilengitide[44]
Signal transduction inhibitor	EGFR	Cetuximab
	MEK	AZD6244 (selumetinib)[45]
	mTOR/dual TORC	INK0128,[46] AZD2014[47]
DNA repair inhibitors	PARP	Olaparib, veliparib
	ATM	KU-55933, KU-60019, AZD0156, AZD1390
	ATR	Dactolisib
	Precursor depletion	Triapine
Angiogenesis inhibitors	VEGF	Bevacizumab, vandetanib,
	EGFR	cediranib[48]
	Other antiangiogenic targets	Erlotinib, cetuximab Endostatin[49]
Multitarget	Via targeting chaperone protein (Hsp90)	Geldanamycin, 17-N-allylamino-17-demethoxygeldanamycin[50–52]
Epigenetic	HDAC inhibitors	Valproic acid,[53] vorinostat, MS-275[54]
Agents altering metabolism	NAD(P)H NAMPT/NAD(P)H	B-lapachone[55]
	Glycolysis	2-Deoxyglucose[56]
	Mitochondrial complex 1	Papaverine[57]

Abbreviations: ATM, ataxia telangiectasia-mutated; FAK, focal adhesion kinase; HDAC, histone deacetylase; MEK, MAPK kinase; mTOR, mammalian target of rapamycin; VEGF, vascular endothelial growth factor.

tumor cell cycling and result in G_0 arrest, further reducing radiation and chemosensitivity.[61,62] Hypoxia and the resulting altered metabolism and pH can additionally affect DNA repair.[63] Several agents that can target these aspects of tumor physiology have been described (see **Table 1**).

RADIATION PROTECTORS AND MITIGATORS

Agents that reduce radiation injury of normal tissues are also radiation modifiers. Normal tissue injury can be modified in a variety of ways, through prevention of a portion of the damage through radioprotection or through postexposure treatment using radiation mitigators or treatments. A full discussion of radiation mitigation and treatment of radiation injury is outside the scope of this article, and the discussion focuses on radioprotectors.

Short-lived free radicals generated by ionizing radiation can be highly damaging to cellular components, such as DNA. Most chemical radioprotectors are antioxidants that reduce cellular damage caused by free radicals.[64] These antioxidants produce a more stable reactive species by donating a hydrogen atom to free radicals. Antioxidants can exist as small molecules, such as ascorbic acid, polyphenols, and thiols, or as enzymes, such as superoxide dismutase, catalase, and glutathione peroxidase.[64] Not every antioxidant has radioprotective effects,[65,66] as not all antioxidants are reactive toward the secondary species generated by radiation.[66] Because chemical radioprotectors scavenge short-lived free radicals, a high local concentration is required at the time of radiation exposure to be effective, as the free radicals that they scavenge have an extremely short half-life, on the order of fractions of a second.

Perhaps the best studied chemical radioprotector is Amifostine, a thiol compound that efficiently scavenges free radicals. Amifostine is the only radioprotector approved by Food and Drug Administration (FDA), which has been used to prevent xerostomia in patients receiving radiotherapy.[67] Amifostine is dephosphorylated by alkaline phosphatase, the active form, and accumulates in normal tissues relative to tumor.[68] The selectivity of amifostine is further enhanced by the physiology of tumors in which low pH, vascular anomalies, and lower expression of alkaline phosphatase reduce activity in tumors.[69]

Although amifostine was tested in numerous clinical trials for reduction in mucositis with radiotherapy, a systematic review of these trials found that data supporting the use of amifostine for oral mucositis was inconclusive.[70] Studies evaluating the capacity for amifostine to reduce esophagitis have been similarly conflicting.[71–75] Additional trials have studied amifostine as a method to prevent proctitis and dermatitis,[76–78] soft tissue fibrosis,[79] and lung fibrosis[79,80] in patients receiving radiation.

Although amifostine is FDA approved for use as a radioprotector, its use is limited. This is in part due to challenges in using the drug: it must be delivered 15 to 30 minutes before each dose of radiation and delivery causes nausea and hypotension. Modern radiotherapeutic modalities, such as intensity-modulated radiation therapy, may provide a greater capacity to shield sensitive organs, such as salivary glands, reducing the benefit achieved with amifostine. Importantly, the concern of protecting tumor with amifostine remains a controversial topic and a concern for many treating physicians, despite preclinical data suggesting a lack of tumor protection. Newer aminothiol agents that exhibit radioprotection without hypotension and nausea have been described in preclinical studies but have yet to be translated to the clinic.[81–83]

Nitroxides

Nitroxides are another class of compounds that have been shown to have the capacity to prevent cytotoxicity induced by radiation. These compounds are recycling antioxidants that convert between the oxidized and reduced form. When in the oxidized form, nitroxides exist as a stable-free radical that can undergo hydrogen reductions to hydroxylamines. Although both nitroxide radicals and hydroxylamine have antioxidant functions,[66,84] only nitroxides exhibit radioprotective effects. Nitroxides can reduce DNA damage and cell death induced by radiation in vitro[85,86] and reduce the lethality of total body radiation exposures in vivo.[87,88]

Tempol (4-hydroxy-2,2,6,6-tetramethylpiperidine-1-oxyl) is a nitroxide radioprotector that has been shown to have efficacy in both topical[89,90] and systemic administration.[87,88,91] Tempol has been shown to selectively protect normal tissues relative to tumor in animal models,[91,92] which is thought to relate to faster reduction to the hydroxylamine metabolite in tumor compared with normal tissues.[92] Tempol in its oxidized form can also act as a contrast agent in MRI, thus allowing imaging of the reduction of tempol to the hydroxylamine form in tissues.[93] Thus, individual patients could be imaged to determine the optimal timing of Tempol delivery in relation to radiotherapy in their specific tumor relative to their normal tissues. Initial studies of Tempol as a method to prevent alopecia with topical application have been promising with minimal evidence of systemic leak.[94]

FUTURE DIRECTIONS

The introduction of molecular tumor subtyping and genomic predictors of prognosis and response offers unique opportunities for the development of radiation modifiers. A knowledge of which patients are at the highest risk for local recurrence based on these markers will allow selection of patients for treatment intensification with a radiation sensitizer in the setting where additional toxicity may be warranted. Similarly, knowledge of underlying normal tissue sensitivity to the deleterious effects of ionizing radiation may provide an opportunity to introduce radioprotectors in only those at highest risk of severe toxicity. Perhaps most importantly, molecular characterization may allow the development of sensitizers based on target presence, pathway activation, or proposed sensitivity instead of solely on primary tumor location or histology, as has been prior practice. Integration of radiation modifiers with other developing fields, such as immunotherapy and nanotechnology, may also provide unique opportunities moving forward.

The role of radiation modifiers in the setting of increasing popular ablative techniques, such as stereotactic ablative radiation therapy (SBRT), will likely evolve as the comfort with these techniques and indications for their use continues to grow. Because local control is exceptional with some SBRT regimens, it is unlikely that addition of a radiation sensitizer would improve outcomes. However, when dose is limited due to nearby critical structures, or local recurrence remains a concern despite ablative dosing, an agent that selectively targets tumor relative to normal tissues may conceivable provide a therapeutic opportunity. Ablative treatments may provide a unique setting in which normal tissue protection can be accomplished through more invasive methods, such as instillation of protective agents in adjacent organs, a technique that is more burdensome to patient and care-giving team with conventionally fractionated approaches.

SUMMARY

Radiation therapy is an ever-evolving field, in which technologic improvements have led to substantially reduced toxicity with an enhanced capacity for cure. A growing knowledge of the molecular biology of tumors, tumor physiology, and normal tissue biology have allowed the development of agents that can selectively enhance radiation killing in tumor or reduce injury of normal tissues. Description of molecular predictors of sensitization may allow eventual translation based on an individual patient's expected benefit.

REFERENCES

1. Bi Y, Verginadis II, Dey S, et al. Radiosensitization by the PARP inhibitor olaparib in BRCA1-proficient and deficient high-grade serous ovarian carcinomas. Gynecol Oncol 2018;150(3):534–44.
2. Chatterjee P, Choudhary GS, Sharma A, et al. PARP inhibition sensitizes to low dose-rate radiation TMPRSS2-ERG fusion gene-expressing and PTEN-deficient prostate cancer cells. PLoS One 2013;8(4):e60408.
3. Liu Q, Gheorghiu L, Drumm M, et al. PARP-1 inhibition with or without ionizing radiation confers reactive oxygen species-mediated cytotoxicity preferentially to cancer cells with mutant TP53. Oncogene 2018;37(21):2793–805.
4. Senra JM, Telfer BA, Cherry KE, et al. Inhibition of PARP-1 by olaparib (AZD2281) increases the radiosensitivity of a lung tumor xenograft. Mol Cancer Ther 2011; 10(10):1949–58.
5. Kuban DA, Tucker SL, Dong L, et al. Long-term results of the M. D. Anderson randomized dose-escalation trial for prostate cancer. Int J Radiat Oncol Biol Phys 2008;70(1):67–74.
6. Chan JL, Lee SW, Fraass BA, et al. Survival and failure patterns of high-grade gliomas after three-dimensional conformal radiotherapy. J Clin Oncol 2002;20(6): 1635–42.
7. Bradley JD, Paulus R, Komaki R, et al. Standard-dose versus high-dose conformal radiotherapy with concurrent and consolidation carboplatin plus paclitaxel with or without cetuximab for patients with stage IIIA or IIIB non-small-cell lung cancer (RTOG 0617): a randomised, two-by-two factorial phase 3 study. Lancet Oncol 2015;16(2):187–99.
8. Russo A, Mitchell J, Kinsella T, et al. Determinants of radiosensitivity. Semin Oncol 1985;12(3):332–49.
9. Stupp R, Mason WP, van den Bent MJ, et al. Radiotherapy plus concomitant and adjuvant temozolomide for glioblastoma. N Engl J Med 2005;352(10):987–96.
10. Keys HM, Bundy BN, Stehman FB, et al. Cisplatin, radiation, and adjuvant hysterectomy compared with radiation and adjuvant hysterectomy for bulky stage IB cervical carcinoma. N Engl J Med 1999;340(15):1154–61.
11. Rose PG, Bundy BN, Watkins EB, et al. Concurrent cisplatin-based radiotherapy and chemotherapy for locally advanced cervical cancer. N Engl J Med 1999; 340(15):1144–53.
12. Curran WJ Jr, Paulus R, Langer CJ, et al. Sequential vs. concurrent chemoradiation for stage III non-small cell lung cancer: randomized phase III trial RTOG 9410. J Natl Cancer Inst 2011;103(19):1452–60.
13. Calais G, Alfonsi M, Bardet E, et al. Randomized trial of radiation therapy versus concomitant chemotherapy and radiation therapy for advanced-stage oropharynx carcinoma. J Natl Cancer Inst 1999;91(24):2081–6.
14. A multi-institutional comparative trial of radiation therapy alone and in combination with 5-fluorouracil for locally unresectable pancreatic carcinoma. The Gastrointestinal Tumor Study Group. Ann Surg 1979;189(2):205–8.
15. Mierzwa ML, Nyati MK, Morgan MA, et al. Recent advances in combined modality therapy. Oncologist 2010;15(4):372–81.

16. Lawrence TS, Davis MA, Maybaum J. Dependence of 5-fluorouracil-mediated radiosensitization on DNA-directed effects. Int J Radiat Oncol Biol Phys 1994;29(3): 519–23.

17. Ostruszka LJ, Shewach DS. The role of cell cycle progression in radiosensitization by 2',2'-difluoro-2'-deoxycytidine. Cancer Res 2000;60(21):6080–8.

18. Cornelius J, McGinn TSL, Mark M, et al. On the development of gemcitabine-based chemoradiotherapy regimens in pancreatic cancer. Cancer 2002;95(S4): 933–40.

19. Rao S, Krauss NE, Heerding JM, et al. 3'-(p-azidobenzamido)taxol photolabels the N-terminal 31 amino acids of beta-tubulin. J Biol Chem 1994;269(5):3132–4.

20. Cornforth MN, Bedford JS. A quantitative comparison of potentially lethal damage repair and the rejoining of interphase chromosome breaks in low passage normal human fibroblasts. Radiat Res 1987;111(3):385–405.

21. Citrin DE, Mitchell JB. Altering the response to radiation: sensitizers and protectors. Semin Oncol 2014;41(6):848–59.

22. Hengel SR, Spies MA, Spies M. Small-molecule inhibitors targeting DNA repair and DNA repair deficiency in research and cancer therapy. Cell Chem Biol 2017;24(9):1101–19.

23. Chalmers AJ, Lakshman M, Chan N, et al. Poly(ADP-ribose) polymerase inhibition as a model for synthetic lethality in developing radiation oncology targets. Semin Radiat Oncol 2010;20(4):274–81.

24. Thoms J, Bristow RG. DNA repair targeting and radiotherapy: a focus on the therapeutic ratio. Semin Radiat Oncol 2010;20(4):217–22.

25. Choudhury A, Cuddihy A, Bristow RG. Radiation and new molecular agents part I: targeting ATM-ATR checkpoints, DNA repair, and the proteasome. Semin Radiat Oncol 2006;16(1):51–8.

26. McMahon M, Frangova TG, Henderson CJ, et al. Olaparib, monotherapy or with ionizing radiation, exacerbates DNA damage in normal tissues: insights from a new p21 reporter mouse. Mol Cancer Res 2016;14(12):1195–203.

27. de Murcia JM, Niedergang C, Trucco C, et al. Requirement of poly(ADP-ribose) polymerase in recovery from DNA damage in mice and in cells. Proc Natl Acad Sci U S A 1997;94(14):7303–7.

28. Moding EJ, Lee CL, Castle KD, et al. Atm deletion with dual recombinase technology preferentially radiosensitizes tumor endothelium. J Clin Invest 2014; 124(8):3325–38.

29. Ben-Hur E, Utsumi H, Elkind MM. Inhibitors of poly(ADP-ribose) synthesis enhance X-ray killing of log-phase Chinese hamster cells. Radiat Res 1984; 97(3):546–55.

30. Chabot P, Hsia TC, Ryu JS, et al. Veliparib in combination with whole-brain radiation therapy for patients with brain metastases from non-small cell lung cancer: results of a randomized, global, placebo-controlled study. J Neurooncol 2017; 131(1):105–15.

31. Terasima T, Tolmach LJ. Changes in x-ray sensitivity of HeLa cells during the division cycle. Nature 1961;190:1210–1.

32. Mitchell JB, Choudhuri R, Fabre K, et al. In vitro and in vivo radiation sensitization of human tumor cells by a novel checkpoint kinase inhibitor, AZD7762. Clin Cancer Res 2010;16(7):2076–84.

33. Cuneo KC, Nyati MK, Ray D, et al. EGFR targeted therapies and radiation: Optimizing efficacy by appropriate drug scheduling and patient selection. Pharmacol Ther 2015;154:67–77.

34. Schmidt-Ullrich RK, Mikkelsen RB, Dent P, et al. Radiation-induced proliferation of the human A431 squamous carcinoma cells is dependent on EGFR tyrosine phosphorylation. Oncogene 1997;15(10):1191–7.

35. Chung EJ, Urick ME, Kurshan N, et al. MEK1/2 inhibition enhances the radiosensitivity of cancer cells by downregulating survival and growth signals mediated by EGFR ligands. Int J Oncol 2013;42(6):2028–36.

36. Urick ME, Chung EJ, Shield WP 3rd, et al. Enhancement of 5-fluorouracil-induced in vitro and in vivo radiosensitization with MEK inhibition. Clin Cancer Res 2011; 17(15):5038–47.

37. Bonner JA, Harari PM, Giralt J, et al. Radiotherapy plus cetuximab for squamous-cell carcinoma of the head and neck. N Engl J Med 2006;354(6):567–78.

38. Bonner JA, Harari PM, Giralt J, et al. Radiotherapy plus cetuximab for locoregionally advanced head and neck cancer: 5-year survival data from a phase 3 randomised trial, and relation between cetuximab-induced rash and survival. Lancet Oncol 2010;11(1):21–8.

39. Ang KK, Zhang Q, Rosenthal DI, et al. Randomized phase III trial of concurrent accelerated radiation plus cisplatin with or without cetuximab for stage III to IV head and neck carcinoma: RTOG 0522. J Clin Oncol 2014;32(27):2940–50.

40. Gillison ML, Trotti AM, Harris J, et al. Radiotherapy plus cetuximab or cisplatin in human papillomavirus-positive oropharyngeal cancer (NRG Oncology RTOG 1016): a randomised, multicentre, non-inferiority trial. Lancet 2019;393(10166): 40–50.

41. Mehanna H, Robinson M, Hartley A, et al. Radiotherapy plus cisplatin or cetuximab in low-risk human papillomavirus-positive oropharyngeal cancer (De-ESCALaTE HPV): an open-label randomised controlled phase 3 trial. Lancet 2019; 393(10166):51–60.

42. Steglich A, Vehlow A, Eke I, et al. alpha integrin targeting for radiosensitization of three-dimensionally grown human head and neck squamous cell carcinoma cells. Cancer Lett 2015;357(2):542–8.

43. Hehlgans S, Eke I, Cordes N. Targeting FAK radiosensitizes 3-dimensional grown human HNSCC cells through reduced Akt1 and MEK1/2 signaling. Int J Radiat Oncol Biol Phys 2012;83(5):e669–76.

44. Albert JM, Cao C, Geng L, et al. Integrin alpha v beta 3 antagonist Cilengitide enhances efficacy of radiotherapy in endothelial cell and non-small-cell lung cancer models. Int J Radiat Oncol Biol Phys 2006;65(5):1536–43.

45. Chung EJ, Brown AP, Asano H, et al. In vitro and in vivo radiosensitization with AZD6244 (ARRY-142886), an inhibitor of mitogen-activated protein kinase/extracellular signal-regulated kinase 1/2 kinase. Clin Cancer Res 2009;15(9):3050–7.

46. Hayman TJ, Wahba A, Rath BH, et al. The ATP-competitive mTOR inhibitor INK128 enhances in vitro and in vivo radiosensitivity of pancreatic carcinoma cells. Clin Cancer Res 2014;20(1):110–9.

47. Kahn J, Hayman TJ, Jamal M, et al. The mTORC1/mTORC2 inhibitor AZD2014 enhances the radiosensitivity of glioblastoma stem-like cells. Neuro Oncol 2014;16(1):29–37.

48. Abdollahi A, Lipson KE, Sckell A, et al. Combined therapy with direct and indirect angiogenesis inhibition results in enhanced antiangiogenic and antitumor effects. Cancer Res 2003;63(24):8890–8.

49. Itasaka S, Komaki R, Herbst RS, et al. Endostatin improves radioresponse and blocks tumor revascularization after radiation therapy for A431 xenografts in mice. Int J Radiat Oncol Biol Phys 2007;67(3):870–8.

50. Dote H, Burgan WE, Camphausen K, et al. Inhibition of hsp90 compromises the DNA damage response to radiation. Cancer Res 2006;66(18):9211–20.
51. Russell JS, Burgan W, Oswald KA, et al. Enhanced cell killing induced by the combination of radiation and the heat shock protein 90 inhibitor 17-allylamino-17- demethoxygeldanamycin: a multitarget approach to radiosensitization. Clin Cancer Res 2003;9(10 Pt 1):3749–55.
52. Bisht KS, Bradbury CM, Mattson D, et al. Geldanamycin and 17-allylamino-17-de-methoxygeldanamycin potentiate the in vitro and in vivo radiation response of cervical tumor cells via the heat shock protein 90-mediated intracellular signaling and cytotoxicity. Cancer Res 2003;63(24):8984–95.
53. Camphausen K, Cerna D, Scott T, et al. Enhancement of in vitro and in vivo tumor cell radiosensitivity by valproic acid. Int J Cancer 2005;114(3):380–6.
54. Camphausen K, Scott T, Sproull M, et al. Enhancement of xenograft tumor radio-sensitivity by the histone deacetylase inhibitor MS-275 and correlation with his-tone hyperacetylation. Clin Cancer Res 2004;10(18 Pt 1):6066–71.
55. Li LS, Reddy S, Lin ZH, et al. NQO1-mediated tumor-selective lethality and radio-sensitization for head and neck cancer. Mol Cancer Ther 2016;15(7):1757–67.
56. Rashmi R, Huang X, Floberg JM, et al. Radioresistant cervical cancers are sen-sitive to inhibition of glycolysis and redox metabolism. Cancer Res 2018;78(6): 1392–403.
57. Benej M, Hong X, Vibhute S, et al. Papaverine and its derivatives radiosensitize solid tumors by inhibiting mitochondrial metabolism. Proc Natl Acad Sci U S A 2018;115(42):10756–61.
58. Brown JM. Tumor microenvironment and the response to anticancer therapy. Cancer Biol Ther 2002;1(5):453–8.
59. Thomlinson RH, Gray LH. The histological structure of some human lung cancers and the possible implications for radiotherapy. Br J Cancer 1955;9(4):539–49.
60. Bristow RG, Hill RP. Hypoxia and metabolism. Hypoxia, DNA repair and genetic instability. Nat Rev Cancer 2008;8(3):180–92.
61. Liebmann J, Cook JA, Fisher J, et al. In vitro studies of Taxol as a radiation sensi-tizer in human tumor cells. J Natl Cancer Inst 1994;86(6):441–6.
62. Teicher BA, Holden SA, al-Achi A, et al. Classification of antineoplastic treatments by their differential toxicity toward putative oxygenated and hypoxic tumor sub-populations in vivo in the FSaIIC murine fibrosarcoma. Cancer Res 1990; 50(11):3339–44.
63. Bailey KM, Wojtkowiak JW, Hashim AI, et al. Targeting the metabolic microenvi-ronment of tumors. Adv Pharmacol 2012;65:63–107.
64. Citrin D, Cotrim AP, Hyodo F, et al. Radioprotectors and mitigators of radiation-induced normal tissue injury. Oncologist 2010;15(4):360–71.
65. Camphausen K, Citrin D, Krishna MC, et al. Implications for tumor control during protection of normal tissues with antioxidants. J Clin Oncol 2005;23(24):5455–7.
66. Xavier S, Yamada K, Samuni AM, et al. Differential protection by nitroxides and hydroxylamines to radiation-induced and metal ion-catalyzed oxidative damage. Biochim Biophys Acta 2002;1573(2):109–20.
67. Kouvaris JR, Kouloulias VE, Vlahos LJ. Amifostine: the first selective-target and broad-spectrum radioprotector. Oncologist 2007;12(6):738–47.
68. Yuhas JM. Active versus passive absorption kinetics as the basis for selective protection of normal tissues by S-2-(3-aminopropylamino)-ethylphosphorothioic acid. Cancer Res 1980;40(5):1519–24.

69. Giatromanolaki A, Sivridis E, Maltezos E, et al. Down-regulation of intestinal-type alkaline phosphatase in the tumor vasculature and stroma provides a strong basis for explaining amifostine selectivity. Semin Oncol 2002;29(6 Suppl 19):14–21.

70. Nicolatou-Galitis O, Sarri T, Bowen J, et al. Systematic review of amifostine for the management of oral mucositis in cancer patients. Support Care Cancer 2013; 21(1):357–64.

71. Werner-Wasik M, Axelrod RS, Friedland DP, et al. Phase II: trial of twice weekly amifostine in patients with non-small cell lung cancer treated with chemoradiotherapy. Semin Radiat Oncol 2002;12(1 Suppl 1):34–9.

72. Antonadou D. Radiotherapy or chemotherapy followed by radiotherapy with or without amifostine in locally advanced lung cancer. Semin Radiat Oncol 2002; 12(1 Suppl 1):50–8.

73. Komaki R, Lee JS, Milas L, et al. Effects of amifostine on acute toxicity from concurrent chemotherapy and radiotherapy for inoperable non-small-cell lung cancer: report of a randomized comparative trial. Int J Radiat Oncol Biol Phys 2004;58(5):1369–77.

74. Movsas B, Scott C, Langer C, et al. Randomized trial of amifostine in locally advanced non-small-cell lung cancer patients receiving chemotherapy and hyperfractionated radiation: radiation therapy oncology group trial 98-01. J Clin Oncol 2005;23(10):2145–54.

75. Sarna L, Swann S, Langer C, et al. Clinically meaningful differences in patient-reported outcomes with amifostine in combination with chemoradiation for locally advanced non-small-cell lung cancer: an analysis of RTOG 9801. Int J Radiat Oncol Biol Phys 2008;72(5):1378–84.

76. Kouvaris J, Kouloulias V, Kokakis J, et al. The cytoprotective effect of amifostine in acute radiation dermatitis: a retrospective analysis. Eur J Dermatol 2002;12(5): 458–62.

77. Singh AK, Menard C, Guion P, et al. Intrarectal amifostine suspension may protect against acute proctitis during radiation therapy for prostate cancer: a pilot study. Int J Radiat Oncol Biol Phys 2006;65(4):1008–13.

78. Simone NL, Menard C, Soule BP, et al. Intrarectal amifostine during external beam radiation therapy for prostate cancer produces significant improvements in Quality of Life measured by EPIC score. Int J Radiat Oncol Biol Phys 2008; 70(1):90–5.

79. Koukourakis MI, Panteliadou M, Abatzoglou IM, et al. Postmastectomy hypofractionated and accelerated radiation therapy with (and without) subcutaneous amifostine cytoprotection. Int J Radiat Oncol Biol Phys 2013;85(1):e7–13.

80. Antonadou D, Coliarakis N, Synodinou M, et al. Randomized phase III trial of radiation treatment +/- amifostine in patients with advanced-stage lung cancer. Int J Radiat Oncol Biol Phys 2001;51(4):915–22.

81. Copp RR, Peebles DD, Soref CM, et al. Radioprotective efficacy and toxicity of a new family of aminothiol analogs. Int J Radiat Biol 2013;89(7):485–92.

82. Peebles DD, Soref CM, Copp RR, et al. ROS-scavenger and radioprotective efficacy of the new PrC-210 aminothiol. Radiat Res 2012;178(1):57–68.

83. Soref CM, Hacker TA, Fahl WE. A new orally active, aminothiol radioprotector-free of nausea and hypotension side effects at its highest radioprotective doses. Int J Radiat Oncol Biol Phys 2012;82(5):e701–7.

84. Samuni A, Goldstein S, Russo A, et al. Kinetics and mechanism of hydroxyl radical and OH-adduct radical reactions with nitroxides and with their hydroxylamines. J Am Chem Soc 2002;124(29):8719–24.

85. Soule BP, Hyodo F, Matsumoto K, et al. Therapeutic and clinical applications of nitroxide compounds. Antioxid Redox Signal 2007;9(10):1731–43.

86. Soule BP, Hyodo F, Matsumoto K, et al. The chemistry and biology of nitroxide compounds. Free Radic Biol Med 2007;42(11):1632–50.

87. Hahn SM, Tochner Z, Krishna CM, et al. Tempol, a stable free radical, is a novel murine radiation protector. Cancer Res 1992;52(7):1750–3.

88. Hahn SM, Krishna CM, Samuni A, et al. Potential use of nitroxides in radiation oncology. Cancer Res 1994;54(7 Suppl):2006s–10s.

89. Cuscela D, Coffin D, Lupton GP, et al. Protection from radiation-induced alopecia with topical application of nitroxides: fractionated studies. Cancer J Sci Am 1996; 2(5):273–8.

90. Goffman T, Cuscela D, Glass J, et al. Topical application of nitroxide protects radiation-induced alopecia in guinea pigs. Int J Radiat Oncol Biol Phys 1992; 22(4):803–6.

91. Cotrim AP, Hyodo F, Matsumoto K, et al. Differential radiation protection of salivary glands versus tumor by Tempol with accompanying tissue assessment of Tempol by magnetic resonance imaging. Clin Cancer Res 2007;13(16):4928–33.

92. Hahn SM, Sullivan FJ, DeLuca AM, et al. Evaluation of tempol radioprotection in a murine tumor model. Free Radic Biol Med 1997;22(7):1211–6.

93. Davis RM, Mitchell JB, Krishna MC. Nitroxides as cancer imaging agents. Anticancer Agents Med Chem 2011;11(4):347–58.

94. Metz JM, Smith D, Mick R, et al. A phase I study of topical Tempol for the prevention of alopecia induced by whole brain radiotherapy. Clin Cancer Res 2004; 10(19):6411–7.

Immunotherapy and Radiation

Charting a Path Forward Together

Vishwajith Sridharan, MD, MBA[a],
Jonathan D. Schoenfeld, MD, MPhil, MPH[b],*

KEYWORDS

- Radiation therapy • Immunotherapy • Clinical trials • Abscopal
- Immune checkpoint • PD-1

KEY POINTS

- Preclinical and clinical data suggest that radiation significantly alters the tumor immune microenvironment by producing effects including: up-regulating cytokines, causing immunogenic cell death, and potentiating tumor-specific immune responses.
- Key radiation parameters, including dose, fractionation, and timing relative to immunotherapy, play a critical role in affecting the outcome and may be tumor specific or context specific.
- Structural challenges to further developing radiation/immunotherapy combination therapy include the need for coordination among disciplines during trial design, and execution and variable radiation access and quality.

INTRODUCTION

Immune checkpoint inhibitors (ICPIs) targeting programmed cell death protein (PD-1), PD-L1, or cytotoxic T-lymphocyte–associated antigen 4 (CTLA-4) receptors have transformed oncology due to proved survival benefit across multiple malignancies.[1-6] Recent decades have also witnessed significant advances in radiation therapy (RT), allowing for more targeted treatments in fewer fractions using stereotactic radiosurgery (SRS) or stereotactic ablative radiotherapy (SABR).[7,8] Only a minority of solid

Conflict of Interest: Dr J.D. Schoenfeld reports grants, personal fees, and nonfinancial support from Bristol-Myers Squibb; grants from Merck; personal fees and nonfinancial support from AstraZeneca; personal fees and nonfinancial support from Debiopharm; personal fees from Nanobiotix; personal fees from Tilos Therapeutics; and grants from Regeneron. Mr V. Sridharan reports consulting fees from Takeda Pharmaceuticals and Volcano Capital Management.

[a] Department of Medicine, Massachusetts General Hospital, 75 Fruit Street, Boston, MA 02114, USA; [b] Department of Radiation Oncology, Brigham and Women's Hospital/Dana-Farber Cancer Institute, 75 Francis Street, L2, Boston, MA 02115, USA
* Corresponding author. Department of Radiation Oncology, Dana-Farber/Brigham and Women's Cancer Center, 450 Brookline Avenue, DA L2-57, Boston, MA 02114.
E-mail address: jdschoenfeld@partners.org

Hematol Oncol Clin N Am 33 (2019) 1057–1069
https://doi.org/10.1016/j.hoc.2019.08.001
0889-8588/19/© 2019 Elsevier Inc. All rights reserved.

tumor patients (approximately 1 in 4–5 patients), however, benefit from currently approved ICPIs, and existing biomarkers are unable to predict which patients will benefit. The benefits of RT vary widely, and use in the metastatic setting historically has been focused on palliative treatment with the goal of providing short-term symptom relief.[9] Only recently have studies started to examine the ability of RT to meaningfully alter disease course in select patients with metastatic disease.[10,11]

Intriguingly, preclinical data demonstrate pronounced synergies between ICPIs and RT, and this has generated intense interest in translating these findings to clinical practice.[12] Despite large numbers of ongoing clinical trials, there are important questions that have an impact on study design and outcome, including:

1. How can preclinical data be best translated to clinical testing?
2. What radiation parameters might have an impact on combined treatment outcome?
3. What study designs and outcome measures are most likely to advance patient care?

In this article, the authors highlight the existing data and address some of the structural and economic challenges that are relevant to executing combination RT immunotherapy trials.

TRANSLATING PRECLINICAL DATA

Preclinical studies are critical to identifying signals that two distinct therapies may work well together, and preclinical studies have suggested that this combination can lead to increased rates of systemic and local (within the RT field) responses.[13,14] These effects extend across multiple disease types and specific model systems, arguing against an idiosyncratic effect.

With regard to mechanism, preclinical studies have suggested that RT may be a particularly appealing partner for immunotherapy given its ability to engender immunogenic cell death.[13,15] This specific phenotype is marked by translocation of calreticulin from the endoplasmic reticulum to the cell surface, the release of extracellular ATP, and alterations in major histocompatibility complex-1 and intercellular adhesion molecule-1 expression that can enhance T-cell–mediated killing.[16–21] This immunogenic cell death can give rise to tumor-specific immune responses that are critical to the success of current immunotherapies. For instance, RT has been shown to activate the cytosolic DNA-sensing stimulator of interferon genes (STING) pathway, leading to the induction of type I interferon, which is essential for $CD8^+$ antitumor responses.[22] Enhancing the STING pathway with exogenous cyclic guanosine monophosphate–adenosine monophosphate enhanced the antitumor effort of radiation, whereas STING loss prevented the regression of tumors in the content of RT + IO.[22,23] In addition, RT causes up-regulation of proinflammatory cytokines (ie, interleukin [IL]-1, IL-6, and tumor necrosis factor [TNF]-α) and chemokines (CXCL10 and CXCL16) to levels that are detectable in circulating serum[24–27] (**Fig. 1**).

Less clear is the ability to translate specifics gleaned from preclinical studies to their clinical counterparts. For example, preclinical models suggest hypofractionated RT doses of approximately 6 Gy to 10 Gy may be optimal to generate tumor-specific immunity.[28–30] Dose effects of RT tend to be more model specific, however, and it can be challenging to adapt a specific RT dose used in animal models to human patients, where the number of tumor cells treated is orders of magnitude greater.[31] Perhaps more straightforward is the ability to draw on mechanisms identified in preclinical studies to guide the development of biomarkers in human studies. For instance,

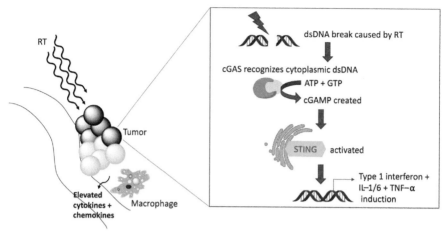

Fig. 1. Radiation causes activation of the STING pathway, promoting the release of type I interferon, inflammatory cytokines, and chemokines that attract CD8$^+$ T cells to the tumor microenvironment. ATP, adenosine tri-phosphate; cGAS, Cyclic GMP-AMP synthase; GTP, guanine triphosphate.

preclinical studies have suggested that RT can give rise to tumor antigen–specific immune responses.[32] Recently, this was confirmed in human studies combining RT and immune checkpoint blockade.[33] RT, in combination with ICPI, also was found to increase the diversity and frequency of common T-cell receptor clones, expand specific T-cell populations, and reverse T-cell exhaustion.[34] There are simultaneous changes, however, in immune-suppressive cell populations (regulatory T cells and myeloid-derived suppressor cells), suggesting that combination RT + ICPI could tip the balance toward a proimmune state.[35,36]

CRITICAL RADIATION THERAPY PARAMETERS

These preclinical studies along with early clinical experience can provide guidance to developing a successful combinatorial strategy.

Sequencing radiation therapy with immune checkpoint inhibitors

Recent studies have indicated that tumors that have an inflamed phenotype, or have significant tumor-infiltrating T lymphocytes (TILs), may respond better to ICPIs relative to cold tumors.[37,38] RT is known to increase TILs in the tumor microenvironment as well as promote the recognition of tumor-associated antigens to potentiate ICPIs.[32,39] Even with robust T-cell infiltration, however, up-regulation of immune checkpoint expression that occurs within the tumor can limit antitumor immunity. As such, appropriate sequencing of RT with ICPIs could have a significant impact on clinical outcomes.

Several studies have attempted to elucidate optimal timing of RT when given in combination with immunotherapy. Murine studies of colon carcinoma, melanoma, and triple-negative breast cancer irradiated to 10 Gy in 5 fractions, and given anti–PD-1 or anti–PD-L1 antibodies, indicated that concurrent but not sequential therapy was effective at improving local control and survival.[40] These data revealed that PD-L1 expression were increased in tumor cells in the 24 hours to 7 days post–fractionated RT delivery, suggesting that early inhibition of the PD-1 axis may be necessary to generate appropriate antitumor responses. A similar benefit for concurrent RT and immune therapy was seen in a study of 75 melanoma patients treated with SRS (to median 20 Gy) and ICPIs (anti-CTLA4 or anti-PD1) for brain metastases, where patients receiving concurrent therapy had a greater reduction in lesion size at 6 months compared with nonconcurrent therapy.[41] A separate retrospective analysis of more than 750 patients treated with ICPIs and RT across a range of metastatic solid tumors showed improvement in overall survival (OS) with concurrent RT + ICPIs.[42]

Less clear, however, is the benefit of concurrent versus sequential radiation and immune checkpoint blockade in the definitive or locally advanced setting. Initial results from the PACIFIC trial demonstrated a significant improvement in progression-free survival (PFS) and OS in patients with stage III non–small cell lung cancer (NSCLC) who were treated with chemoradiation, followed by consolidation durvalumab (anti–PD-L1) starting 1 day to 42 days post-RT.[43,44] Although treatment was administered sequentially, post hoc analyses demonstrated patients who received ICPIs closer to chemoradiation (within 14 days) tended to derive greater benefit from anti–PD-L1 therapy compared with those who received ICPIs later.

Preclinical trials have suggested that optimal timing of RT and immunotherapy may depend on the type of immunotherapy administered. For example, in murine colorectal cancer models treated to 20 Gy in a single fraction in combination with anti-CTLA4 or OX40-stimulating agents, the optimal timing of anti-CTLA4 therapy was 7 days prior to RT, whereas the optimal timing for OX40-directed therapy was 1 day after RT.[45] The mechanism of action of the particular immunotherapy agent combined with radiotherapy will likely have an impact on the appropriate timing of therapy for optimal response.

Dose and Fractionation Schedule

Recent decades have witnessed a shift in practice patterns toward shorter RT courses and higher-dose stereotactic treatments. Conventional fractionation schedules (ie, 1.8–2 Gy given over several weeks) remains common, however, especially when administering upfront treatment. The fractionation most suited to use in combination with ICPIs remains an open question and is likely dependent on the clinical setting.[46] Preclinical melanoma mice models treated to either 15 Gy in a single fraction or 3 Gy in 5 fractions both showed the capacity to enhance T-cell trafficking into the tumor microenvironment, but the single-dose fraction resulted in a greater number of TILs.[47] When combined with ICPIs, mouse models of breast carcinoma treated to distinct regimens (20 Gy × 1, 8 Gy × 3, and 6 Gy × 5) alongside anti-CTLA4 have indicated that the abscopal effect was elicited only in fractionated and not single-dose RT regimens.[29] Recently, the DNA exonuclease Trex1 was identified as a negative regulator of RT-induced tumor immunogenicity that counteracts the STING pathway by degrading double-stranded DNA (dsDNA). In cancer cell lines, Trex1 is induced at approximately 12 Gy to 18 Gy.[30] At RT doses that avoid Trex1 induction (ie, 8 Gy × 3), dsDNA accumulates inside cancer cells and activates the type I interferon pathway via STING and promotes antitumor immunity. At higher doses (ie, 20 Gy ×1), however, Trex1 is activated, causing dsDNA to be cleared from the cytosol and prevents interferon beta release by the tumor. As these preclinical studies demonstrate, RT dose and fractionation significantly influence the immune effects of targeted radiotherapy.

There also are concerns that conventionally fractionated RT may induce peripheral lymphopenia that could limit the efficacy of ICPIs, especially RT fields incorporate the draining lymph nodes. For instance, patients receiving both RT and ICPIs without intervening chemotherapy often were found to have decreases in absolute lymphocyte count, and patients who developed severe lymphopenia prior to ICPIs initiation had inferior survival.[48] In addition, preclinical models demonstrate that when draining lymph nodes are included in the treatment field, the absolute number of TILs in tumor microenvironment is reduced.[49]

Selecting Appropriate Disease Types and Disease Burden

At present, multiple efforts are working to combine RT and immune therapy in both early-stage and metastatic disease, and it is unclear in which settings the combination will prove most efficacious. Currently, SABR is used predominantly for patients with advanced metastatic disease or in stage I nonoperable NSCLC.[7] As such, a majority of ongoing combination SABR and ICPI trials assessing safety and efficacy are conducted in the metastatic setting. There is evidence to suggest, however, that patients with earlier-stage disease and reduced tumor burden may be particularly responsive to ICPIs. For instance, melanoma and head and neck cancer patients with higher tumor burden have been shown to respond more poorly to ICPIs[50,51] and preoperative studies conducted in patients with limited burden of disease also have demonstrated promising response rates (RRs) in patients with NSCLC and bladder cancer.[52,53]

The relationship between burden of disease and immunotherapy response may be explained by a study that examined factors affecting reinvigoration of exhausted T cells in patients with metastatic melanoma on anti–PD-1 therapy.[54] Their finding that the ratio of T-cell reinvigoration to tumor burden was directly correlated to PFS suggests that patients with lower tumor burden have more active antitumor immunity compared with those with higher tumor burden. This effect may also, at least in part, explain the deviations from proportional hazards assumptions observed in immunotherapy trials, because there likely exists a population of nonresponding patients who demonstrate early progression as a result of more massive and quickly progressive disease.[55] This suggests a potential value to more tumoricidal therapies, such as RT or chemotherapy, preceding or in conjunction with the start of ICPIs as a means to increase the opportunity for ICPIs' effectiveness.[56]

Thus, there is significant opportunity to expand the range of patients who may benefit from RT when paired with an effective class of systemic therapy, such as immunotherapy. RT is playing a more important role in the treatment of patients with oligometastatic disease.[10,11,57] RT also could be systematically tested in combination with ICPIs in cases of oligoprogression, where patients exhibit isolated sites of progression while receiving immune checkpoint blockade.[58] For instance, in the authors' retrospective experience, 25 of 59 (42%) patients who received palliative RT after progressing on PD-1 therapy were found able to remain on anti–PD-1 therapy for a median of 5.9 months. Patients who remained on ICPIs after palliative RT demonstrated prolonged survival.[59] In such patients, RT could address acquired or isolated resistance by ablating focal areas of ICPI resistance, thereby allowing for continued effective systemic immune therapy.[60,61]

Monitoring Patterns of Response and Toxicity

Patterns of response to ICPIs also are distinct compared with chemotherapy or RT. Approximately 10% of melanoma patients treated with ICPIs were seen to exhibit pseudoprogression, where the tumor appears radiologically larger after initiation of therapy and then shrinks on subsequent scans.[62] This is likely related to tumor-associated edema, but the true rates of pseudoprogression were noted to be much lower in other malignancies (ie, NSCLC and head and neck squamous cell carcinoma).[51,63] In trials where the primary or metastatic lesion is receiving RT + ICPIs, the rates of pseudoprogression may change given RT can elicit a significant inflammatory response at the targeted site.[64]

RT often is administered with the goal of achieving locoregional control either as the primary treatment or in the adjuvant setting. When the aim of RT is to elicit systemic antitumor immunity, however, combination RT + ICPI trials may assess improvements in RRs, PFS, and OS.[65] Although OS is the gold standard, the shorter follow-up is needed to make RR and PFS attractive surrogates. PFS endpoints, however, often do not adequately capture the benefits offered by ICPIs, even when there is an ultimate benefit in OS.[66] Combination trials also should clearly delineate how irradiated lesions are incorporated into these measurements because it is important to identify potential synergies in local as well as systemic responses.

Regulatory agencies also are increasingly mandating the inclusion of patient-reported outcomes in oncology trials. Given the significant toxicity that can result from definitive RT or chemoradiation approaches, the inclusion of patient-reported outcomes may help establish a role for immunotherapy-based approaches based on their potential to decrease toxicity. For instance, in CheckMate 141, there were significant decreases in toxicity reported by patients (dyspnea, appetite loss, and social functioning) in using nivolumab compared with chemotherapy (methotrexate, docetaxel, or cetuximab).[67]

With further regard to toxicity, there is a growing literature that suggests that the combination of RT and ICPI is generally well tolerated.[58] For example, large retrospective series of 133 patients receiving focal palliative RT (median 22.5 Gy in 1–6 doses) and CTLA-4 and/or PD-1 blockade indicated that combined therapy did not suggest a higher rate of key immune-mediated toxicities, such as pneumonitis or colitis, even when RT was administered in conjunction with ICPIs and the RT fields overlapped the lung or bowel.[68] Other retrospective studies have been similarly reassuring in terms of rates of immune-mediated toxicity.[69,70] Similarly, a growing number of prospective trials have also demonstrated ICPIs is well tolerated when given in combination with conventional RT fractionation, hypofractionation, and higher-dose SBRT.[34,44,71] Specifically, in the PACIFIC trial, sequential administration of the PD-L1 inhibitor durvalumab after definitive intent chemoradiation administered to stage III NSCLC patients showed rates of pneumonitis were slightly higher in the durvalumab group (4.8%) compared with placebo (2.6%), but the rates of radiation pneumonitis were similar (1.3%).[44]

Although these safety data generally are reassuring, there remain few data in regard to long-term or RT-specific toxicities. For example, the authors observed a potential increase in symptomatic brain necrosis after the combination of SRS and ICPIs, particularly when ipilimumab was administered in melanoma patients that receive SRS.[72] Another recent study identified higher than expected rates of toxicity when hypofractionated RT was administered in combination with ICPIs in bladder cancer.[73] Additionally, there have been RT recall effects reported when ICPI is administered after the completion of RT.[74]

BARRIERS TO FURTHER DEVELOPMENT OF RADIATION THERAPY AND IMMUNOTHERAPY COMBINATIONS

Given the number of RT parameters and variables related to the immunotherapy agent, trial designs can become unwieldy and impractical. Alternative and novel study designs and biomarker driven trials, therefore, may be helpful to maximize efficiency. For example, innovative dual-agent combination trial designs, such as Product of

Independent beta Probabilities dose Escalation (PIPE) design, can be used to identify optimal doses of agents to be used in combination to advance to phase II studies.[75] PIPE uses probabilities of toxicity for each individual agent and updates them as patient toxicity data are added to arrive at the optimal doses for future study.

There are appreciable economic and structural barriers that hinder combination RT and ICPI development. A majority of ICPI trials are industry sponsored, and designing and conducting RT + ICPIs trials incur higher costs (to provide RT to trial patients) and add complexity (in coordinating care across different providers). A recent analysis of all open trials that administered RT showed that industry-sponsored trials were far less likely to have radiation oncology principal investigators and that radiation oncologists were also far less likely to lead RT + immunotherapy trials.[76] Lack of radiation oncology involvement in the design and execution of RT immunotherapy trials can lead to less input regarding the interplay between radiobiology and ICPI agents. For example, it is difficult to accurately attribute toxicity, such as pneumonitis, without a detailed understanding of the location of the RT fields and RT plan.

Moreover, given the rapid pace of advancement in cancer immunotherapy and the regulatory and oversight burden inherent in running large trials, contract research organizations often are employed to oversee multicenter protocols. Contract research organizations often employ trial monitors with limited cancer or RT expertise and exhibit high personnel turnover.[77] These issues pose difficulty for effective data collection to assess toxicities or identify biomarkers when following patients longitudinally in complex combination protocols across different specialties. Many immunotherapy trials have not collected all the relevant RT information, including sites targeted, doses and fractionation schedules, RT dosing to normal tissues, and so forth. Ensuring appropriate RT quality also is a significant hurdle, and noncompliant RT plans can have substantial effects on OS. For instance, in the TROG 02.02 trial, deficient RT plans were associated with a 20% reduction in OS.[78] In addition, pharmaceutical companies often are seeking regulatory approval across multiple countries. Therefore, RT + ICPI protocols may presuppose easy access to RT in different geographies, which currently is not the case.[79] Differences in RT equipment and standards for RT dose fractionation regimens may differ substantially between countries.[80]

Many of these issues, however, are surmountable (**Fig. 2**). Radiation oncologists must be encouraged to take greater leadership roles in designing combination RT immunotherapy protocols. National Cancer Institute (NCI)-funded trials and cooperative group trials can remain active proponents of testing RT and immunotherapy strategies together rather than focusing on single-modality and drug-only trials. With regard to trial costs, it has been well established that RT is a cost-effective treatment modality, and SABR has been shown to be even more cost saving, providing benefits for payors and hospitals systems in a value-based reimbursement setting.[81] Innovative trial designs, such as PIPE or flip-flop, also can drive down trial costs to help accelerate enrollment, data collection, and regulatory approval timelines.[82] For instance, in FLIP-FLOP, patients are recruited to 2 parallel streams in which different novels agents (drug A and drug B) are combined with radiation. Closure of a cohort in the drug A study track triggers opening of recruitment to the drug B study track (and vice versa). This design avoids gaps in patient recruitment by ensuring that recruitment to either track is always open as doses are escalated.

These benefits should be emphasized by professional societies in promoting development of combination protocols. During trial enrollment and monitoring, CROs and their representatives should be provided basic knowledge about the radiation oncology workflow. Quality control and assurance procedures should be streamlined

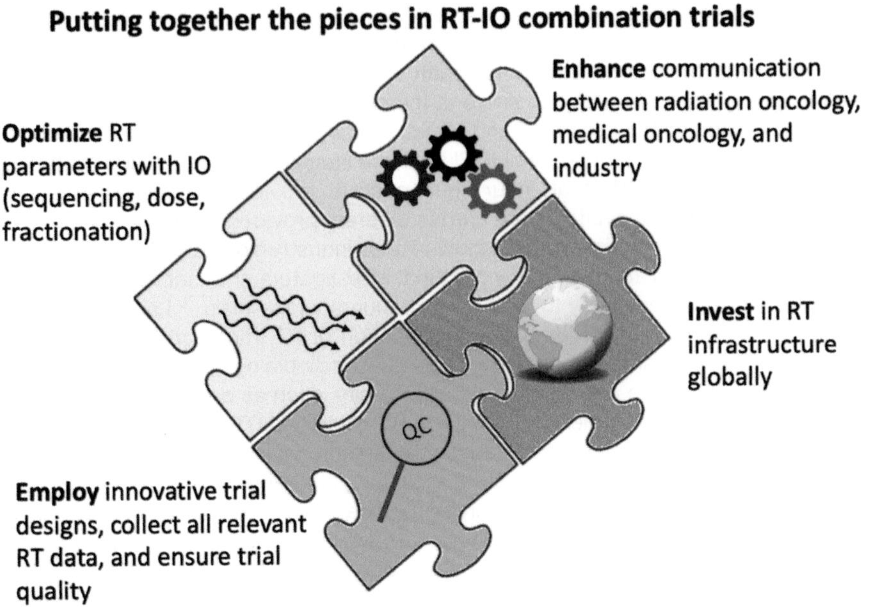

Putting together the pieces in RT-IO combination trials

Optimize RT parameters with IO (sequencing, dose, fractionation)

Enhance communication between radiation oncology, medical oncology, and industry

Invest in RT infrastructure globally

Employ innovative trial designs, collect all relevant RT data, and ensure trial quality

Fig. 2. Key strategies to help ensure the success of future RT-IO combination trials. IO, immuno-oncology; QC, quality control.

and consistent across trial sites and follow recommendations provided by the RT Global Quality Assurance of Radiation Therapy Clinical Trials Group.[83] Lastly, efforts should be undertaken to address the global shortfall in access to RT.[79]

SUMMARY

Rational combination of immunotherapy with RT holds significant promise in improving outcomes for patients. Key to furthering these multimodality treatment strategies will be developing understanding the immunologic and genetic mechanisms that underpin the efficacy of different therapies and developing relevant biomarkers that pinpoint the populations that may derive the greatest benefit from this combined approach.

Questions remain regarding the timing, dose, and fractionation of RT to use in combination with immunotherapy agents and the most preferable disease setting to test combination strategies, but these questions also represent opportunities for future collaborative trials. Collaborative effort between medical oncology, radiation oncology, industry, the NCI, cooperative groups, and other stakeholders is required to address these open questions and to mitigate structural barriers that hinder the execution of combination RT + ICPI trials.

REFERENCES

1. Schadendorf D, Hodi FS, Robert C, et al. Pooled analysis of long-term survival data from phase II and phase III trials of ipilimumab in unresectable or metastatic melanoma. J Clin Oncol 2015;33(17):1889–94.
2. Ferris RL, Blumenschein G Jr, Fayette J, et al. Nivolumab for recurrent squamous-cell carcinoma of the head and neck. N Engl J Med 2016;375(19):1856–67.

3. Motzer RJ, Escudier B, McDermott DF, et al. Nivolumab versus Everolimus in advanced renal-cell carcinoma. N Engl J Med 2015;373(19):1803–13.

4. Garon EB, Rizvi NA, Hui R, et al. Pembrolizumab for the treatment of non-small-cell lung cancer. N Engl J Med 2015;372(21):2018–28.

5. Bellmunt J, de Wit R, Vaughn DJ, et al. Pembrolizumab as second-line therapy for advanced urothelial carcinoma. N Engl J Med 2017;376(11):1015–26.

6. Le DT, Uram JN, Wang H, et al. PD-1 blockade in tumors with mismatch-repair deficiency. N Engl J Med 2015;372(26):2509–20.

7. Bernstein MB, Krishnan S, Hodge JW, et al. Immunotherapy and stereotactic ablative radiotherapy (ISABR): a curative approach? Nat Rev Clin Oncol 2016; 13(8):516–24.

8. Garibaldi C, Jereczek-Fossa BA, Marvaso G, et al. Recent advances in radiation oncology. Ecancermedicalscience 2017;11:785.

9. Topalian SL, Hodi FS, Brahmer JR, et al. Safety, activity, and immune correlates of anti-PD-1 antibody in cancer. N Engl J Med 2012;366(26):2443–54.

10. Gomez DR, Blumenschein GR Jr, Lee JJ, et al. Local consolidative therapy versus maintenance therapy or observation for patients with oligometastatic non-small-cell lung cancer without progression after first-line systemic therapy: a multicentre, randomised, controlled, phase 2 study. Lancet Oncol 2016; 17(12):1672–82.

11. Parker CC, James ND, Brawley CD, et al. Radiotherapy to the primary tumour for newly diagnosed, metastatic prostate cancer (STAMPEDE): a randomised controlled phase 3 trial. Lancet 2018;392(10162):2353–66.

12. Tang J, Yu JX, Hubbard-Lucey VM, et al. Trial watch: The clinical trial landscape for PD1/PDL1 immune checkpoint inhibitors. Nat Rev Drug Discov 2018;17(12): 854–5.

13. Formenti SC, Demaria S. Combining radiotherapy and cancer immunotherapy: a paradigm shift. J Natl Cancer Inst 2013;105(4):256–65.

14. Ngwa W, Irabor OC, Schoenfeld JD, et al. Using immunotherapy to boost the abscopal effect. Nat Rev Cancer 2018;18(5):313–22.

15. Gameiro SR, Jammeh ML, Wattenberg MM, et al. Radiation-induced immunogenic modulation of tumor enhances antigen processing and calreticulin exposure, resulting in enhanced T-cell killing. Oncotarget 2014;5(2):403–16.

16. Gameiro SR, Ardiani A, Kwilas A, et al. Radiation-induced survival responses promote immunogenic modulation to enhance immunotherapy in combinatorial regimens. Oncoimmunology 2014;3:e28643.

17. Leone P, Shin EC, Perosa F, et al. MHC class I antigen processing and presenting machinery: organization, function, and defects in tumor cells. J Natl Cancer Inst 2013;105(16):1172–87.

18. Reits EA, Hodge JW, Herberts CA, et al. Radiation modulates the peptide repertoire, enhances MHC class I expression, and induces successful antitumor immunotherapy. J Exp Med 2006;203(5):1259–71.

19. Garnett CT, Palena C, Chakraborty M, et al. Sublethal irradiation of human tumor cells modulates phenotype resulting in enhanced killing by cytotoxic T lymphocytes. Cancer Res 2004;64(21):7985–94.

20. Wan S, Pestka S, Jubin RG, et al. Chemotherapeutics and radiation stimulate MHC class I expression through elevated interferon-beta signaling in breast cancer cells. PLoS One 2012;7(3):e32542.

21. Sato H, Suzuki Y, Ide M, et al. HLA class I expression and its alteration by preoperative hyperthermo-chemoradiotherapy in patients with rectal cancer. PLoS One 2014;9(9):e108122.

22. Deng L, Liang H, Xu M, et al. STING-dependent cytosolic DNA sensing promotes radiation-induced type I interferon-dependent antitumor immunity in immunogenic tumors. Immunity 2014;41(5):843–52.

23. Harding SM, Benci JL, Irianto J, et al. Mitotic progression following DNA damage enables pattern recognition within micronuclei. Nature 2017;548(7668):466–70.

24. Sridharan V, Margalit DN, Lynch SA, et al. Definitive chemoradiation alters the immunologic landscape and immune checkpoints in head and neck cancer. Br J Cancer 2016;115(2):252–60.

25. Kovacs C. Cytokine profiles in patients receiving wide-field + prostate boost radiotherapy (xRT) for adenocarcinoma of the prostate. Cytokine 2003;23(6):151–63.

26. Miyamoto Y, Hosotani R, Doi R, et al. Interleukin-6 inhibits radiation induced apoptosis in pancreatic cancer cells. Anticancer Res 2001;21(4a):2449–56.

27. Matsumura S, Demaria S. Up-regulation of the pro-inflammatory chemokine CXCL16 is a common response of tumor cells to ionizing radiation. Radiat Res 2010;173(4):418–25.

28. Zhang X, Niedermann G. Abscopal effects with hypofractionated schedules extending into the effector phase of the tumor-specific T-Cell response. Int J Radiat Oncol Biol Phys 2018;101(1):63–73.

29. Dewan MZ, Galloway AE, Kawashima N, et al. Fractionated but not single-dose radiotherapy induces an immune-mediated abscopal effect when combined with anti-CTLA-4 antibody. Clin Cancer Res 2009;15(17):5379–88.

30. Vanpouille-Box C, Alard A, Aryankalayil MJ, et al. DNA exonuclease Trex1 regulates radiotherapy-induced tumour immunogenicity. Nat Commun 2017;8:15618.

31. Koontz BF, Verhaegen F, De Ruysscher D. Tumour and normal tissue radiobiology in mouse models: how close are mice to mini-humans? Br J Radiol 2017;90(1069):20160441.

32. Sharabi AB, Nirschl CJ, Kochel CM, et al. Stereotactic radiation therapy augments antigen-specific PD-1-mediated antitumor immune responses via cross-presentation of tumor antigen. Cancer Immunol Res 2015;3(4):345–55.

33. Formenti SC, Rudqvist NP, Golden E, et al. Radiotherapy induces responses of lung cancer to CTLA-4 blockade. Nat Med 2018;24(12):1845–51.

34. Twyman-Saint Victor C, Rech AJ, Maity A, et al. Radiation and dual checkpoint blockade activate non-redundant immune mechanisms in cancer. Nature 2015;520(7547):373–7.

35. Parikh F, Duluc D, Imai N, et al. Chemoradiotherapy-induced upregulation of PD-1 antagonizes immunity to HPV-related oropharyngeal cancer. Cancer Res 2014;74(24):7205–16.

36. Schmidt MA, Fortsch C, Schmidt M, et al. Circulating regulatory T cells of cancer patients receiving radiochemotherapy may be useful to individualize cancer treatment. Radiother Oncol 2012;104(1):131–8.

37. Galon J, Costes A, Sanchez-Cabo F, et al. Type, density, and location of immune cells within human colorectal tumors predict clinical outcome. Science 2006;313(5795):1960–4.

38. Hellmann MD, Ciuleanu TE, Pluzanski A, et al. Nivolumab plus Ipilimumab in lung cancer with a high tumor mutational burden. N Engl J Med 2018;378(22):2093–104.

39. Morisada M, Clavijo PE, Moore E, et al. PD-1 blockade reverses adaptive immune resistance induced by high-dose hypofractionated but not low-dose daily fractionated radiation. Oncoimmunology 2018;7(3):e1395996.

40. Dovedi SJ, Adlard AL, Lipowska-Bhalla G, et al. Acquired resistance to fractionated radiotherapy can be overcome by concurrent PD-L1 blockade. Cancer Res 2014;74(19):5458–68.

41. Qian JM, Yu JB, Kluger HM, et al. Timing and type of immune checkpoint therapy affect the early radiographic response of melanoma brain metastases to stereotactic radiosurgery. Cancer 2016;122(19):3051–8.

42. Samstein R, Rimner A, Barker CA, et al. Combined immune checkpoint blockade and radiation therapy: timing and dose fractionation associated with greatest survival duration among over 750 treated patients. Int J Radiat Oncol Biol Phys 2017; 99(2):S129–30.

43. Antonia SJ, Villegas A, Daniel D, et al. Durvalumab after chemoradiotherapy in stage III non-small-cell lung cancer. N Engl J Med 2017;377(20):1919–29.

44. Antonia SJ, Villegas A, Daniel D, et al. Overall survival with durvalumab after chemoradiotherapy in stage III NSCLC. N Engl J Med 2018;379(24):2342–50.

45. Young KH, Baird JR, Savage T, et al. Optimizing timing of immunotherapy improves control of tumors by hypofractionated radiation therapy. PLoS One 2016;11(6):e0157164.

46. Wang Y, Deng W, Li N, et al. Combining immunotherapy and radiotherapy for cancer treatment: current challenges and future directions. Front Pharmacol 2018;9:185.

47. Lugade AA, Moran JP, Gerber SA, et al. Local radiation therapy of B16 melanoma tumors increases the generation of tumor antigen-specific effector cells that traffic to the tumor. J Immunol 2005;174(12):7516–23.

48. Pike LRG, Bang A, Mahal BA, et al. The impact of radiation therapy on lymphocyte count and survival in metastatic cancer patients receiving pd-1 immune checkpoint inhibitors. Int J Radiat Oncol Biol Phys 2019;103(1):142–51.

49. Marciscano AE, Nirschl TR, Francica BJ, et al. Does prophylactic nodal irradiation inhibit potential synergy between radiation therapy and immunotherapy? Int J Radiat Oncol Biol Phys 2016;96(2):S88.

50. Wang X, Feng Y, Bajaj G, et al. Quantitative characterization of the exposure-response relationship for cancer immunotherapy: a case study of nivolumab in patients with advanced melanoma. CPT Pharmacometrics Syst Pharmacol 2017;6(1):40–8.

51. Sridharan V, Rahman RM, Huang RY, et al. Radiologic predictors of immune checkpoint inhibitor response in advanced head and neck squamous cell carcinoma. Oral Oncol 2018;85:29–34.

52. Necchi A, Anichini A, Raggi D, et al. Pembrolizumab as neoadjuvant therapy before radical cystectomy in patients with muscle-invasive urothelial bladder carcinoma (PURE-01): an open-label, single-arm, phase II study. J Clin Oncol 2018; 36(34):3353–60.

53. Forde PM, Chaft JE, Smith KN, et al. Neoadjuvant PD-1 blockade in resectable lung cancer. N Engl J Med 2018;378(21):1976–86.

54. Huang AC, Postow MA, Orlowski RJ, et al. T-cell invigoration to tumour burden ratio associated with anti-PD-1 response. Nature 2017;545(7652):60–5.

55. Alexander BM, Schoenfeld JD, Trippa L. Hazards of hazard ratios - deviations from model assumptions in immunotherapy. N Engl J Med 2018;378(12):1158–9.

56. Schoenfeld JD. We are all connected: modeling the tumor-immune ecosystem. Trends Cancer 2018;4(10):655–7.

57. Iyengar P, Wardak Z, Gerber DE, et al. Consolidative radiotherapy for limited metastatic non-small-cell lung cancer: a phase 2 randomized clinical trial. JAMA Oncol 2018;4(1):e173501.

58. Bang A, Schoenfeld JD. Immunotherapy and radiotherapy for metastatic cancers. Ann Palliat Med 2019;8(3):312–25.

59. Pike LRG, Bang A, Ott P, et al. Radiation and PD-1 inhibition: favorable outcomes after brain-directed radiation. Radiother Oncol 2017;124(1):98–103.

60. Mansfield AS, Aubry MC, Moser JC, et al. Temporal and spatial discordance of programmed cell death-ligand 1 expression and lymphocyte tumor infiltration between paired primary lesions and brain metastases in lung cancer. Ann Oncol 2016;27(10):1953–8.

61. Anagnostou V, Smith KN, Forde PM, et al. Evolution of neoantigen landscape during immune checkpoint blockade in non-small cell lung cancer. Cancer Discov 2017;7(3):264–76.

62. Hodi FS, Hwu WJ, Kefford R, et al. Evaluation of immune-related response criteria and RECIST v1.1 in patients with advanced melanoma treated with pembrolizumab. J Clin Oncol 2016;34(13):1510–7.

63. Nishino M, Dahlberg SE, Adeni AE, et al. Tumor response dynamics of advanced non-small cell lung cancer patients treated with PD-1 inhibitors: imaging markers for treatment outcome. Clin Cancer Res 2017;23(19):5737–44.

64. Sridharan V, Schoenfeld JD. Immune effects of targeted radiation therapy for cancer. Discov Med 2015;19(104):219–28.

65. Sharma RA, Plummer R, Stock JK, et al. Clinical development of new drug-radiotherapy combinations. Nat Rev Clin Oncol 2016;13(10):627–42.

66. Hodi FS, O'Day SJ, McDermott DF, et al. Improved survival with ipilimumab in patients with metastatic melanoma. N Engl J Med 2010;363(8):711–23.

67. Harrington KJ, Ferris RL, Blumenschein G Jr, et al. Nivolumab versus standard, single-agent therapy of investigator's choice in recurrent or metastatic squamous cell carcinoma of the head and neck (CheckMate 141): health-related quality-of-life results from a randomised, phase 3 trial. Lancet Oncol 2017;18(8):1104–15.

68. Bang A, Wilhite TJ, Pike LRG, et al. Multicenter evaluation of the tolerability of combined treatment with PD-1 and CTLA-4 immune checkpoint inhibitors and palliative radiation therapy. Int J Radiat Oncol Biol Phys 2017;98(2):344–51.

69. Shaverdian N, Lisberg AE, Bornazyan K, et al. Previous radiotherapy and the clinical activity and toxicity of pembrolizumab in the treatment of non-small-cell lung cancer: a secondary analysis of the KEYNOTE-001 phase 1 trial. Lancet Oncol 2017;18(7):895–903.

70. Hwang WL, Niemierko A, Hwang KL, et al. Clinical outcomes in patients with metastatic lung cancer treated with PD-1/PD-L1 inhibitors and thoracic radiotherapy. JAMA Oncol 2018;4(2):253–5.

71. Luke JJ, Lemons JM, Karrison TG, et al. Safety and clinical activity of pembrolizumab and multisite stereotactic body radiotherapy in patients with advanced solid tumors. J Clin Oncol 2018;36(16):1611–8.

72. Martin AM, Cagney DN, Catalano PJ, et al. Immunotherapy and symptomatic radiation necrosis in patients with brain metastases treated with stereotactic radiation. JAMA Oncol 2018;4(8):1123–4.

73. Tree AC, Jones K, Hafeez S, et al. Dose-limiting urinary toxicity with pembrolizumab combined with weekly hypofractionated radiation therapy in bladder cancer. Int J Radiat Oncol Biol Phys 2018;101(5):1168–71.

74. Shibaki R, Akamatsu H, Fujimoto M, et al. Nivolumab induced radiation recall pneumonitis after two years of radiotherapy. Ann Oncol 2017;28(6):1404–5.

75. Mander AP, Sweeting MJ. A product of independent beta probabilities dose escalation design for dual-agent phase I trials. Stat Med 2015;34(8):1261–76.

76. Giacalone NJ, Milani N, Rawal B, et al. Funding support and principal investigator leadership of oncology clinical trials using radiation therapy. Int J Radiat Oncol Biol Phys 2018;102(1):34–43.
77. Roberts DA, Kantarjian HM, Steensma DP. Contract research organizations in oncology clinical research: challenges and opportunities. Cancer 2016;122(10):1476–82.
78. Peters LJ, O'Sullivan B, Giralt J, et al. Critical impact of radiotherapy protocol compliance and quality in the treatment of advanced head and neck cancer: results from TROG 02.02. J Clin Oncol 2010;28(18):2996–3001.
79. Atun R, Jaffray DA, Barton MB, et al. Expanding global access to radiotherapy. Lancet Oncol 2015;16(10):1153–86.
80. Zubizarreta E, Van Dyk J, Lievens Y. Analysis of global radiotherapy needs and costs by geographic region and income level. Clin Oncol 2017;29(2):84–92.
81. Hodges JC, Lotan Y, Boike TP, et al. Cost-effectiveness analysis of stereotactic body radiation therapy versus intensity-modulated radiation therapy: an emerging initial radiation treatment option for organ-confined prostate cancer. J Oncol Pract 2012;8(3 Suppl):e31s–7s.
82. Harrington KJ, Billingham LJ, Brunner TB, et al. Guidelines for preclinical and early phase clinical assessment of novel radiosensitisers. Br J Cancer 2011;105(5):628–39.
83. Melidis C, Bosch WR, Izewska J, et al. Radiation therapy quality assurance in clinical trials–Global Harmonisation Group. Radiother Oncol 2014;111(3):327–9.

Nanotechnology in Radiation Oncology

Bo Sun, PhD[a], C. Tilden Hagan IV, BSE[b], Joseph Caster, MD, PhD[c],
Andrew Z. Wang, MD[d],*

KEYWORDS

- Nanoparticles • Radiosensitization • Radiotherapy • Tumor imaging
- Cancer biomarkers • Liquid biopsy • Circulating tumor cells • Circulating tumor DNA

KEY POINTS

- Nanoparticles can facilitate the delivery of contrast agents and thus obtain better radiographic imaging with high sensitivity and specificity.
- Nanotherapeutics serves as a complement to conventional radiotherapy by providing high antitumor efficacy with manageable toxicities.
- Nanoparticles made with high Z materials can serve as radiosensitizers and improve the therapeutic outcomes of radiotherapy.
- CapioCyte is a system that integrates nanotechnology and biomimicry, which significantly improve the sensitivity and specificity of the capture of circulating tumor cells in clinical pilot studies.
- Analysis of circulating tumor cells can have a profound impact on conventional cancer management, and its clinical translation as an indispensable assay to current methodologies is rapidly approaching.

INTRODUCTION

Clinical medicine has been a continually progressing branch of science that incorporates breakthrough technologies from multiple disciplines. Nanotechnology, the manipulation of matter on atomic and molecular scales, has made remarkable contributions in clinical oncology over the past decades. Nanoscale materials bear unique

Disclosure Statement: A.Z. Wang is a cofounder of Capio Biosciences Inc, a biotech startup that is commercializing biomimetic circulating tumor cells detection technology (CapioCyte.
[a] Radiation Oncology, The University of North Carolina at Chapel Hill, 125 Mason Farm Road, Marsico 2236, Chapel Hill, NC 27599, USA; [b] UNC/NCSU Joint Department of Biomedical Engineering, 125 Mason Farm Road, Marsico 2120, Chapel Hill, NC 27599, USA; [c] Radiation Oncology, University of Iowa Carver College of Medicine, 200 Hawkins Drive, Iowa City, IA 52242, USA; [d] Radiation Oncology, The University of North Carolina at Chapel Hill, 101 Manning Drive, Chapel Hill, NC 27599, USA
* Corresponding author.
E-mail address: zawang@med.unc.edu

Hematol Oncol Clin N Am 33 (2019) 1071–1093
https://doi.org/10.1016/j.hoc.2019.08.002
0889-8588/19/© 2019 Elsevier Inc. All rights reserved.

hemonc.theclinics.com

physical and chemical properties that distinguish them from bulk materials and small molecules. Therapeutics and diagnostic tools made with nanomaterials inherit those distinctive properties, including versatile surface functionalization, controlled release, enhanced tumor accumulation, tunable biodistribution, metabolism, and excretion. The surface of nanoparticles (NPs) enables functionalization to achieve tumor targeting effects and better stability in the bloodstream. NPs can be engineered with specific structures and dimensions such that they can encapsulate a variety of poorly water-soluble molecules and also control the in vivo release of payloads. Because of their larger size, NPs preferentially accumulate in tumor tissues with permeable vasculature accompanied by poor lymphatics and are mostly cleared from systemic circulation via hepatic or renal excretion and mononuclear phagocytosis, whereas small molecules are widely distributed to many organs. These characteristics grant NPs superior abilities to deliver therapeutics or imaging agents for radiation oncology.

The development of minimally invasive techniques to detect and monitor cancers remains a major challenge in different stages of cancer management. The study of liquid biopsies has shown great promise in the era of personalized medicine. Compared with tissue biopsies and radiographic imaging approaches, the analysis of circulating tumor cells (CTCs) is a much less invasive method to monitor the dynamic molecular profiles of tumors. Advancing biotechnology has enabled the analysis of CTCs at a higher sensitivity and specificity than before. The translational potential of CTCs as a novel cancer biomarker has been demonstrated in several clinically relevant studies. In this article, the authors summarize the clinical applications of nanomaterials in radiation oncology and discuss the implications of CTCs in cancer detection and monitoring.

NANOTECHNOLOGY IN IMAGING

Medical imaging has been reshaped by advances in nanotechnology. A wide range of materials has been engineered such that they can be incorporated into NPs to deliver or serve as contrast agents for various imaging paradigms. For example, carbon nanotubes (CNTs) have been studied as a versatile nanoplatform for imaging and drug delivery.[1,2] CNTs have been used as vehicles for contrast agents, such as chelated paramagnetic metal ions (Gd^{3+}, Mn^{2+}, and so forth), iron oxide NPs, high Z materials (I^-, Bi^{3+}), and radionuclides ($^{64}Cu^{2+}$, ^{99m}Tc), for different imaging techniques. The application of CNTs has mainly been in preclinical settings owing to the in vivo toxicity of CNTs, which still requires further investigation before significant clinical translation can take place.[2–5] In the past 2 decades, several iron oxide NP products (one of the most extensively investigated contrast agents for MRI and multimodal imaging)[6] have been approved by the Food and Drug Administration (FDA) and European Medicines Agency for imaging of bowel, liver lesions, and lymph node metastases and for therapy for adult anemia with chronic kidney disease. These early compounds are rarely encountered in current practice because most were discontinued because of regulatory and marketing issues after 2005.[6,7] However, there has been a recent resurgence of interest in using iron oxide NPs in ongoing clinical trials attempting to improve the imaging of primary or metastatic tumors with MRI or combined with other imaging techniques (**Table 1**).

Metastases to lymph nodes are one of the most important prognostic indicators for patients with melanoma. Early staging of lymphatic metastases would be critical for the determination of therapeutic strategies and patients' outcomes. However, several drawbacks are associated with current techniques of mapping sentinel lymph nodes (SLNs). Noninvasive imaging techniques, such as computed tomography (CT), MRI,

Table 1
Clinical trials using inorganic nanoparticles

Name	Material/Functionality	Application/Indication	Clinical Trial ID
Feraheme; Rienso; Ferumoxytol	Iron oxide NPs coated with polyglucose sorbitol carboxymethyl ether. Magnetic-field responsive NPs for MRI and multimodal imaging	Childhood brain neoplasm, brain tumors or cerebral metastases	NCT00978562, NCT00103038, NCT00659126
		Bone sarcomas and osteomyelitis	NCT01336803
		Triple-negative breast	NCT01770353
		Head and neck cancer	NCT01895829
		Lymph nodes	NCT01815333
		Lymph node metastases in prostate, bladder and kidney cancers	NCT02141490
		Thyroid cancer	NCT01927887
		Esophageal cancer	NCT02253602
		Whole-body imaging for cancer staging	NCT01542879
Ferumoxtran-10; Combidex; Sineren	Iron oxide NPs coated with dextran. Magnetic-field responsive for MRI imaging	Lymph node metastasis in advanced cervical cancer or endometrial cancer	NCT00416455
AuroLase	Silica-gold nanoshells coated with PEG. Laser responsive	Thermal ablation of solid tumors: head/neck cancer. Primary and/or metastatic lung tumors	NCT00848042, NCT01679470
Sienna+	Iron oxide particles coated with carboxydextran. Magnetic responsive particles use with SentiMag device	Mark and locate cancerous lymph nodes before surgery	NCT01790399, NCT02249208
Magnablate	Iron NPs. Magnetic-field responsive for thermal ablation	Prostate cancer	NCT2033447
Sensors functionalized with gold NPs	Organic functionalized gold NPs	Detection of gastric lesions	NCT01420588

Adapted from Anselmo AC, Mitragotri S. A Review of Clinical Translation of Inorganic Nanoparticles. AAPS J 2015;17(5):1044; with permission.

single-photon emission CT, and PET, are commonly used to locate lymph nodes with abnormal dimensions or increased metabolic activity before surgery.[8,9] However, these imaging methods cannot provide precise 3-dimensional locations of lymph nodes for surgical procedures or differentiate real metastases from abnormalities caused by infection or inflammation. Radionuclide-labeled sulfur colloid and isosulfan blue have also been injected locally to visualize SLNs intraoperatively, but they fail to provide adequate visualization because of their inefficient tissue distribution. Therefore, a new imaging platform for SLN mapping is highly needed.

A silica-based nanoplatform has been developed for cancer imaging with PET.[10] Silica cores were coated with polyethylene glycol (PEG) chains, which were partially end-capped with cyclo-(Arg-Gly-Asp-Tyr) peptides (cRGDY) that target integrin $\alpha_v\beta_3$ expressed by various types of tumors. A positron-emitting radionuclide [124]I was further conjugated to the peptide ligand for quantitative imaging by PET.[11] The clearance half-life of the particles was longer than 30 hours in tumors and major organs in an M21 tumor xenograft murine model. Because of the small size (~7 nm), nearly 50% of the particles were excreted in the first 24 hours after intravenous (IV) injection via renal clearance, and up to 72% was excreted in the next 3 days. Particle accumulation in tumors reached a maximum ~4 hours after injection, and the concentration in tumors was 3-fold higher than with nontargeting control NPs. More particles remained in tumors than muscles 1 to 4 days after injection. When used in a spontaneous melanoma mini-swine model, [124]I-cRGDY-silica NPs showed a higher sensitivity in detecting metastatic nodules and draining lymphatic channels after subdermal injection than fludeoxyglucose F18 (^{18}F-FDG).[9] In addition, [124]I-cRGDY-silica NPs were able to discriminate metastatic tumor burdens from inflammatory and other metabolically active tissues identified by ^{18}F-FDG in mini-swines. These preclinical findings underscored the specific targeting effect of the [124]I-cRGDY-silica NPs in staging metastatic tumors.

The silica-based nanoplatform was further assessed in a microdosing study in patients with metastatic melanoma and malignant brain tumors (NCT01266096).[10] The systemic clearance half-lives ranged from 13 to 21 hours without notable accumulation in the reticuloendothelial system. Consistent with the preclinical study, a large fraction of the particles was cleared via renal excretion over 72 hours. A liver

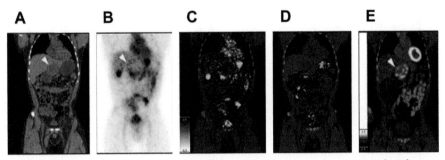

Fig. 1. Whole-body PET-CT imaging of particle biodistribution and tumor uptake after systemic injection of [124]I-cRGDY-PEG-C dots. (*A*) Coronal CT in patient 1 shows hepatic metastasis (*arrowhead*). (*B*) Coronal PET image at 4 hours after injection demonstrates particle activity along the peripheral aspect of the tumor (*arrowhead*). Coregistered PET-CT at (*C*) 4 hours and (*D*) 24 hours after injection. (*E*) Corresponding ^{18}F-FDG PET-CT image showing the hepatic metastasis in (*A*) (*arrowhead*). (*From* Phillips E, Penate-Medina O, Zanzonico PB, et al. Clinical translation of an ultrasmall inorganic optical-PET imaging nanoparticle probe. Sci Transl Med 2014;6(260):149-260; with permission.)

metastasis was seen 4 hours after IV injection of ^{124}I-cRGDY-silica NPs in patient 1, which was consistent with the ^{18}F-FDG PET image (**Fig. 1**). A cystic lesion in the pituitary gland was located in the brain of patient 2, confirming the finding on previous MRI scans (**Fig. 2**). The toxicity of these particle tracers was assessed based on clinical symptoms and laboratory analysis of urine and blood samples. No substantial changes in liver and renal functions were found related to particle injection over 2 weeks of the study. The data in this trial warranted further evaluation in the context of image-guided surgeries and interventions. Currently, these targeted silica NPs loaded with the fluorescent probe Cy5.5 are being evaluated in a phase 1/2 trial for real-time imaging of SLNs during surgical procedures in patients with breast or colorectal cancer or melanoma (NCT02106598).

NANOTHERAPEUTICS TO IMPROVE CHEMORADIOTHERAPY

Chemoradiotherapy (CRT) has played a significant role in the battle against many human cancers but does have limitations. Nanotherapeutics has demonstrated great potential to overcome the limitations in conventional CRT. For example, Abraxane is a nanoparticle albumin-bound paclitaxel (nab-PTX), which was developed to improve

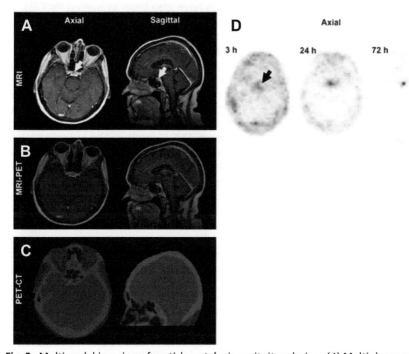

Fig. 2. Multimodal imaging of particle uptake in a pituitary lesion. (*A*) Multiplanar contrast-enhanced MR axial and sagittal images of patient 2 at 72 hours after injection demonstrate a subcentimeter cystic focus (*arrows*) within the right aspect of the anterior pituitary gland. (*B*) Coregistered axial and sagittal MRI-PET images reveal increased focal activity (*red*; 124I-cRGDY-PEG-C dots) localized to the lesion site. (*C*) Axial and sagittal PET-CT images localize activity to the right aspect of the sella. (*D*) Axial PET images of ^{124}I-cRGDY-PEG-C dots in the brain at 3, 24, and 72 hours after injection demonstrate progressive accumulation of activity within the sellar region. (*Adapted from* Phillips E, Penate-Medina O, Zanzonico PB, et al. Clinical translation of an ultrasmall inorganic optical-PET imaging nanoparticle probe. Sci Transl Med 2014;6(260):149-260; with permission.)

the antitumor efficacy of PTX by using enhanced permeability and retention (EPR) effects in tumor tissue while avoiding the excipient-related toxicities of Taxol. nab-PTX has been used concurrently with cisplatin and radiotherapy (RT) in a phase 2 trial (ChiCTR-ONC-12002615) in patients with locally advanced nasopharyngeal carcinoma.[12] Thirty complete responses and 6 partial responses were observed among 36 patients after 2 cycles of concurrent CRT using nab-PTX. The progression-free survival and cancer-specific survival rates were 86% and 92%, respectively, at the median follow-up time of 45 months. The combination of nab-PTX and CRT showed encouraging antitumor efficacy with manageable toxicities, warranting phase 3 trials of this regimen. nab-PTX plus gemcitabine has also been evaluated in an early phase 1 trial to determine the recommended dose with concurrent RT for patients with borderline resectable pancreatic cancer.[13] Carboplatin was administered together with nab-PTX weekly for 6 weeks to patients with advanced non–small cell lung cancer (NSCLC) in a phase 1 trial.[14] Thoracic RT was given concurrently at 2 Gy every weekday for the same period of time. Ten out of 14 patients achieved partial response with tolerable toxicity, and 12 patients survived to the median follow-up time of 13 months. Because of these promising outcomes, recent clinical trials have been focused on the treatment paradigm of CRT using nab-PTX (**Table 2**).

Other nanoformulations of anticancer drugs have also been evaluated for CRT. A lipid-mitomycin C (MMC) prodrug was encapsulated in PEGylated liposomes as a radiation-responsive formulation (Promitil) for use in CRT.[15] MMC could be liberated from liposomes after cleavage of a lipid linker in the prodrug by radiation-induced increase in reducing agents in tumors, such as dithiothreitol or cysteine. In a preclinical study using human rectal tumor xenografts, Promitil was combined with RT and 5-fluorouracil (5-FU) and showed more improved antitumor effects than an equivalent dose of free MMC. All mice treated with Promitil and RT survived to the end of this study, whereas all of those treated with the combination of free MMC and RT did not, indicating the attenuated toxicity of liposomal MCC prodrug. The improved tolerance of Promitil was affirmed by a phase 1 clinical study (NCT01705002) in solid tumor patients.[16] A phase 1 clinical study (NCT03823989) is recruiting patients with cancer for combined therapy with Promitil and external beam RT. Nanotherapeutics, such as liposomal doxorubicin and polymer-PTX conjugates, was assessed in clinical trials of CRT; however, they were not adopted in CRT regimens because of a lack of significantly improved outcomes compared with standard therapy and dose-limiting toxicities respectively.[17]

The importance of radiosensitizers has been widely recognized in RT. Some potent radiosensitizers, such as the anticancer drug camptothecin (CPT)[18] and DNA repair inhibitors KU55933[15] and wortmannin (Wtmn),[19] are very toxic when delivered systemically in their free forms. Therefore, NP platforms were developed for these molecules, aiming to evaluate their synergisms with CRT against tumors. Wtmn has been encapsulated in biodegradable NPs together with docetaxel (DTX) or cisplatin to facilitate CRT against lung and prostate cancer.[20] DTX/Wtmn coencapsulated NPs remarkably prolonged the survival time of mice with PC3 xenografts that received RT simultaneously, in contrast to other groups treated with single-drug–loaded NPs or a mixture of 2 single-drug–loaded NPs. In a similar study, Wtmn-loaded NPs reversed Platinum resistance and inhibited tumor growth of A2780 cis xenograft tumors without inducing any significant off-target toxicity.[21] CPT NP-drug conjugates (CRLX101) have also been evaluated as radiosensitizers in murine models grafted with human colorectal cancer cells HT-29 or SW480.[18] When combined with RT, CRLX101 inhibited tumor progress better than 5-FU plus RT in SW480 xenografts. As expected, the combination of CRLX101, 5-FU, and RT showed a higher therapeutic index compared with

Table 2
Clinical trials of nanoparticle albumin-bound paclitaxel combined with radiotherapy

Trial ID	Status	Study Phase	Study Design	Condition	Intervention and Arms
NCT03600623	Recruiting	Early phase 1	Nonrandomized, parallel assignment	Locally advanced pancreatic cancer, borderline pancreatic inoperable cancer, pancreatic cancer	Folfirinox followed by stereotactic body radiotherapy (SBRT); Gemcitabine nab-PTX followed by SBRT
NCT02394535	Recruiting	Phase 1	Single group assignment	Pancreatic adenocarcinoma, stage III pancreatic cancer American Joint Committee on Cancer 6th & 7th editions	Capecitabine, nab-PTX, radiation therapy
NCT03257033	Recruiting	Phase 4	Randomized, parallel assignment	Locally advanced pancreatic cancer	RT followed by intraarterial gemcitabine; RT followed by IV gemcitabine and nab-PTX
NCT02427841	Recruiting	Phase 2	Single group assignment	Pancreatic adenocarcinoma, Resectable pancreatic carcinoma	Preoperative chemotherapy: nab-PTX, gemcitabine HCl, image-guided intensity-modulated radiation therapy, FU Surgical resection Postoperative chemotherapy: nab-PTX, gemcitabine HCl
NCT02207465	Recruiting	Phase 1	Single group assignment	Locally advanced unresectable pancreatic cancer treated with CRT, borderline resectable pancreatic cancer treated with CRT	RT, gemcitabine, nab-PTX
NCT01847326	Recruiting	Phase 1	Single group assignment	Recurrent head and neck cancer	nab-PTX combined with 5-FU and hydroxyurea and radiation for good induction responders; nab-PTX and hypofractionated RT for poor responders
NCT02318095	Active, not recruiting	Not applicable	Single group assignment	Resectable pancreatic cancer	Gemcitabine, nab-PTX, hypofractionated image-guided intensity-modulated radiation therapy, surgical resection
NCT02723331	Recruiting	Phase 2	Nonrandomized, parallel assignment	Pancreatic cancer, Pancreatic adenocarcinoma, Pancreas ductal adenocarcinoma	nab-PTX and gemcitabine followed by SBRT for resectable pancreatic ductal adenocarcinoma; nab-PTX and gemcitabine followed by SBRT for borderline-resectable pancreatic ductal adenocarcinoma

CRLX101 plus RT in HT-29 xenografts. Additional results suggested that CRLX101 was synergistic with 5-FU and outperformed the combination of oxaliplatin and 5-FU in suppressing tumor growth in both HT-29 and SW480 murine xenograft models undergoing RT. Furthermore, CRLX101 had decreased hair and gastrointestinal toxicity in mice compared with CPT. Encouraged by the preclinical study, a phase 1b/2 clinical study (NCT02010567) was carried out to evaluate the toxicity of CRLX101 and its ability to improve therapeutic responses when combined with capecitabine and RT for locally advanced rectal cancer.[22] The results showed that capecitabine-based CRT combined with CRLX101 at 15 mg/m^2 per week was well tolerated with moderate to complete therapeutic responses in 24/32 patients, justifying this regimen for a larger phase 2 trial.[23]

With the advance of immunotherapy, antibody-based approaches have also been combined with RT against cancers. A novel 2-step radioimmunotherapy paradigm has been evaluated preclinically for the treatment of non-Hodgkin lymphoma.[24] In the pretargeting step, Dibenzocyclooctyne (DBCO) functionalized anti-CD20 antibodies (Rituximab) were used to specifically bind Raji B-cell lymphoma cells overexpressing CD20 antigens. Azide-functionalized dendrimers conjugated with radionuclide ^{90}Y were administered to tag those prelabeled lymphoma cells via click chemistry between DBCO and azide in vivo. This pretargeted system achieved a highly specific delivery of radionuclides to tumor cells and concomitantly enhanced the complement-dependent cytotoxicity of antibodies, which inhibited tumor progress in both xenograft and disseminated non-Hodgkin lymphoma xenotransplant murine models. This 2-step pretargeting strategy overcame the challenges in conventional radioimmunotherapy and bears great potential for clinical translation.

INORGANIC NANOPARTICLES AS RADIOSENSITIZERS

Another strategy to improve CRT is to deliver inorganic NPs made of materials with high atomic numbers (Z) into tumor tissues as radiosensitizers. Gold NPs (Z = 79) have been extensively evaluated as a multimodal imaging agent and radiosensitizer with photon, proton, and carbon RT.[25] Despite promising results from preclinical studies, the path toward clinical translation remains a challenge, and the clinical evaluation of gold NPs as radiosensitizers has not begun.

Hafnium NPs (Z = 72), have also been investigated as radiosensitizers and show promise for clinical translation. Hafnium oxide NPs (NBTXR3) are potent radiosensitizers in murine models of sarcoma and colorectal cancers.[26] Nanobiotix has finished a phase 1 clinical trial of NBTXR3 crystalline NPs (NCT01433068), in which all the patients well tolerated NBTXR3 and subsequent RT, demonstrating a good safety profile and encouraging antitumor effect in patients with locally advanced soft tissue sarcoma (STS).[27] Currently, NBTXR3 NPs are being evaluated in a phase 2/3 clinical trial in advanced STS (NCT02379845). Several phase 1/2 clinical trials of NBTXR3 have been conducted for different cancers, such as a combination of NBTXR3 with RT and chemotherapy for patients with rectal cancer and head and neck cancer (NCT02465593, NCT02901483), NBTXR3 and RT for liver cancers (NCT02721056), and NBTXR3 combined with brachytherapy for prostate cancer (NCT02805894).

Gadolinium (Gd, Z = 64)-based NPs (AGuIX) have been constructed with a polysiloxane core and Gd chelated on the surface, aiming to facilitate MRI-guided RT on multiple brain melanoma metastases.[28] These ~3-nm particles were mainly eliminated via renal clearance, and a single bolus injection of AGuIX accumulated quickly in mouse kidneys and was retained in kidneys for less than a week. Weekly IV injections for 3 consecutive weeks only caused transient perturbation on renal function and insignificant tissue alterations in mice. Similar safety profiles were observed in rats and monkeys after weekly IV injections for 2 weeks, suggesting a promising clinical translation.[29–31] When combined with RT, AGuIX demonstrated strong radiosensitizing effects in preclinical animal models with pancreatic cancer, brain melanoma metastases, glioblastoma, head and neck cancer, and lung cancer.[28,30,32–34] Currently, AGuIX NPs are being evaluated in phase 1 and 2 trials for their safety and radiosensitizing effects with whole brain RT for patients with multiple brain melanoma metastases (NCT02820454, NCT03818386).[35]

RADIATION-ENHANCED DRUG DELIVERY USING NANOPARTICLES

Radiation therapy has frequently been used in combination with both chemotherapy and immunotherapeutic NPs. However, several challenges have hindered the transport of NPs through tumor microenvironment (TME), such as long transport distances in tumor extracellular matrix, heterogenous tumor vasculature, and elevated interstitial fluid pressure.[36,37] Local tumor RT has the potential to facilitate the delivery of nanotherapeutics by changing the endothelial architecture, increasing the vascular permeability, and reducing the interstitial fluid pressure in tumor tissues, which collectively enhance the EPR effect.[38] In addition to the primed EPR effect, Miller and colleagues[39,40] have demonstrated that irradiation of tumors could recruit tumor-associated macrophages (TAMs), which would serve as reservoirs of NPs. Radiation-induced TAM enrichment was found near microvasculature in tumor xenografts, eliciting vascular burst and particle uptake in the neighboring tumor cells. When combined with the DNA alkylating agent cyclophosphamide, radiation improved the tumor accumulation of PLGA-BODIPY630, liposomal doxorubicin, and liposomal irinotecan in 4T1 orthotopic tumor models. Improved accumulation was translated into remarkable synergistic inhibiting effects in HT1080 human fibrosarcoma murine models treated with liposomal irinotecan and a 5-Gy dose of radiation compared with each single treatment. However, radiation-enhanced NP delivery would be attenuated if TAMs were depleted with liposomal clodronate from tumor tissues. This study demonstrated that radiation altered the TME and facilitated NP delivery in a TAM-dependent approach. However, the possibility of radioresistance in tumors under fractionated radiation has not been fully evaluated in this study. Furthermore, polarization of TAMs and their interactions with surviving tumor cells, stroma cells, and other immune cells after radiation therapy still needs further investigation.[41]

NANOTECHNOLOGY IN THE DEVELOPMENT OF CANCER BIOMARKERS

Cancer biomarkers are generally defined as biomolecules generated by either tumor cells or other tissues as a response to cancers, and even more broadly they can be biological processes, including angiogenesis, proliferation, and apoptosis.[42,43] Cancer-related biomarkers encompass a broad spectrum of molecules, such as peptides, proteins, metabolites, nucleotides, and lipids, which could be detected in blood, secretions, or biological fluids produced by many organs.[43,44] Even though a large number of candidate biomarkers have been identified and evaluated preclinically, the FDA has only approved approximately 20 cancer biomarkers for clinical use. Most of these are proteins that can be detected in serum, plasma, urine, or feces, with only a small number requiring solid tissue biopsies.[42] Among cancer biomarkers, the tumor circulome is a collection of tumor-derived elements found in the blood circulation, which includes proteins, nucleic acids (DNA and RNA), exosomes, tumor-related platelets, and CTCs.[45,46] The significance of the tumor circulome has been widely recognized in recent decades because it could provide valuable information about primary and metastatic tumors, resistance-related mutations, and therapeutic responses from blood in patients with cancer. Here, the authors highlight the significant applications of circulome in clinical oncology.

CIRCULATING TUMOR DNA AND EXOSOMES

Circulating tumor DNA (ctDNA) is fragmented DNA originated from tumor cells, and its level in the blood is directly correlated with the presence of malignant diseases.[45] ctDNA could be actively secreted by tumor cells or simply liberated from dead tumor cells as free nucleic acids or being encapsulated in extracellular vesicles. CTCs were thought to be another source of ctDNA.[47] Similar to CTCs, ctDNA can be obtained in less invasive methods compared with tissue biopsies, which allows longitudinal monitoring of tumor heterogeneity and multiclonality with high specificity. In addition, ctDNA yields high detection rates and can be found when detectable CTCs are absent in patients.[48,49] Tumor-derived cell-free DNA could also be detected in various bodily fluids other than blood, such as cerebrospinal fluid, saliva, sputum, pleural effusions, urine, and stool,[50] suggesting the presence of local or distant tumors. Because tumor-associated cell-free DNA has multiple sources, preanalytical processing of the sample could be critical for an accurate and sensitive detection. Before sequencing, ctDNA needs enrichment or extraction, which could be accomplished with various commercial kits.[51] The detection of ctDNA usually aims at the alterations in DNA sequence, DNA methylation, and variations of DNA copy number.[52] ctDNA sequencing technologies[51,53] and recent clinical studies[45] have been summarized in the literature.

Tumor-derived exosomes are nanovesicles composed of phospholipid, proteins, and encapsulated nucleic acids.[54] They are secreted by dividing cancer cells and hence carry abundant proteomic and genetic information on primary tumor and TME.[55] Similar to ctDNA, exosomes can be found in large quantities in various bodily fluids and even from tumors, which release sparse amount of CTCs, such as those in the central nervous system.[56–58] The conventional methods of exosome isolation include ultracentrifugation and density-gradient separation, which require extensive processing, making them impractical for clinical implications. Novel techniques can be categorized into size-dependent microfluidic platforms[59] and immunoaffinity-based systems, which isolate exosomes by their specific surface markers.[60] Further characterization and analysis of biomolecules in exosomes were thoroughly discussed in recent reviews.[54,61]

CIRCULATING TUMOR CELLS

Around 90% of the mortality among patients with solid tumors is caused by the formation of metastases rather than primary tumors.[62] The metastatic process starts with the journey of CTCs. After detaching from a primary tumor mass, CTCs migrate toward blood vasculature and intravasate into the circulation where they have to evade immune detection on their way to distant organs. Only surviving CTCs can settle within a favorable tissue and become micrometastases/macrometastases (**Fig. 3**).[63] Preclinical studies suggested that less than 0.01% of CTCs had the chance to survive and eventually form secondary tumors.[64,65] Accumulating evidence has proven a good correlation between CTC counts in blood samples and the disease progression of patients with cancer[66–68] and therefore demonstrated the clinical value of CTCs as a significant biomarker for diagnosis and prognosis of various cancers, including breast,[69] prostate,[70] lung,[71,72] colorectal,[73,74] liver,[75] and pancreatic cancers[76] as well as melanoma.[77]

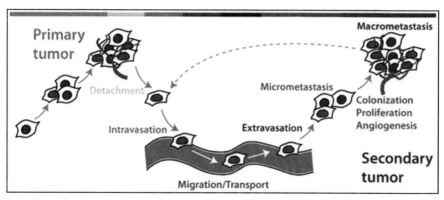

Fig. 3. Metastatic progression of a malignant tumor. (*From* Divoli A, Mendonça EA, Evans JA, et al. Conflicting Biomedical Assumptions for Mathematical Modeling: The Case of Cancer Metastasis. PLOS Comput Biol 2011;7(10): e1002132; with permission.)

Liquid biopsies for CTCs or ctDNA of blood of patients with cancer have remarkable advantages over medical imaging techniques and solid tissue biopsies for cancer diagnosis and prognosis.[47,78] The analysis of the blood sample can be conducted more frequently for patients with cancer than imaging techniques.[79–81] Liquid biopsy samples are collected with a less invasive method from patients and at a lower cost than solid biopsies, which usually generate discomfort, pain, and the possibility of bleeding and infection. Furthermore, CTC analysis can better represent the tumor heterogeneity and real-time information from primary and metastatic tumors than solid biopsies from a single location.[82–84]

However, detection of CTCs is much easier said than done because of their rarity among blood cells. The number of CTCs could be as low as 1 to 10 cells per 10 mL of whole blood from most patients with cancer, which demands detection technologies with high sensitivity and specificity.[85–87] Enrichment of CTCs is a preceding step of detection, and CTCs can be enriched on the basis of their biological and physical properties (**Fig. 4**).[88] CTCs from epithelial tumors can be distinguished from normal blood cells by their surface markers, such as epithelial cell adhesion molecule (EpCAM) and proteins that appear after epithelial-to-mesenchymal transition.[89,90] Anti-epithelial (E) and anti-mesenchymal (M) antibodies are widely used to positively select CTCs from blood cells (see **Fig. 4**A). In addition, CTCs from certain tumors or tissues can be captured by antibodies targeting highly expressed tumor or tissue-specific markers. For example, antibody-dendrimer conjugates were used for the capture of CTCs expressing human epidermal growth factor receptor 2 (HER2) or prostate-specific antigen (PSA) in human blood spiked with breast cancer and prostate cancer cells.[91] A capture efficiency of 82% and purity of 50% to 90% of captured cells had been achieved from blood samples with 1×10^5 tumor cells per milliliter. An alternative approach to select CTCs is based on their physical properties, such as size, deformability, density, and surface charge, in specific media. CTCs are usually larger and stiffer than normal blood cells, allowing them to be trapped in microfilters (see **Fig. 4**C, D).[92] Another size-based cell separation was achieved by flowing samples through a spiral microchannel, where larger CTCs were gradually separated from blood cells by inertial lift and the Dean drag force (see **Fig. 4**G).[93] Furthermore, hematological cells, such as leukocytes and granulocytes, could be separated from CTCs by immunomagnetic beads against leukocyte antigen CD45 or granulocyte marker CD15 (see **Fig. 4**B) after

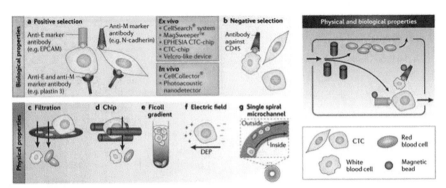

Fig. 4. (*A–G*) CTC enrichment approaches. DEP, dielectrophoresis. (*From* Alix-Panabières C, Pantel K. Challenges in circulating tumour cell research. Nat Rev Cancer 2014;14(9):623-631; with permission.)

red blood cells have been removed by density gradient centrifugation (see **Fig. 4E**).[94] Because of the higher surface area and larger capacitance of CTCs in contrast to normal blood cells, CTCs usually exhibit negative dielectrophoresis and hence could be isolated under a given electric field frequency (see **Fig. 4F**).[95] CTC enrichment technologies and their pros and cons have been summarized previously in literature.[96]

An efficient enrichment of CTCs can be achieved by a combination of biological and physical property-based techniques. Ozkumur and colleagues[97] have developed a microfluidic CTC capture device (CTC-iChip) (**Fig. 5B**), integrating hydrodynamic cell sorting, inertial focusing, and magnetophoresis (**Fig. 5A**). A whole blood sample was first incubated with anti-EpCAM (aEpCAM), anti-CD45, or anti-CD15 antibody conjugated magnetic beads. Red blood cells and platelets were then separated using deterministic lateral displacement based on their size (**Fig. 5C**). The remaining CTCs and white blood cells were aligned after flowing through a microchannel by inertial focusing and entered the channel under magnetic field for further sorting (**Fig. 5D**). Two immunomagnetic sorting options were available for the final isolation, which included positive selection of CTCs and depletion of leukocytes and granulocytes from the presorted blood sample. CTC-iChip outperformed the CellSearch system when used to capture CTCs in patient specimens with low CTC burdens (<4 CTCs per milliliter).

Another new CTC detection platform was built by integrating biomimetic cell rolling and multivalent binding via antibody-dendrimer conjugates.[98] E-selectin is a single-chain transmembrane glycoprotein on the vascular endothelium, which plays a significant role in cell rolling and adhesion with surface ligands on various tumor cells (**Fig. 6A**).[99,100] aEpCAM, a widely used CTC capturing antibody, was immobilized together with recombinant human E-selectin Fc chimera proteins on the capture surface to recruit CTCs and hematological cells from the bulk flow. The addition of E-selectin improved the ability of aEpCAM to recognize and bind tumor cells by greater than 3-fold compared with aEpCAM alone, with hematological cells rolling on the E-selectin surface but not binding aEpCAM. To strengthen the binding and stability between CTCs and aEpCAM or other tumor specific antibodies, such as anti-PSA (aPSA) and anti-HER2 (aHER2), antibodies were conjugated to nanoscale poly(amidoamine) dendrimers anchored on the capture surface instead of direct immobilization on the surface via conventional PEGylation

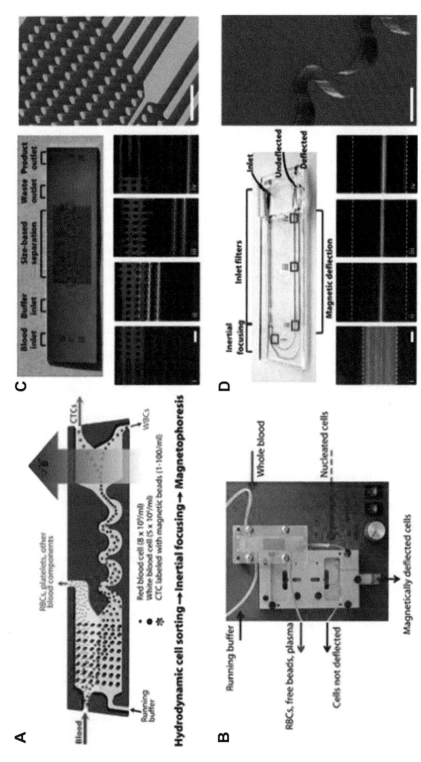

Fig. 5. CTC-iChip. (A) Three microfluidic components of the CTC-iChip are shown schematically. The debulking array sits in a custom polycarbonate manifold that enables fluidic connections to the inputs, waste line, and second-stage microfluidic channels. The inertial

(**Fig. 6**B). To validate this combined technology, MDA-PCa-2b, MCF-7 (low HER2 expression), and MDA-MB-361 (high HER2 expression) cells were added in human blood samples and injected to the flow chamber (**Fig. 6**C). More than 80% capture efficiency and nearly 90% purity were achieved, approximately 10-fold higher than a surface without E-selectin and dendrimers (**Fig. 6**D, E).[91] The result demonstrated a highly efficient CTC enrichment technique with clinical translatability. This CTC capture device (named as CapioCyte), equipped with aEpCAM, aHER2, and aEGFR, has already been used in a clinical study aiming to monitor CTC changes during and after therapy.[101] CapioCyte detected CTCs in all 24 patients and showed a significant decline of median CTC counts in 18 patients, from 113 counts per milliliter before treatment to 32 counts per milliliter at the completion of RT, which demonstrated the sensitivity, specificity, and reliability of CapioCyte. In addition to therapeutic outcomes monitoring, captured CTCs could be expanded and analyzed in vitro, facilitating the discovery of CTC biomarkers and the establishment of in vitro CTC models. CapioCyte is currently a prototype undergoing optimization. This biomimetic platform needs to be validated with more types of cancer and their therapeutic responses. Diverse combinations of capturing agents should be established to tackle tumor heterogeneity and even other biomarkers, including nucleic acids, exosomes, and proteins from patients' specimens.

CLINICAL UTILITY OF CIRCULATING TUMOR CELLS

CTCs can be exploited in many clinical contexts. A direct correlation has been established between the number of CTCs in peripheral blood and the survival of patients with advanced cancers.[66,67,102] The FDA has approved the CellSearch system for the detection of CTCs in clinical specimens from patients with colorectal, prostate, and metastatic breast cancer.[103] Regardless of therapies that patients received, decreased progression-free survival and overall survival were associated with the relatively high level of CTCs in patients' blood samples before treatment. The potential utility of CTCs was expanded to detection and monitoring of melanoma[104] and lung cancer lately.[105–107] In addition, molecular profiling of CTCs can serve as a noninvasive method to genotype tumor during treatment and hence guide the future selection of therapy.[108] In an initial clinical study, DNA analysis of EGFR mutation was performed on CTCs from patients with NSCLC.[109] EGFR activating mutation was detected in CTCs from 92% of patients, among whom drug-resistant mutation

◄─────────────────────────────────────

focusing and magnetophoresis chip is placed in an aluminum manifold that houses the quadrupole magnetic circuit. Magnetically deflected cells are collected in a vial. (*C*) Hydrodynamic size-based sorting. A mixture of 2-mm (*red*) and 10-mm (*green*) beads enters the channel (*i*). Whereas the 2-mm beads remain in laminar flow and follow the fluid streamlines, the 10-mm spheres interact with the postarray (*ii* and *iii*) as shown in the scanning electron microscope (SEM) image (*right panel*). Larger beads are fully deflected into the coincident running buffer stream by the end of the array (*iv*). Scale bars, 100 mm. (*D*) Cell focusing and magnetophoretic sorting. Magnetically labeled SKBR3 (*red*) and unlabeled PC3-9 (*green*) cell populations are mixed and enter the channel in random distribution (*i*). After passing through 60 asymmetric focusing units (pictured in the SEM; *right panel*), the cells align in a single central stream (*ii*). Magnetically tagged cells are then deflected (*iii*) using an external magnetic field, and separation is achieved by the end of the channel (*iv*). Scale bars, 100 mm. RBCs, red blood cells; WBCs, white blood cells. (*From* Ozkumur E, Shah AM, Ciciliano JC, et al. Inertial Focusing for Tumor Antigen-Dependent and -Independent Sorting of Rare Circulating Tumor Cells. Sci Transl Med 2013;5(179):179ra147; with permission.)

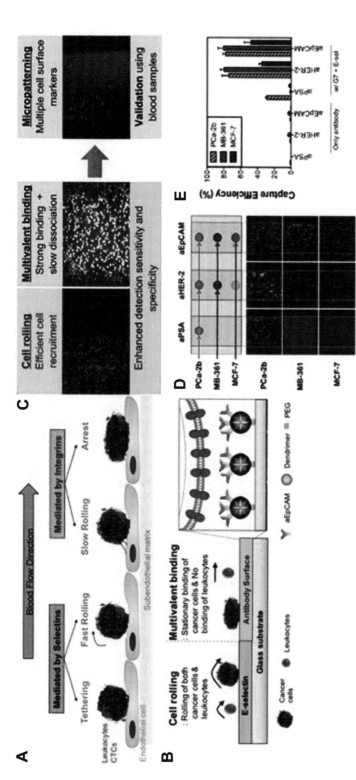

Fig. 6. (*A*) Cell rolling and (*B*) multivalent binding in the CapioCyte system. (*C*) The surface marker-dependent cell capture using aPSA, aHER-2, and aEpCAM. (*D*) The capture patterns of the 3 cell lines labeled with 3 different fluorescent colors. The lower capture efficiency of MCF-7 cells for aHER-2 due to low HER-2 expression of MCF-7 cells. (*E*) A combination of dendrimers and E-selectin (a cell rolling inducing agent), along with multiple antibodies achieved highly sensitive differential detection of tumor cells (up to 82%; Error bars: standard error [n = 4]). aPSA, anti-prostate specific antigen; aHER-2, anti-human epidermal growth factor receptor 2; aEpCAM, anti-Epithelial cell adhesion molecule. (*From* [*A–C*] Myung JH, Park SJ, Wang AZ, et al. Integration of biomimicry and nanotechnology for significantly improved detection of circulating tumor cells (CTCs). Advanced Drug Delivery Reviews 2018;125:36-47, with permission; and [*D–E*] *From* Myung JH, Gajjar KA, Chen J, et al. Differential detection of tumor cells using a combination of cell rolling, multivalent binding, and multiple antibodies. Anal Chem 2014;86(12):6091; with permission. Link- https://pubs.acs.org/doi/abs/10.1021/ac501243a.)

T790M became detectable after treatment with gefitinib or erlotinib. The presence of T790M mutation was associated with the reduction of progression-free survival from 16.5 months to 7.7 months. CTC enumeration was positively correlated with tumor progression and emerging EGFR mutations. In addition, recent study has demonstrated the correlation between programmed death-ligand 1 (PD-L1) expression in CTCs and tumor tissue from NSCLC patients, indicating the potential implication of CTCs as a noninvasive and real-time biopsy to monitor the dynamic change of PD-L1 in patients with cancer.[110] In an effort to identify responders to immune checkpoint regulators, CTCs were collected from patients with HER2-negative breast cancer and analyzed for PD-L1 expression on the CTCs.[111] PD-L1-positive CTCs were found in 11 out of 16 patients, and the percentage of PD-L1 expressing CTCs could range from 0.2% to 100% in different patients. This study demonstrated the existence of PD-L1 on CTCs, which could benefit patient selection and monitoring for immune checkpoint blockade therapy. In another study, CTCs were isolated from patients with nonmetastatic NSCLC, and PD-L1 expression in CTCs was monitored before, during, and after RT or CRT.[112] The fraction of PD-L1-positive CTCs was elevated after RT, suggesting the upregulated expression of PD-L1 in tumor cells. Similar to other clinical reports, higher level of PD-L1 in CTCs was associated with shorter progression-free survival.[113] This study not only demonstrated the prognostic value of CTCs but also provided a rationale for combined therapies with immune checkpoint blockade and RT.

FUTURE PERSPECTIVES

Emerging more than 3 decades ago, nanotechnology has made a great impact on the development of diagnostics and therapeutics for patients with cancer. The clinical development of many novel nanotechnologies is still in its infancy. Clinical gains with first-generation NPs that mainly relied on passive tumor targeting via the EPR effect (which is dynamic and heterogenous because of different tumor types and stages) have been modest and inconsistent compared with those predicted by preclinical studies.[114] This issue could be resolved through a better understanding of tumor biology and the development of novel technologies to address these shortcomings. In addition, most NPs used for imaging and radiosensitization are produced with heavy metals or other inorganic materials, which could pose health risks. Although no evidence of immediate liver injury was found in the aforementioned studies in this review, long-term exposure of inorganic NPs to the liver could pose risks owing to their lack of biodegradability, nonspecific interactions with endogenous proteins, and hepatic oxidative damage.[115] Further efforts should be directed to improve colloidal stability in systemic circulation, penetration/accumulation at target tissues, and most importantly, biocompatibility by manipulating the properties of inorganic NPs.[25,115]

Liquid biopsies are expected to play a vital role in precision medicine and personalized therapy against various cancers. CTCs have been validated as a prognostic biomarker in metastatic and nonmetastatic cancers.[48] Other applications of CTCs are being extensively studied, aiming to benefit the current practice in screening for malignancy, therapeutic outcomes monitoring, and surveillance after treatment. With the advance of CTC isolation techniques, more CTC detection platforms will enter clinical trials and expand the applications of CTCs in the clinic in the foreseeable future.

ACKNOWLEDGMENTS

This work was supported by funding from National Institutes of Health/National Cancer Institute (U54CA198999 and R01 EB25651), Department of Defense

(W81XWH-16-1-0530), and The University of North Carolina's Research Opportunities Initiative grant.

REFERENCES

1. Hernández-Rivera M, Zaibaq NG, Wilson LJ. Toward carbon nanotube-based imaging agents for the clinic. Biomaterials 2016;101:229–40.
2. Amenta V, Aschberger K. Carbon nanotubes: potential medical applications and safety concerns. Wiley Interdiscip Rev Nanomed Nanobiotechnol 2015; 7(3):371–86.
3. Jing W, Yuanzhi X, Zhi Y, et al. Toxicity of carbon nanotubes. Curr Drug Metab 2013;14(8):891–9.
4. Liu Y, Zhao Y, Sun B, et al. Understanding the toxicity of carbon nanotubes. Acc Chem Res 2013;46(3):702–13.
5. Zhao X, Liu R. Recent progress and perspectives on the toxicity of carbon nanotubes at organism, organ, cell, biomacromolecule levels. Environ Int 2012;40: 244–55.
6. Anselmo AC, Mitragotri S. A review of clinical translation of inorganic nanoparticles. AAPS J 2015;17(5):1041–54.
7. Pellico J, Llop J, Fern, et al. Iron oxide nanoradiomaterials: combining nanoscale properties with radioisotopes for enhanced molecular imaging. Contrast Media Mol Imaging 2017;2017:24.
8. Bradbury MS, Pauliah M, Zanzonico P, et al. Intraoperative mapping of sentinel lymph node metastases using a clinically translated ultrasmall silica nanoparticle. Wiley Interdiscip Rev Nanomed Nanobiotechnol 2016;8(4):535–53.
9. Bradbury MS, Phillips E, Montero PH, et al. Clinically-translated silica nanoparticles as dual-modality cancer-targeted probes for image-guided surgery and interventions. Integr Biol (Camb) 2013;5(1):74–86.
10. Phillips E, Penate-Medina O, Zanzonico PB, et al. Clinical translation of an ultrasmall inorganic optical-PET imaging nanoparticle probe. Sci Transl Med 2014; 6(260):260ra149.
11. Benezra M, Penate-Medina O, Zanzonico PB, et al. Multimodal silica nanoparticles are effective cancer-targeted probes in a model of human melanoma. J Clin Invest 2011;121(7):2768–80.
12. Ke L-R, Xia W-X, Qiu W-Z, et al. A phase II trial of induction NAB-paclitaxel and cisplatin followed by concurrent chemoradiotherapy in patients with locally advanced nasopharyngeal carcinoma. Oral Oncol 2017;70:7–13.
13. Takahashi H, Akita H, Ioka T, et al. Phase I trial evaluating the safety of preoperative gemcitabine/nab-paclitaxel with concurrent radiation therapy for borderline resectable pancreatic cancer. Pancreas 2018;47(9):1135–41.
14. Kaira K, Tomizawa Y, Imai H, et al. Phase I study of nab-paclitaxel plus carboplatin and concurrent thoracic radiotherapy in patients with locally advanced non-small cell lung cancer. Cancer Chemother Pharmacol 2017;79(1):165–71.
15. Tian X, Lara H, Wagner KT, et al. Improving DNA double-strand repair inhibitor KU55933 therapeutic index in cancer radiotherapy using nanoparticle drug delivery. Nanoscale 2015;7(47):20211–9.
16. Golan T, Grenader T, Ohana P, et al. Pegylated liposomal mitomycin C prodrug enhances tolerance of mitomycin C: a phase 1 study in advanced solid tumor patients. Cancer Med 2015;4(10):1472–83.
17. Wang AZ, Tepper JE. Nanotechnology in radiation oncology. J Clin Oncol 2014; 32(26):2879–85.

18. Tian X, Nguyen M, Foote HP, et al. CRLX101, a nanoparticle–drug conjugate containing camptothecin, improves rectal cancer chemoradiotherapy by inhibiting DNA repair and HIF1α. Cancer Res 2017;77(1):112.

19. Karve S, Werner ME, Sukumar R, et al. Revival of the abandoned therapeutic wortmannin by nanoparticle drug delivery. Proc Natl Acad Sci 2012;109(21):8230.

20. Au KM, Min Y, Tian X, et al. Improving cancer chemoradiotherapy treatment by dual controlled release of wortmannin and docetaxel in polymeric nanoparticles. ACS Nano 2015;9(9):8976–96.

21. Zhang M, Hagan CT, Min Y, et al. Nanoparticle co-delivery of wortmannin and cisplatin synergistically enhances chemoradiotherapy and reverses platinum resistance in ovarian cancer models. Biomaterials 2018;169:1–10.

22. Wang A, McRee AJ, Blackstock AW, et al. Phase Ib/II study of neoadjuvant chemoradiotherapy with CRLX101 and capecitabine for locally advanced rectal cancer. J Clin Oncol 2017;35(15_suppl):e15144.

23. Sanoff HK, Moon DH, Moore DT, et al. Phase I/II trial of nano-camptothecin CRLX101 with capecitabine and radiotherapy as neoadjuvant treatment for locally advanced rectal cancer. Nanomedicine 2019;18:189–95.

24. Au KM, Tripathy A, Lin CP-I, et al. Bespoke pretargeted nanoradioimmunotherapy for the treatment of non-Hodgkin lymphoma. ACS Nano 2018;12(2):1544–63.

25. Her S, Jaffray DA, Allen C. Gold nanoparticles for applications in cancer radiotherapy: mechanisms and recent advancements. Adv Drug Deliv Rev 2017;109:84–101.

26. Maggiorella L, Barouch G, Devaux C, et al. Nanoscale radiotherapy with hafnium oxide nanoparticles. Future Oncol 2012;8(9):1167–81.

27. Bonvalot S, Le Pechoux C, De Baere T, et al. Phase I study of NBTXR3 nanoparticles, in patients with advanced soft tissue sarcoma (STS). J Clin Oncol 2014;32(15_suppl):10563.

28. Kotb S, Detappe A, Lux F, et al. Gadolinium-based nanoparticles and radiation therapy for multiple brain melanoma metastases: proof of concept before phase I trial. Theranostics 2016;6(3):418–27.

29. Sancey L, Kotb S, Truillet C, et al. Long-term in vivo clearance of gadolinium-based AGuIX nanoparticles and their biocompatibility after systemic injection. ACS Nano 2015;9(3):2477–88.

30. Verry C, Dufort S, Barbier EL, et al. MRI-guided clinical 6-MV radiosensitization of glioma using a unique gadolinium-based nanoparticles injection. Nanomedicine 2016;11(18):2405–17.

31. Kotb S, Piraquive J, Lamberton F, et al. Safety evaluation and imaging properties of gadolinium-based nanoparticles in nonhuman primates. Sci Rep 2016;6:35053.

32. Detappe A, Kunjachan S, Sancey L, et al. Advanced multimodal nanoparticles delay tumor progression with clinical radiation therapy. J Control Release 2016;238:103–13.

33. Dufort S, Bianchi A, Henry M, et al. Nebulized gadolinium-based nanoparticles: a theranostic approach for lung tumor imaging and radiosensitization. Small 2015;11(2):215–21.

34. Miladi I, Aloy M-T, Armandy E, et al. Combining ultrasmall gadolinium-based nanoparticles with photon irradiation overcomes radioresistance of head and neck squamous cell carcinoma. Nanomedicine 2015;11(1):247–57.

35. Lux F, Tran VL, Thomas E, et al. AGuIX® from bench to bedside—transfer of an ultrasmall theranostic gadolinium-based nanoparticle to clinical medicine. Br J Radiol 2019;92(1093):20180365.
36. Nichols JW, Bae YH. EPR: evidence and fallacy. J Control Release 2014;190: 451–64.
37. Balasubramanian V, Liu Z, Hirvonen J, et al. Bridging the knowledge of different worlds to understand the big picture of cancer nanomedicines. Adv Healthc Mater 2018;7(1):1700432.
38. Stapleton S, Jaffray D, Milosevic M. Radiation effects on the tumor microenvironment: implications for nanomedicine delivery. Adv Drug Deliv Rev 2017;109: 119–30.
39. Miller MA, Chandra R, Cuccarese MF, et al. Radiation therapy primes tumors for nanotherapeutic delivery via macrophage-mediated vascular bursts. Sci Transl Med 2017;9(392):eaal0225.
40. Miller MA, Zheng Y-R, Gadde S, et al. Tumour-associated macrophages act as a slow-release reservoir of nano-therapeutic Pt(IV) pro-drug. Nat Commun 2015;6: 8692.
41. Russell J, Brown J. The irradiated tumor microenvironment: role of tumor-associated macrophages in vascular recovery. Front Physiol 2013;4:157.
42. Füzéry AK, Levin J, Chan MM, et al. Translation of proteomic biomarkers into FDA approved cancer diagnostics: issues and challenges. Clin Proteomics 2013;10(1):13.
43. Mordente A, Meucci E, Martorana GE, et al. Cancer biomarkers discovery and validation: state of the art, problems and future perspectives. In: Scatena R, editor. Advances in Cancer Biomarkers: from biochemistry to clinic for a critical revision. Dordrecht (the Netherlands): Springer Netherlands; 2015. p. 9–26.
44. Srivastava A, Creek DJ. Discovery and validation of clinical biomarkers of cancer: a review combining metabolomics and proteomics. Proteomics 2019;19(10). 1700448.
45. De Rubis G, Krishnan SR, Bebawy M. Circulating tumor DNA–current state of play and future perspectives. Pharmacol Res 2018;136:35–44.
46. Kanikarla-Marie P, Lam M, Menter DG, et al. Platelets, circulating tumor cells, and the circulome. Cancer Metastasis Rev 2017;36(2):235–48.
47. Crowley E, Di Nicolantonio F, Loupakis F, et al. Liquid biopsy: monitoring cancer-genetics in the blood. Nat Rev Clin Oncol 2013;10:472.
48. Moon DH, Lindsay DP, Hong S, et al. Clinical indications for, and the future of, circulating tumor cells. Adv Drug Deliv Rev 2018;125:143–50.
49. Bettegowda C, Sausen M, Leary RJ, et al. Detection of circulating tumor DNA in early- and late-stage human malignancies. Sci Transl Med 2014;6(224):224ra24.
50. Peng M, Chen C, Hulbert A, et al. Non-blood circulating tumor DNA detection in cancer. Oncotarget 2017;8(40):69162–73.
51. Fettke H, Kwan EM, Azad AA. Cell-free DNA in cancer: current insights. Cell Oncol 2019;42(1):13–28.
52. Heitzer E, Ulz P, Geigl JB, et al. Non-invasive detection of genome-wide somatic copy number alterations by liquid biopsies. Mol Oncol 2016;10(3):494–502.
53. Gorgannezhad L, Umer M, Islam MN, et al. Circulating tumor DNA and liquid biopsy: opportunities, challenges, and recent advances in detection technologies. Lab Chip 2018;18(8):1174–96.
54. Ko J, Carpenter E, Issadore D. Detection and isolation of circulating exosomes and microvesicles for cancer monitoring and diagnostics using micro-/nano-based devices. Analyst 2016;141(2):450–60.

55. Shao H, Chung J, Issadore D. Diagnostic technologies for circulating tumour cells and exosomes. Biosci Rep 2016;36(1):e00292.

56. Shao H, Chung J, Balaj L, et al. Protein typing of circulating microvesicles allows real-time monitoring of glioblastoma therapy. Nat Med 2012;18(12):1835–40.

57. Graner MW, Alzate O, Dechkovskaia AM, et al. Proteomic and immunologic analyses of brain tumor exosomes. FASEB J 2009;23(5):1541–57.

58. Skog J, Würdinger T, van Rijn S, et al. Glioblastoma microvesicles transport RNA and proteins that promote tumour growth and provide diagnostic biomarkers. Nat Cell Biol 2008;10(12):1470–6.

59. Liu C, Guo J, Tian F, et al. Field-free isolation of exosomes from extracellular vesicles by microfluidic viscoelastic flows. ACS Nano 2017;11(7):6968–76.

60. Dudani JS, Gossett DR, Tse HTK, et al. Rapid inertial solution exchange for enrichment and flow cytometric detection of microvesicles. Biomicrofluidics 2015;9(1):014112.

61. Bu H, He D, He X, et al. Exosomes: isolation, analysis, and applications in cancer detection and therapy. Chembiochem 2019;20(4):451–61.

62. Gupta GP, Massagué J. Cancer metastasis: building a framework. Cell 2006; 127(4):679–95.

63. Divoli A, Mendonça EA, Evans JA, et al. Conflicting biomedical assumptions for mathematical modeling: the case of cancer metastasis. PLoS Comput Biol 2011; 7(10):e1002132.

64. Langley RR, Fidler IJ. The seed and soil hypothesis revisited–the role of tumor-stroma interactions in metastasis to different organs. Int J Cancer 2011;128(11): 2527–35.

65. Fidler IJ. Metastasis: quantitative analysis of distribution and fate of tumor emboli labeled with 125 I-5-iodo-2'-deoxyuridine. J Natl Cancer Inst 1970; 45(4):773–82.

66. Cristofanilli M, Budd GT, Ellis MJ, et al. Circulating tumor cells, disease progression, and survival in metastatic breast cancer. N Engl J Med 2004;351(8): 781–91.

67. Cohen SJ, Punt CJA, Iannotti N, et al. Relationship of circulating tumor cells to tumor response, progression-free survival, and overall survival in patients with metastatic colorectal cancer. J Clin Oncol 2008;26(19):3213–21.

68. Hayes DF, Cristofanilli M, Budd GT, et al. Circulating tumor cells at each follow-up time point during therapy of metastatic breast cancer patients predict progression-free and overall survival. Clin Cancer Res 2006;12(14):4218.

69. Zhang L, Riethdorf S, Wu G, et al. Meta-analysis of the prognostic value of circulating tumor cells in breast cancer. Clin Cancer Res 2012;18(20):5701.

70. Scher HI, Jia X, de Bono JS, et al. Circulating tumour cells as prognostic markers in progressive, castration-resistant prostate cancer: a reanalysis of IMMC38 trial data. Lancet Oncol 2009;10(3):233–9.

71. Hou J-M, Krebs MG, Lancashire L, et al. Clinical significance and molecular characteristics of circulating tumor cells and circulating tumor microemboli in patients with small-cell lung cancer. J Clin Oncol 2012;30(5):525–32.

72. Krebs MG, Sloane R, Priest L, et al. Evaluation and prognostic significance of circulating tumor cells in patients with non–small-cell lung cancer. J Clin Oncol 2011;29(12):1556–63.

73. Aggarwal C, Mitchell E, Miller MC, et al. Relationship among circulating tumor cells, CEA and overall survival in patients with metastatic colorectal cancer. Ann Oncol 2012;24(2):420–8.

74. Denève E, Riethdorf S, Ramos J, et al. Capture of viable circulating tumor cells in the liver of colorectal cancer patients. Clin Chem 2013;59(9):1384.
75. Fan ST, Yang ZF, Ho DWY, et al. Prediction of posthepatectomy recurrence of hepatocellular carcinoma by circulating cancer stem cells: a prospective study. Ann Surg 2011;254(4):569–76.
76. Khoja L, Backen A, Sloane R, et al. A pilot study to explore circulating tumour cells in pancreatic cancer as a novel biomarker. Br J Cancer 2011;106:508.
77. Xu X, Zhong JF. Circulating tumor cells and melanoma progression. J Invest Dermatol 2010;130(10):2349–51.
78. Pantel K, Alix-Panabières C. Real-time liquid biopsy in cancer patients: fact or fiction? Cancer Res 2013;73(21):6384.
79. Saslow D, Boetes C, Burke W, et al. American Cancer Society Guidelines for Breast Screening with MRI as an adjunct to mammography. CA Cancer J Clin 2007;57(2):75–89.
80. Lehman CD, Gatsonis C, Kuhl CK, et al. MRI evaluation of the contralateral breast in women with recently diagnosed breast cancer. N Engl J Med 2007; 356(13):1295–303.
81. Bar-Shalom R, Yefremov N, Guralnik L, et al. Clinical performance of PET/CT in evaluation of cancer: additional value for diagnostic imaging and patient management. J Nucl Med 2003;44(8):1200–9.
82. Gerlinger M, Rowan AJ, Horswell S, et al. Intratumor heterogeneity and branched evolution revealed by multiregion sequencing. N Engl J Med 2012; 366(10):883–92.
83. Swanton C. Intratumor heterogeneity: evolution through space and time. Cancer Res 2012;72(19):4875.
84. Shackleton M, Quintana E, Fearon ER, et al. Heterogeneity in cancer: cancer stem cells versus clonal evolution. Cell 2009;138(5):822–9.
85. Hong B, Zu Y. Detecting circulating tumor cells: current challenges and new trends. Theranostics 2013;3(6):377–94.
86. Lalmahomed ZS, Kraan J, Gratama JW, et al. Circulating tumor cells and sample size: the more, the better. J Clin Oncol 2010;28(17):e288–9.
87. Zieglschmid V, Hollmann C, Böcher O. Detection of disseminated tumor cells in peripheral blood. Crit Rev Clin Lab Sci 2005;42(2):155–96.
88. Alix-Panabières C, Pantel K. Challenges in circulating tumour cell research. Nat Rev Cancer 2014;14:623.
89. Pantel K, Alix-Panabières C, Riethdorf S. Cancer micrometastases. Nat Rev Clin Oncol 2009;6:339.
90. Pantel K, Alix-Panabières C. Circulating tumour cells in cancer patients: challenges and perspectives. Trends Mol Med 2010;16(9):398–406.
91. Myung JH, Gajjar KA, Chen J, et al. Differential detection of tumor cells using a combination of cell rolling, multivalent binding, and multiple antibodies. Anal Chem 2014;86(12):6088–94.
92. Lin HK, Zheng S, Williams AJ, et al. Portable filter-based microdevice for detection and characterization of circulating tumor cells. Clin Cancer Res 2010; 16(20):5011.
93. Hou HW, Warkiani ME, Khoo BL, et al. Isolation and retrieval of circulating tumor cells using centrifugal forces. Sci Rep 2013;3:1259.
94. Yang L, Lang JC, Balasubramanian P, et al. Optimization of an enrichment process for circulating tumor cells from the blood of head and neck cancer patients through depletion of normal cells. Biotechnol Bioeng 2009;102(2):521–34.

95. Low WS, Wan Abas WAB. Benchtop technologies for circulating tumor cells separation based on biophysical properties. Biomed Research International 2015; 2015:239362.

96. Kowalik A, Kowalewska M, Góźdź S. Current approaches for avoiding the limitations of circulating tumor cells detection methods—implications for diagnosis and treatment of patients with solid tumors. Translational Res 2017;185: 58–84.e15.

97. Ozkumur E, Shah AM, Ciciliano JC, et al. Inertial focusing for tumor antigen-dependent and -independent sorting of rare circulating tumor cells. Sci Transl Med 2013;5(179):179ra147.

98. Myung JH, Park SJ, Wang AZ, et al. Integration of biomimicry and nanotechnology for significantly improved detection of circulating tumor cells (CTCs). Adv Drug Deliv Rev 2018;125:36–47.

99. Tedder TF, Steeber DA, Chen A, et al. The selectins: vascular adhesion molecules. FASEB J 1995;9(10):866–73.

100. Köhler S, Ullrich S, Richter U, et al. E-/P-selectins and colon carcinoma metastasis: first in vivo evidence for their crucial role in a clinically relevant model of spontaneous metastasis formation in the lung. Br J Cancer 2009;102:602.

101. Myung JH, Eblan MJ, Caster JM, et al. Multivalent binding and biomimetic cell rolling improves the sensitivity and specificity of circulating tumor cell capture. Clin Cancer Res 2018;24(11):2539.

102. de Bono JS, Scher HI, Montgomery RB, et al. Circulating tumor cells predict survival benefit from treatment in metastatic castration-resistant prostate cancer. Clin Cancer Res 2008;14(19):6302–9.

103. Welinder C, Jansson B, Lindell G, et al. Cytokeratin 20 improves the detection of circulating tumor cells in patients with colorectal cancer. Cancer Lett 2015; 358(1):43–6.

104. De Souza LM, Robertson BM, Robertson GP. Future of circulating tumor cells in the melanoma clinical and research laboratory settings. Cancer Lett 2017;392: 60–70.

105. Zhou J, Kulasinghe A, Bogseth A, et al. Isolation of circulating tumor cells in non-small-cell-lung-cancer patients using a multi-flow microfluidic channel. Microsyst Nanoeng 2019;5(1):8.

106. Hiltermann TJ, Liesker J, Schouwink H, et al. Circulating tumor cells (CTC) in small cell lung cancer (SCLC), a promising prognostic factor. J Clin Oncol 2010;28(15_suppl):7630.

107. Kapeleris J, Kulasinghe A, Warkiani ME, et al. The prognostic role of circulating tumor cells (CTCs) in lung cancer. Front Oncol 2018;8:311.

108. Sequist LV, Nagrath S, Toner M, et al. The CTC-Chip: an exciting new tool to detect circulating tumor cells in lung cancer patients. J Thorac Oncol 2009; 4(3):281–3.

109. Maheswaran S, Sequist LV, Nagrath S, et al. Detection of mutations in EGFR in circulating lung-cancer cells. N Engl J Med 2008;359(4):366–77.

110. Ilié M, Szafer-Glusman E, Hofman V, et al. Detection of PD-L1 in circulating tumor cells and white blood cells from patients with advanced non-small-cell lung cancer. Ann Oncol 2017;29(1):193–9.

111. Mazel M, Jacot W, Pantel K, et al. Frequent expression of PD-L1 on circulating breast cancer cells. Mol Oncol 2015;9(9):1773–82.

112. Wang Y, Kim TH, Fouladdel S, et al. PD-L1 expression in circulating tumor cells increases during radio(chemo)therapy and indicates poor prognosis in non-small cell lung cancer. Sci Rep 2019;9(1):566.

113. Kallergi G, Vetsika E-K, Aggouraki D, et al. Evaluation of PD-L1/PD-1 on circulating tumor cells in patients with advanced non-small cell lung cancer. Ther Adv Med Oncol 2018;10. 1758834017750121.
114. Maeda H. Toward a full understanding of the EPR effect in primary and metastatic tumors as well as issues related to its heterogeneity. Adv Drug Deliv Rev 2015;91:3–6.
115. Tee JK, Peng F, Ho HK. Effects of inorganic nanoparticles on liver fibrosis: optimizing a double-edged sword for therapeutics. Biochem Pharmacol 2019;160: 24–33.

Artificial Intelligence in Radiation Oncology

Christopher R. Deig, MD[a], Aasheesh Kanwar, MD[a], Reid F. Thompson, MD, PhD[a,b,*]

KEYWORDS

- Artificial intelligence • Machine learning • Deep learning

KEY POINTS

- Artificial intelligence may aid in pretreatment disease outcome and toxicity prediction.
- Artificial intelligence may aid in the treatment planning process with autosegmentation and enhanced dose optimization.
- Artificial intelligence may optimize the quality assurance process and support a higher level of safety, quality, and efficiency of care.

INTRODUCTION

Artificial intelligence (AI) is a broad area of computer science that can be thought of as a computer's ability to recognize patterns and make decisions based on existing data and statistical models. For focused tasks, AI has shown superiority to professionals, for instance, in playing intricate games, such as Go,[1] and it is the foundation of facial and voice recognition algorithms. It is currently used in the industrial and business sectors for monitoring of systems and processes, quality control by automating fault detection, business forecasting and planning, factory automation, and in autonomous vehicles.[2] Out of demand for AI expertise and consulting in the health care sector, companies are now creating tools to rapidly analyze clinical data and are developing and deploying machine learning tools to improve processes in health care and insurance. AI is rapidly increasing in terms of the depth and breadth of its use and it has become a transformative global force, with potential implications for health care.

Radiation oncology, as a profession, has rapidly evolved with the advent of more precise, highly conformal treatments (ie, intensity-modulated radiation therapy

Disclosure Statement: The authors have nothing to disclose.
Disclaimer: The contents do not represent the views of the U.S. Department of Veterans Affairs or the United States Government.
[a] Radiation Medicine, Oregon Health & Science University, 3181 Southwest Sam Jackson Park Road, Portland, OR 97239, USA; [b] Hospital & Specialty Medicine, VA Portland Healthcare System, 3710 SW US Veterans Hospital Road, Portland, OR 97239, USA
* Corresponding author.
E-mail address: thompsre@ohsu.edu
twitter: @thompson_lab (R.F.T.)

Hematol Oncol Clin N Am 33 (2019) 1095–1104
https://doi.org/10.1016/j.hoc.2019.08.003
0889-8588/19/Published by Elsevier Inc.

[IMRT], stereotactic ablative radiation therapy, and stereotactic radiosurgery [SRS]), and the subsequent increase of complexity within the treatment planning, quality assurance (QA), and delivery processes. The integration of AI within the radiation oncologist's workflow has great promise to improve patient care and outcomes. Radiation oncologists, like many physicians, aim to maximize face-to-face time with patients to establish trust and thoughtfully engage in shared decision making; too often, this critical human connection is encroached on, not only by administrative demands, but also by the growing technical complexity of safe radiation delivery.[3]

Beginning from the initial patient encounter, AI may aid in pretreatment disease outcome and toxicity prediction. AI may also aid in the treatment planning process with auto-segmentation of both normal structures (ie, organs at risk [OARs]) and target structures, and enhanced dose optimization. Finally, AI may optimize the QA process and support a higher level of safety, quality, and efficiency of care.[4–6] In this article, the authors describe various components of the radiation consultation, planning, and treatment process and how the thoughtful integration of AI may improve shared decision making, planning efficiency, planning quality, patient safety, and ultimately patient outcomes (**Fig. 1**).

DEFINING ARTIFICIAL INTELLIGENCE

Broadly, AI refers to the use of a machine (computer) to perform tasks that typically require human thought. The idea of AI dates back to the 1950s but has seen significant interest in the last decade owing to computational and mathematical advances. Often, AI is used interchangeably with the terms machine learning and deep learning. Machine learning refers to a set of computational algorithms that take a set of input data and produce a desired output without being explicitly programmed to do so, but instead through the recognition of patterns not readily appreciated by the human operator. The term learning refers to the training or adaptation of the algorithm using a set of input data. The trained algorithm is then applied to new, unseen data to produce a desired output. Machine learning is often separated into two broad categories, namely, supervised and unsupervised learning. In supervised machine learning, the input data are structured and labeled with a known output and the algorithm works to learn a rule to produce a desired output. Image classification is a common example of supervised learning that is currently being used in radiology to detect and characterize suspicious lesions, for instance, in lung imaging.[7,8] In unsupervised learning, only the input data are labeled by the human operator and the algorithm finds patterns within. A number of supervised and unsupervised learning algorithms have been proposed over the past several decades, but the recent advances in AI have been driven in large part by advances in convolutional neural networks or so-called deep learning.

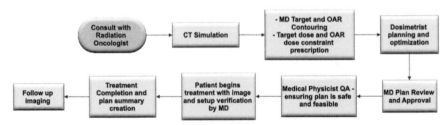

Fig. 1. The radiation oncologist's workflow with each step representing areas for potential use of AI. CT, computed tomography; MD, medical doctor; QA, quality assurance.

Artificial neural networks are modeled on the way in which biological nervous systems process information. These consist of an input layer, an output layer, and hidden layers consisting of multiple interconnected nodes. Each node performs a calculation based on its input signals and its connection to other nodes, similar to the way a neuron processes stimuli. Data are fed into the input layer and is processed through nodes of the hidden layers to yield a result in the output layer (**Fig. 2**). Artificial neural networks have been used to process more complex problems, such as medical imaging and speech recognition, but training effective deep learning models requires substantial computer resources.

SHARED DECISION-MAKING TOOLS

During the initial patient consultation, it is the radiation oncologist's duty to provide an accurate estimate of the relative risks, benefits, and alternatives to enable true shared decision making. It is well-known that the shared decision making process empowers patients to feel in control of their oncologic care and improves the patient-provider relationship.[9-11] Conversely, the absence of shared decision making creates anxiety, depression, and fatigue in radiation oncology patients who desire but did not perceive to have control of their care.[12] AI has the potential to enhance the quality of shared decision making via delivery of more accurate and comprehensive outcomes and toxicity predictions.

Predicting outcomes and complication rates are often inherently difficult in the pretreatment setting, particularly in radiation oncology, owing to the wide variation in tumor and normal tissue responses to radiation, variations in normal anatomy and the relative position and size of the target volume, radiosensitization with adjuvant therapies, and treatment planning and delivery variability. In addition, there are typically more than a single OAR at risk, each OAR has a variable response to radiation,

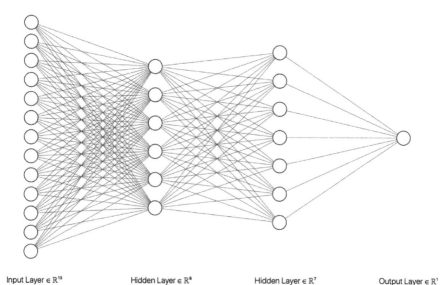

Input Layer ∈ R¹³   Hidden Layer ∈ R⁸   Hidden Layer ∈ R⁷   Output Layer ∈ R¹

Fig. 2. A conceptual schematic displaying how a deep learning neural network, including numerous hidden layers, helps produce a desired output. As illustrated, the increased number of connections between layers allows for more nuanced decisions.

and there is a complex, heterogeneous dose distribution in normal tissues, making predictions of early and late toxicities nearly impossible in its current state (Machine Learning in Radiation Oncology).[13] Further, radiation oncologists aggregate an OAR into a single homogenous volume with the assumption that each subsite within that volume has equal radiation sensitivity and consequence for toxicity. This is obviously not the case for structures such as the heart where coronary artery radiation toxicity has a disproportionate impact on outcomes compared with the myocardium.[14] Currently, dose constraints are used based on volumetric data during treatment planning. A common spinal cord constraint, for example, is to keep the maximum dose received at less than 45 Gy.

Toxicity Prediction

AI has the potential to transform the clinician's ability to predict complications by integrating higher level information, such as detailed clinical and comorbidity data, in addition to complex dosimetric data, into a more comprehensive and quantitative model. For example, machine learning approaches have demonstrated the ability to aid in the prediction of radiation pneumonitis, recently illustrated in a cohort of 201 patients undergoing lung stereotactic ablative radiation therapy using 61 different patient-specific clinical features.[15] In a similar fashion, machine learning and the use of artificial neural networks has been shown to accurately predict gastrointestinal and genitourinary toxicity in patients undergoing definitive prostate external beam radiotherapy with a relatively high sensitivity and specificity (area under the curve, 0.7).[16] Using convolutional neural networks, one team demonstrated the ability to predict hepatobiliary toxicity after stereotactic body radiotherapy. When combining the convolutional neural network predicted model with a 3-dimensional dose plan analysis, this technique produced an area under the curve of 0.85 for toxicity prediction.[17] These advanced decision-making tools further have the potential to enhance clinical trial design, including via nuanced patient randomization (eg, pretreatment subgrouping of patients who are at high risk of toxicity).

Further, the external validity of toxicity outcomes data is frequently suspect, largely extrapolated from nonmodern era radiation delivery techniques in a dissimilar patient population or treatment setting. By leveraging existing data sources and models in an efficient, accessible way, the treating physician can personalize treatment decisions, allowing for an enhanced shared decision making process, improving satisfaction, and facilitating adaptive modifications of treatment.

Outcome Prediction

Clinicians are frequently overly optimistic when estimating patient survival, and individual survival estimations are often nonreproducible.[18] In a study evaluating the associations between life expectancy and aggressive end-of-life care, only 32% of patients met the criteria for having received aggressive treatment, with younger age, female sex, primary cancer diagnosis, no brain metastases, and having private insurance being independent factors. Among oncologists, 22% inaccurately predicted a patient life expectancy of less than 12 months, and patients with longer estimated life expectancies often received more aggressive end-of-life treatment.[19] A fully automated machine learning model demonstrated superior performance at predicting survival for patients with metastatic disease receiving palliative radiotherapy.[20]

In a single-center study from the Netherlands, AI-driven decision support tools were used and compared with physician-predicted and European Organization for Research and Treatment of Cancer guideline-based recommendations of 2-year survival, dyspnea, and dysphagia outcomes for lung patients with cancer being treated with chemoradiation. Interestingly, the AI decision support tools, which used information based on sex, performance status, forced expiratory volume in 1 second, gross tumor volume, and number of positive lymph nodes, significantly outperformed experienced radiation oncologist's predictions and European Organization for Research and Treatment of Cancer guideline-based recommendations currently in use in clinical practice.[21] As illustrated, limiting radiation dose to specific OARs to reduce complications is only part of the story, and AI may afford physicians access to powerful clinical decision tools to help guide decisions.

Artificial Intelligence in Medical Imaging and Predicting Treatment Response

Beyond clinical characteristics, other domains of information such as imaging can provide useful insights for the shared decision-making process. Indeed, the field of radiomics is one of the more active areas of research in AI that has shown applicability throughout oncology. Using different forms of AI to gauge prognosis or predict treatment response can be meaningful to both the physician and the patient. The potential for this approach has been studied in multiple disease sites where imaging plays an essential role of the clinical workup and treatment planning process. Although basic quantitative metrics such as tumor size are used for clinical staging of most solid cancers, there exists a breadth of information in clinical images that may better predict disease outcomes and behavior. For example, Aerts and colleagues[22] have constructed radiomic signatures to discriminate overall survival probability in non-small cell lung and patients with head and neck cancer and were able to validate their findings using multiple external datasets. Kwan and colleagues[23] have shown that the addition of radiomic data to standard risk models can improve prognostication of distant metastases in human papilloma virus-related oropharyngeal cancers. Among patients with lung adenocarcinoma, Dou and colleagues[24] have shown that radiomic analysis of the 3 mm peritumoral volume can discriminate patients at high risk for distant metastasis.

Beyond radiation therapy, using imaging analysis to predict response to immune checkpoint inhibitor therapy is also an area of active research. Recently, Trebeschi and colleagues[25] showed that radiomic analysis of pretreatment noncontrast imaging of metastatic lesions from melanoma and non-small cell lung cancer in patients receiving anti-PD1 therapy can distinguish between lesions likely to respond to therapy and those that do not. This burgeoning field of research is relevant for patients with cancer throughout all oncologic subspecialties.

TREATMENT PLANNING EFFICIENCY AND QUALITY

One of the major roles of the radiation oncologist is target delineation. This time-intensive process involves manual delineation of the gross tumor volume and the clinical target volume on a slice-by-slice basis on the planning computed tomography (CT) scan. To make this process more efficient, many software developers in the treatment planning domain have created tools for automated delineation of OARs. Traditionally, these have been using an atlas-based approach, which matches the patient's anatomy with that of a patient within a larger cohort. This atlas-based auto-segmentation approach has inherent limitations owing to the amount of intersubject anatomic variation that is seen on CT scans, and it can be difficult to generalize because of the limited number of subjects that are typically included in such atlases. To that end, researchers have leveraged deep learning techniques (eg, convolutional neural networks) to delineate various targets on a voxel-by-voxel basis, even in the most anatomically complex disease sites, such as the head and neck. Cardenas and colleagues[26] trained a deep learning algorithm using information from with the treatment plans from 52 patients oropharyngeal cancer to conduct a voxel-based classification of the high-risk clinical target volume, which typically includes a combination of cervical nodal levels and the gross tumor volume. Using a crowd-sourcing framework for algorithm development, Mak and colleagues[27] cultivated a suite of algorithms designed to perform autosegmentation of lung cancers. Although these software-generated contours often need manual review, Walker and colleagues[28] showed that this revision approach can lead to a 30% reduction in time requirement compared with de novo manual segmentation.

Among genitourinary cancers, radiation therapy is often used in the definitive treatment of intermediate-risk and high-risk prostate adenocarcinoma. Recently, Vu and colleagues[29] reported on the training of a convolutional neural network for automated segmentation of the prostate gland, seminal vesicles, bladder, and rectum using CT imaging data from 114 patients. The validity of the machine contours was assessed against contours manually generated by resident physicians using by the calculating the dice similarity coefficient (DSC). For the prostate, the DSC was comparable for machine contours (0.82) and resident physician contours (DSC, 0.75–0.81), and a similar pattern was seen in the OARs.[29] Other researchers have also looked at applying similar techniques using multiparametric MR imaging. Wang and colleagues[30] recently published a study on prostate autosegmentation using a fully convolutional network, which yielded a DSC of 0.86 ± 0.04. Of note, the model was also assessed using a publicly available dataset of prostate MR imaging (PROMISE12) and yielded a DSC of 0.88 ± 0.05 when compared with manual contours from experienced radiation oncologists.[30] As this class of tools is developed further, it is foreseeable that they will integrate into the standard workflow of the radiation oncology clinic.

In the CT-guided planning era, where targets are drawn volumetrically and delivery can be highly conformal, there can be wide variation among treatment centers. This potential variation warrants rigorous development of high-quality standards that are generalizable across institutions. Knowledge-based treatment planning (KBTP), which uses a database of prior patient and treatment planning information, has been shown to homogenize and improve IMRT planning quality. In 1 compelling study, which assembled a knowledge base from 132 patients with prostate cancer, 40% of KBTP plans spared more bladder and rectal volume, met the femoral head constraints more often, and 90% of KBTP plans had more uniform planning target volume coverage compared with the original (ie, manually derived) plans.[31] Volumetric arc therapy is a specific form of IMRT that can involve multiple iterative steps to create an optimal treatment plan that fulfills OAR and target dose constraints. This process was expedited by using machine learning to analyze anatomic similarities, arc directions, collimator patterns, optimization constraints, and isocenter positions from 83 different volumetric arc therapy plans in prostate patients with cancer. With the use of an improved start point for optimization, the new plans only required simple modifications, which significantly decreased the dosimetrist's planning time.[32] Similarly, SRS involves inherent planning complexity owing to prescribing a large radiation dose within a small volume, with a small tolerance for treatment variation. One group created a KBTP library from 121 patients who underwent brain SRS based on anatomic, dosimetric, and planning considerations and found that the KBTP plans consistently fulfilled predefined OAR dose cutoffs in significantly less time compared with manual treatment planning.[33]

The rapid initiation of a complex radiation plan is often necessary to obtain optimal oncologic outcomes, for example, in head and neck malignancies, which involve delicate OAR and target volume delineation. Contouring OARs is a time intensive and tedious process, and deep learning-based AI methods have been shown to quickly contour complicated head and neck OARs in less than 10 seconds per patient.[34] With the implementation of KBTP and deep learning-based AI tools, these patients would benefit from a rapid creation of a safe and reproducible treatment plan. Perhaps from a practical perspective, the majority of radiation oncology patients would also benefit from a decreased time from consultation to treatment completion out of convenience.

PATIENT SAFETY

After the treatment planning process, medical physicists ensure the safe and accurate delivery of the desired radiation dose through rigorous QA methods. Machine learning has the potential to enhance the QA process and decrease the risk of rare but serious errors that could result in serious harm to a patient. This risk can be mitigated with the use of machine learning anomaly detection methods, which have been preliminarily validated during the QA process for lung stereotactic ablative radiation therapy planning with a high level of sensitivity and specificity (Machine learning in Radiation Oncology).[13] Another potential application of machine learning is to help prioritize physicists' time and energy on IMRT plans that are at the highest risk of failure, rather than performing the same QA checks on every plan. One study describes a novel, virtual IMRT QA framework that was designed and optimized using nearly 500 IMRT plans, which was able to predict QA failure within 3.5% of accuracy at multiple institutions.[35] This novel approach may allow staff to more quickly and rigorously perform QA checks on plans at risk for failure, and prevent treatment delays by detecting major plan flaws early in the planning and QA process.

During treatment delivery of a modern IMRT, volumetric arc therapy, or SRS plan, a symphony of complex movements within the treatment machine occurs, which allows room for errors to occur. One source of error can come from multileaf collimator positioning during the treatment, the object that dynamically shapes the radiation beam as the gantry head rotates around the patient. Carlson and colleagues[36] presented a method to decrease the risk of positional errors in this process using machine-learning. This AI-driven model better predicted the actual multileaf collimator position during treatment delivery, compared with the predicted multileaf collimator position during the standard planning process. There was an improvement in head and neck plan pass rate, and they found that the inclusion of predictions during dose calculation lead to closer representation during plan delivery.[36]

Further, in rapidly responding tumors, such as small cell lung cancer or human papilloma virus-positive squamous cell carcinoma, the tumor volume can decrease significantly in size during a course of treatment, resulting in unnecessary tissue irradiation. Additionally, weight loss can affect the accuracy of treatment delivery. Adaptive replanning is an active area of research that has the potential to precisely tailor radiation treatments to patient's dynamic anatomy during a course of treatment. A unique machine learning tool was created to predict a benefit to adaptive replanning in patients with head and neck cancers. As an example, parotid glands show significant structural change during treatment, occasionally migrating toward high-dose regions as the tumor responds. In this multicenter study, a machine learning tool was able to classify patients with either set-up variations and/or significant anatomic variation from the original treatment plan; prompting physician evaluation and adaptive replanning.[37]

SUMMARY AND NEXT STEPS

AI is transforming the world we live in, and radiation oncology is not immune to this change. As a profession, we are faced with a tremendous opportunity to create sweeping, positive changes in how we counsel patients, design radiation treatment plans, and the ways in which we ensure safe and effective delivery of treatment. Accordingly, there is a growing wave of commercial and academic research interest and applications in this space, particularly in the diagnostic image interpretation realm. However, there remain numerous caveats to the wider adoption and clinical use of AI. As with any other medical device, AI algorithms must undergo QA testing through a standardized and thorough process, of which external validation is an important part. Further research is also necessary to address the challenges of AI interpretability and bias, which remain substantial barriers to broader clinical uptake. The US Food and Drug Administration approval and oversight mechanisms to support this type of algorithmic validation are currently in flux, but currently stratify AI software into risk categories based on the state of the health care situation or condition (ie, critical, serious, nonserious) and the impact on medical decision making, for example, to treat or diagnose, drive clinical management, or inform clinical management. With this risk stratification, the US Food and Drug Administration will differentially use requirements for rigorous testing and validation before clinical adoption.[38] In addition, education of the workforce, beginning with incorporation into national residency curriculums, is essential to uptake of this technology. Improvements in the quality of data input, education surrounding the use of AI technology, and the use of open source data sharing and standardization platforms, will aid in the realization of AI's potential. Although seemingly futuristic, AI is beginning to find its way into the radiation oncologist's standard toolbox.

REFERENCES

1. Silver D, Huang A, Maddison CJ, et al. Mastering the game of Go with deep neural networks and treesearch. Nature 2016;529(7587):484–9.
2. Charrington S. Cloudpulse. Artificial intelligence for industrial applications. Artificial Intelligence for Industrial Applications, Bonsai; 2017.
3. Woolhandler S, Himmelstein DU. Administrative work consumes one-sixth of U.S. physicians' working hours and lowers their career satisfaction. Int J Health Serv 2014;44(4):635–42.
4. Thompson RF, Valdes G, Fuller CD, et al. Artificial intelligence in radiation oncology: a specialty-widedisruptive transformation? Radiother Oncol 2018; 129(3):421–6.
5. Feng M, Valdes G, Dixit N, et al. Machine learning in radiation oncology: opportunities, requirements, and needs. Front Oncol 2018;8:110.
6. Kann BH, Thompson R, Thomas CR Jr, et al. Artificial intelligence in oncology: current applications and future directions. Oncology (Williston Park) 2019;33(2): 46–53.
7. Erickson BJ. Machine learning: discovering the future of medical imaging. J Digit Imaging 2017;30(4):391.
8. Wong KKL, Wang L, Wang D. Recent developments in machine learning for medical imaging applications. Comput Med Imaging Graph 2017;57:1–3.
9. Rao JK, Anderson LA, Inui TS, et al. Communication interventions make a difference in conversations between physicians and patients: a systematic review of the evidence. Med Care 2007;45(4):340–9.

10. Steinhauser KE, Christakis NA, Clipp EC, et al. Factors considered important at the end of life by patients, family, physicians, and other care providers. JAMA 2000;284(19):2476–82.

11. Austin CA, Mohottige D, Sudore RL, et al. Tools to promote shared decision making in serious illness: a systematic review. JAMA Intern Med 2015;175(7): 1213–21.

12. Shabason JE, Mao JJ, Frankel ES, et al. Shared decision-making and patient control in radiationoncology: implications for patient satisfaction. Cancer 2014; 120(12):1863–70.

13. Naqa EI, Ruijang L, Murphy MJ, editors. Machine learning in radiation oncology: theory and applications. Springer International Publishing; 2015.

14. Dilworth JT, Zamdborg L, Blas KG, et al. Left anterior descending artery avoidance for patients receiving breast irradiation. Int J Radiat Oncol Biol Phys 2016;96(2).

15. Valdes G, Solberg TD, Heskel M, et al. Using machine learning to predict radiation pneumonitis in patients with stage I non-small cell lung cancer treated with stereotactic body radiationtherapy. Phys Med Biol 2016;61(16):6105–20.

16. Pella A, Cambria R, Riboldi M, et al. Use of machine learning methods for prediction of acute toxicity in organs at risk following prostate radiotherapy. Med Phys 2011;38(6):2859–67.

17. Ibragimov B, Toesca D, Chang D, et al. Development of deep neural network for individualized hepatobiliary toxicity prediction after liver SBRT. Med Phys 2018; 45(10):4763–74.

18. Clément-Duchêne C, Carnin C, Guillemin F, et al. How accurate are physicians in the prediction of patient survival in advanced lung cancer? Oncologist 2010; 15(7):782–9.

19. Sborov K, Giaretta S, Koong A, et al. Impact of accuracy of survival predictions on quality of end-of-life care among patients with metastatic cancer who receive radiation therapy. J Oncol Pract 2019;15(3):e262–70.

20. Gensheimer MF, Henry AS, Wood DJ, et al. Automated survival prediction in metastatic cancer patients using high-dimensional electronic medical record data. J Natl Cancer Inst 2019;111(6):568–74.

21. Oberije C, Nalbantov G, Dekker A, et al. A prospective study comparing the predictions of doctors versus models for treatment outcome of lung cancer patients: a step toward individualized care and shared decision making. Radiother Oncol 2014;112(1):37–43.

22. Aerts HJWL, Velazquez ER, Leijenaar RTH, et al. Decoding tumour phenotype by noninvasive imaging using a quantitative radiomics approach. Nat Commun 2014;5:4006.

23. Kwan JYY, Su J, Huang SH, et al. Radiomic biomarkers to refine risk models for distant metastasis in HPV-related oropharyngeal carcinoma. Int J Radiat Oncol Biol Phys 2018;102(4):1107–16.

24. Dou TH, Coroller TP, van Griethuysen JJM, et al. Peritumoral radiomics features predict distant metastasis in locally advanced NSCLC. PLoS One 2018;13(11): e0206108.

25. Trebeschi S, Drago SG, Birkbak NJ, et al. Predicting response to cancer immunotherapy using noninvasive radiomic biomarkers. Ann Oncol 2019 [pii:mdz108]. [Epub ahead of print].

26. Cardenas CE, McCarroll RE, Court LE, et al. Deep learning algorithm for autodelineation of high-riskoropharyngeal clinical target volumes with built-in dice

similarity coefficient parameter optimization function. Int J Radiat Oncol Biol Phys 2018;101(2):468–78.

27. Mak RH, Endres MG, Paik JH, et al. Use of crowd innovation to develop an artificial intelligence–based solution for radiation therapy targeting. JAMA Oncol 2019;5(5):654–61.

28. Walker GV, Awan M, Tao R, et al. Prospective randomized double-blind study of atlas-based organ- at-risk autosegmentation-assisted radiation planning in head and neck cancer. Radiother Oncol 2014;112(3):321–5.

29. Vu CC, Z.L., Siddiqui ZA, et al. Automatic segmentation using convolutional neural networks in prostate cancer. IJROBP 2018;102(3):S61.

30. Wang B, Lei Y, Tian S, et al. Deeply supervised 3D fully convolutional networks with group dilated convolution for automatic MRI prostate segmentation. Med Phys 2019;46(4):1707–18.

31. Good D, Lo J, Lee WR, et al. A knowledge-based approach to improving and homogenizing intensity modulated radiation therapy planning quality among treatment centers: an example application to prostate cancer planning. Int J Radiat Oncol Biol Phys 2013;87(1):176–81.

32. Schreibmann E, Fox T. Prior-knowledge treatment planning for volumetric arc therapy using feature-based database mining. J Appl Clin Med Phys 2014; 15(2):4596.

33. Sarkar B, Munshi A, Ganesh T, et al. Standardization of volumetric modulated arc therapy based frameless stereotactic technique using a multidimensional ensemble aided knowledge based planning. Med Phys 2019;46(5):1953–62.

34. van Rooij W, Dahele M, Ribeiro Brandao H, et al. Deep learning-based delineation of head and neck organs-at risk:geometric and dosimetric evaluation. Int J Radiat Oncol Biol Phys 2019;104(3):677–84.

35. Valdes G, Chan MF, Lim SB, et al. IMRT QA using machine learning: a multi-institutional validation. J Appl Clin Med Phys 2017;18(5):279–84.

36. Carlson JN, Park JM, Park SY, et al. A machine learning approach to the accurate prediction of multi-leaf collimator positional errors. Phys Med Biol 2016;61(6): 2514–31.

37. Guidi G, Maffei N, Meduri B, et al. A machine learning tool for re-planning and adaptive RT: a multicenter cohort investigation. Phys Med 2016;32(12):1659–66.

38. FDA. Proposed regulatory framework for modifications to artificial intelligence/machine learning (AI/ML)-based software as a medical device. SaMD); 2019. p. 20.

Patient-Centered Outcomes in Radiation Oncology

Amardeep S. Grewal, MD, Abigail T. Berman, MD MSCE*,[1]

KEYWORDS

- Outcomes • Radiation oncology • Patient-reported outcomes • Quality of life

KEY POINTS

- Traditional outcome measures, including survival and progression, are important metrics but do not address the patient experience during and after cancer treatment.
- Patient-reported outcomes (PROs) provide direct insight and measurements of a patient's experience before, during, or after treatment via validated scales.
- When used in trials and clinical care, PROs can influence changes in treatment guidelines and allow for better patient-centered care.

INTRODUCTION

Patient outcomes are metrics used in oncology practice and research that serve as markers for the quality of care patients receive. Traditionally, such metrics have centered on patient survival, disease progression, and treatment-related morbidity.[1] Other outcomes, including rates of pathologic complete response; mediastinal clearance; and translation outcomes, such as imaging and biomarker endpoints, have also been used in radiation oncology.[2] Although such outcomes reflect whether treatments are successful in achieving disease control without inflicting significant harm, they overlook the experience of the patient throughout and after treatment. Quality of care extends beyond such absolute outcomes because treatments affect the lives of patients in more ways than established metrics, such as survival, can measure.[3] This article focuses on patient-centered outcomes in radiation oncology, including patient-reported outcomes (PROs), health-related quality of life (HRQoL), and cost considerations.

PATIENT-REPORTED OUTCOMES

The value of understanding and appreciating the depth and complexity of the patient experience is reflected in the Institute of Medicine's[4] *Crossing the Quality Chasm*, in

The authors have nothing to disclose.
Department of Radiation Oncology, University of Pennsylvania, 3400 Civic Center Boulevard, TRC-2 Radiation Oncology, Philadelphia, PA 19104, USA
[1] Senior author.
* Corresponding author.
E-mail address: abigail.berman@pennmedicine.upenn.edu

Hematol Oncol Clin N Am 33 (2019) 1105–1116
https://doi.org/10.1016/j.hoc.2019.08.012
0889-8588/19/© 2019 Elsevier Inc. All rights reserved.

hemonc.theclinics.com

which patient-centered care is defined as one of the 6 aims of quality health care. Since the publication of this report, there has been an increased effort to measure the patient experience using PROs.

PROs provide direct insight and measurements of a patient's experience before, during, or after treatment via validated scales that focus on HRQoL, symptoms, physical function, distress, mood, satisfaction, preference, and regret. The US Food and Drug Administration[5] defines PRO as "a measurement based on a report that comes directly from the patient about the status of a patient's health condition without amendment or interpretation of the patient's response by a clinician or anyone else." In the era of digital health, PROs, such as wearable devices and biosensors, strive to provide greater insight on a patient's daily life outside the confines of a clinic or hospital.

Patient-Reported Outcomes in Oncology

Within oncology, PROs have increasingly been used to assess the patient experience during and after treatment. Such measurements have historically been used in the realm of clinical trials, mainly as exploratory endpoints. With time and with the efforts of the National Institute of Health, National Cancer Institute, and cooperative research groups, including the European Organization for Research and Treatment of Cancer (EORTC), PRO scales, have been generated and validated, allowing for such metrics to become incorporated into primary and secondary endpoints of clinical trials. The Prostate Testing for Cancer and Treatment (ProtecT) trial, the largest randomized controlled trial to randomize men with localized prostate cancer to active monitoring, radical prostatectomy, and radiotherapy, used PROs in the domains of quality of life, urinary, bowel, and sexual health to provide greater insight into the lives of subjects based on treatment cohort.[6]

Patient-Reported Outcome Scales

PRO scales can be divided into generic scales and disease-specific or condition-specific scales. Generic scales measure and comprehensively assess patient impact independent of disease type and treatment. Such measurements focus on a patient's physical, psychological, and social wellbeing. In contrast, disease-specific measures focus on symptoms that are unique to a particular disease process or treatment, and can be clinical or experiential.[6] Common instruments used for generic and disease-specific PROs are shown in **Table 1**.

Patient-Reported Outcomes versus Provider-Based Assessment

PROs provide patient-generated health data regarding the patient experience at a greater resolution and with more accuracy than can be collected by a provider directly. Oncologists routinely assign toxicity grades to patients receiving cancer-directed therapy using the Common Terminology Criteria for Adverse Events (CTCAE). In a study of patients receiving chemotherapy for lung cancer, patients and clinicians independently reported 6 CTCAE symptoms.[7] Patients were found to report symptoms earlier than clinicians and, as such, PROs may provide a better real-time picture of the patient experience compared with physician reporting. Furthermore, data from a study by Di Maio and colleagues[8] showed that symptoms tend to be underreported by clinicians compared with patients, highlighting the importance of incorporating PROs in clinical practice to get an accurate representation of the patient experience. Compared with a standard review of systems, which may be subject to provider framing, validated PROs provide a low-friction channel that allows for the collection of health information from the patient without any interpretation bias.

Table 1	
Commonly used patient-reported outcome scales	
PRO Scales	**Description**
Patient-Reported Outcomes of Common Terminology Criteria for Adverse Events (PRO-CTCAE)	Evaluates symptomatic toxicity in subjects in cancer clinical trials 124 items representing 78 symptomatic toxicities
Functional Assessment of Cancer Therapy: Disease Specific (FACT-HN)	Evaluates symptoms specifically associated with different cancer types with unique surveys for each cancer type
MD Anderson Symptom Inventory (MDASI)	Multisymptom measurement of severity of symptoms (eg, pain, fatigue, nausea, dyspnea, xerostomia) and interference with daily living (eg, walking, working, mood)
EORTC disease-specific survey (EORTC QLQ-BM22)	Evaluates symptoms associated with different stages of disease (metastatic disease) and cancer types
Edmonton Symptom Assessment Scale (ESAS)	Assesses severity of pain, fatigue, nausea, depression, anxiety, drowsiness, appetite, wellbeing, and dyspnea on a 0–10 scale
Brief Pain Inventory (BPI)	Rapidly assesses the severity of pain and its affect on functioning Exists in a short form and long form

HEALTH-RELATED QUALITY OF LIFE

An important PRO in oncology is HRQoL, which describes how a patient's health is affected by disease and treatment. Disease and treatment can affect overall patient wellness and HRQoL in different ways, including impairment, functional status, perception of health, social interactions, and duration of life.[9] HRQoL is among the most commonly measured patient-centered outcomes in oncology, and many scales have been created and validated to quantify this vital aspect of care. The most commonly used scales include EORTC QLQ-C30, the 36-item Short Form Health Survey, the Functional Assessment of Chronic Illness Therapy (FACIT) scales, the Nottingham Health Profile, and the Sickness Impact Profile. Domains of HRQoL covered by these scales are shown in **Table 2**.

Health-Related Quality of Life in Radiation Oncology Trials

Subject-reported HRQoL has been found to be prognostic of traditional outcomes, including survival, in several radiation oncology trials. Cognitive functioning measured on the EORTC QLQ-C30 was found to be an independent prognostic factor for survival in subjects with head and neck cancer treated with surgery and/or radiotherapy.[10] Subjects with less than optimal cognitive functioning had a relative risk of disease recurrence of 1.72 (95% CI 1.01–2.93). EORTC Quality of Life Questionnaire (QLQ-C30) was also used by Fang and colleagues[11] to show that baseline fatigue was an independent predictor for survival in subjects with head and neck cancer, with a 10-point increase in fatigue corresponding to a 17% reduction in the likelihood of survival. In a prospective controlled trial of 102 subjects with inoperable non-small cell lung cancer, Kaasa and colleagues[12] found that self-reported psychosocial wellbeing

Table 2
Commonly used health-related quality-of-life scales

HRQoL Scales	Domains Surveyed
EORTC QLQ C30	Physical and emotional functioning, pain, and fatigue
Functional Assessment of Cancer Therapy: General (FACT-G)	Physical, social or family, emotional, and functional wellbeing
European Quality of Life–5 Dimensions	Mobility, self-care, usual activities, pain or discomfort, and anxiety or depression
Short Form Health Survey (SF)-36	Physical, emotional, social functioning, pain, vitality, and overall wellbeing
Nottingham Health Profile	Physical, emotional, and social functioning; pain; and vitality
Sickness Impact Profile	Physical, emotional, cognitive, social functioning, pain, and overall wellbeing

($P = .0002$) and general symptoms ($P = .0006$) were predictive of survival on univariate and multivariate regression analysis. Baseline self-reported quality of life on the EORTC QLQ-C30 scale was also associated with improved survival in subjects with non-small cell lung cancer treated with radiotherapy.[13]

A meta-analysis by Quinten and colleagues[14] of 30 randomized controlled trials from the EORTC analyzed 10,108 subjects who had performed a baseline EORTC QLQ-C30 questionnaire. On multivariate analysis, physical functioning, pain, and appetite loss provided significant prognostic information in regard to overall survival. The addition of HRQoL parameters improved the predictive accuracy of prognosis of overall survival by 6% relative to sociodemographic and clinical characteristics alone.

REAL-TIME MONITORING OF PATIENT-CENTERED OUTCOMES

Many earlier studies included the collection of PROs for research without real-time monitoring of such results by physicians. Given that these data have been found to be prognostic of important oncologic outcomes, there has been a push for providers to integrate the use of PROs into a clinical workflow to improve the patient experience. Such integration and responsiveness to PROs was reported by Basch and colleagues[15] in a trial of subjects with advanced-stage cancer treated with chemotherapy. Subjects randomized to the intervention arm completed electronically captured PROs, which were monitored and acted on by their care team, whereas subjects in the control arm received standard care. Compared with subjects in the control arm, subjects who completed PROs were found to have less quality-of-life deterioration, more quality-of-life improvement, fewer emergency department visits, and improved overall survival. Mooney and colleagues[16] found a similar nursing-monitored, telephone-based PRO reporting system to significantly improve chemotherapy-related symptoms In both these studies, deviations from a patients' baseline PRO scores resulted in triggered check-ins with patients, during which additional supportive care was administered.

TRIAL INCORPORATION OF PATIENT-CENTERED OUTCOMES

The incorporation of PROs in radiation oncology trials has been instrumental in updating best practice recommendations. Many radiation oncology trials use the PROs version of CTCAE (PRO-CTCAE). This version of the CTCAE was established to enable patient self-reporting of symptomatic toxicities. PRO-CTCAE contains 78 symptomatic adverse event terms and, in trials incorporating PRO-CTCAE, subjects are asked fill these out at regular intervals. Each symptom has up to 3 questions on the questionnaire that evaluate symptom frequency, severity, and interference with daily activity. Recently, the North Central Cancer Treatment Group (NCCTG) N1048 and NRG Oncology 1012 trials incorporated PRO-CTCAE and demonstrated the feasibility of this metric within clinical trial design. NCCTG N1048, which compared neoadjuvant chemoradiation with FOLFOX or 5-FU/capecitabine in subjects with locally advanced rectal cancer, aimed to collect PRO-CTCAE from subjects in the preoperative setting. Subjects were allowed to complete the surveys at home between treatments. Compliance with completing PRO-CTCAE on NCCTG N1048 was 92%.[17] In addition to completing PRO-CTCAE at home, the survey can be administered in the waiting room of a clinic. NRG 1012, a trial of prophylactic Manuka honey for reduction of chemoradiation-induced esophagitis-related pain during treatment of lung cancer, also used PRO-CTCAE and the Numerical Rating Pain Scale, and found that 86% of subjects were willing and able to self-report PRO-CTCAE in waiting rooms at scheduled times during treatment.[18] Many subjects completed PRO-CTCAE on tablets given to them by staff in the waiting room. Such trials indicate that patients are willing and able to self-report PRO-CTCAE as frequently as on a weekly basis. Survey collections via the Internet or telephone systems are acceptable to patients, and the results from such surveys have been found to be meaningful for clinical decision-making and adverse event reporting.[19]

Practice Guideline Changes with Trials Incorporating Patient-Reported Outcomes

PROs that have been studied in some radiation oncology trials have been instrumental in allowing for a complete and holistic interpretation of trial results. In the definitive management of prostate cancer, randomized controlled trials of hypofractionation versus conventionally fractionated radiotherapy that included PROs have been performed. The Conventional versus Hypofractionated High-Dose Intensity-Modulated Radiotherapy for Prostate Cancer (CHHiP) trial reported and compared PROs (University of California, Los Angeles [UCLA] Prostate Cancer Index, 36-item Short Form Health Survey, Functional Assessment of Cancer Therapy-Prostate, and Expanded Prostate Index Composite [EPIC]) for subjects receiving both treatment regimens.[20] PRO scales that are tracked over time, such as done in the CHHiP trial, can be interpreted with the use of minimally important differences, thresholds that constitute a clinically relevant change.[21] No significant differences were noted in PROs between the cohorts of subjects over time. These data supported the growing evidence that helped moderately hypofractionated radiotherapy become an evidence-based recommendation for men with localized prostate cancer.[22] PROs were also reported for the ProtecT trial, in which subjects with localized prostate cancer were randomized to active surveillance, surgery, or radiation therapy for the management of their disease.[23] The PROs from ProtecT were reported in a separate article, and showed the urinary, bowel, and sexual functioning side effects of different treatment strategies in men with prostate cancer.[23] In trials such as CHHiP and ProtecT, in which traditional oncologic outcomes, such as survival, are equivalent between treatment arms, PROs offer subjects an insight into what life could look like in different domains years after treatment based on treatment approach. Differences in PRO results can help providers counsel patients so that a patient can make as informed a decision as possible.

Radiation Therapy Oncology Group (RTOG) 0938 incorporated PROs (the EPIC-50 bowel, urinary, and sexual scores) to evaluate 2 ultrahypofractionated regimens for prostate cancer (36.25 Gy in 5 fractions and 51.6 Gy in 12 fractions).[24] At 1 year, a greater than 5-point change in bowel score was seen in 29.8% (P<.01) and 28.4% (P<.01) for the 5-fraction and 12-fraction regimens, respectively. EPIC scores were similarly used to collect PROs in the RTOG 1203, a trial of pelvic intensity-modulated radiotherapy (IMRT) and standard pelvic radiation in subjects with cervical and endometrial cancer. The EPIC bowel score was found to decline by 23.6 points in the standard radiotherapy group and 18.6 points in the IMRT group.[25] Such outcomes led to the conclusion of less gastrointestinal toxicity with IMRT compared with radiotherapy from a patient's perspective. The Breast Cancer Treatment Outcome Scale has also been developed to assess patients with breast cancer for function, cosmetic, and breast-specific pain outcomes, and was used in RTOG 1014, a single-arm study of breast-conserving therapy followed by partial breast irradiation in women with breast cancer recurrence after prior whole breast irradiation.[26] Patient-reported breast cosmetic outcomes correlated well with physician assessments in clinic, and demonstrated that PROs have the potential to act as primary and secondary endpoints in clinical investigations. In the setting of palliative radiation therapy, RTOG 9714 was designed to compare 8 Gy in 1 fraction to 30 Gy in 10 fractions for symptomatic bone metastases.[27] Both radiation regimens were found to be equivalent in terms of subject-reported pain relief at 3 months, with no difference in subject-reported quality of life between the cohorts. Subject-reported pain, function, and symptom frustration were reported in a study by Conway and colleagues[28] of single versus multiple-fraction radiation therapy for bone metastases. Similar to the results from RTOG 9714, improvements in PROs for pain, function, and symptom frustration were similar between single-fraction and multiple-fraction regimens, supporting the use of the single-regimen treatment in select patients. Additional radiation oncology trials that used PROs can be seen in **Table 3**.

INCORPORATION OF PATIENT-CENTERED OUTCOMES IN COST CONSIDERATIONS

Patient-reported HRQoL can be used in cost-effectiveness research while performing cost–utility analysis with quality-adjusted life-years (QALYs). QALYs are used to combine quality and length of life into a single outcome that can be used to determine the value of providing different elements of care.[29] The quality of life used to calculate a QALY is frequently measured using the European Quality of Life–5 Dimensions questionnaire, developed by the EuroQoL Group. In cost–utility analysis, the ratio of the cost of a health-related intervention to the benefit it produces in terms of QALY is called the cost-effectiveness of the intervention. Within radiation oncology, different treatment modalities, including IMRT, stereotactic body radiation therapy, proton therapy, and brachytherapy, can be used to treat the same tumor. The use of the incremental cost-effectiveness ratio, a ratio of the difference in costs to the difference in benefits (QALYs) between 2 treatments, can allow for comparisons between such new treatment modalities, as demonstrated by Amin and colleagues.[30] The cost-effectiveness of $50,000 per QALY gained by using a specific treatment has long served as a benchmark for value.[31] Others have advocated for the use of $50,000 to $100,000 per QALY as still representing a cost-effective intervention.[32]

Such thresholds are often considered arbitrary and, as a result, the willingness-to-pay per QALY threshold has also been used.[33] The willingness-to-pay threshold uses a populations' preferences to determine how much value is associated with services. Within oncology, predicting a patient's future health status can be challenging, complicating the calculation of QALY and cost-effectiveness. A Markov chain model analysis can be used in decision analysis to determine how competing risks of death, cancer

Table 3
Radiation oncology trials with patient reported outcome endpoints

Clinical Trial	Study Arms	PRO Tool Used	Results
NCCTG N1048 (PROSPECT): neoadjuvant FOLFOX vs 5-FU with concurrent radiation for rectal cancer patients	FOLFOX + radiation vs 5-FU or capecitabine with radiation	PRO-CTCAE	High compliance in completion of PROs
NRG 1012: prophylactic Manuka honey for esophagitis in lung cancer patients	Manuka honey daily during radiation therapy	Numerical Rating Pain Scale (NRPS) and PRO-CTCAE	No difference in NRPS between those who did and did not receive honey
ProtecT: monitoring, surgery, or radiotherapy for prostate cancer	Active monitoring vs radical prostatectomy vs radiotherapy	International Consultation on Incontinence Questionnaire (ICIQ), EPIC, SF-12, and EORTC QLQ-C30	Prostatectomy associated with greatest negative effect on sexual and urinary incontinence, bowel function worse in radiation group
CHHiP: Conventional versus Hypofractionated High-Dose Intensity-Modulated Radiotherapy for Prostate Cancer	74 Gy in 37 fractions vs 60–57 Gy in 19–20 fractions	University of California, Los Angeles, Prostate Cancer Index (UCLA-PCI) and EPIC	Low rates of urinary and bowel bother after conventional and hypofractionated radiation therapy
RTOG 0938: Patient Reported Outcomes in NRG Oncology RTOG 0938, Evaluating Two Ultrahypofractionated Regimens for Prostate Cancer	5 fractions (7.25 Gy in 2 wk) or 12 fractions (4.3 Gy in 2.5 wk)	EPIC-50 bowel, urinary, and sexual scores	1-y >5 point change in bowel score of 29.8% and 28/4% in 5 and 12 fraction regimens, respectively
RTOG 1014: Patient Reported Outcomes (PRO) and Cosmesis From a Phase II Study of Repeat Breast Preserving Surgery and 3D Conformal (3D-CRT) Partial Breast Re-Irradiation (PBrI) for In-Breast Recurrence	Lumpectomy with 45 Gy in 1.5 Gy bid fractions	Breast Cancer Treatment Outcome Scale (BCTOS)	Treatment resulted in no change in functional status or pain associated with worsening cosmesis Validated by physician evaluation

(continued on next page)

Table 3
(continued)

Clinical Trial	Study Arms	PRO Tool Used	Results
RTOG 9714: Short versus long course radiation for symptomatic bone metastases	8Gy in 1 fraction vs 30 Gy in 10 fractions	Brief Pain Inventory	Both regimens equivalent in terms of pain relief
RTOG 1203: Patient-Reported Toxicity During Pelvic Intensity-Modulated Radiation Therapy	IMRT vs standard pelvic radiation for endometrial or cervical cancer	EPIC	Mean EPIC bowel score decline of 23.6 and 18.6 points in standard vs IMRT arms
RTOG 0232: A Phase III Study Comparing Combined External Beam Radiation and Transperineal Interstitial Permanent Brachytherapy with Brachytherapy alone in Prostate Cancer	45 Gy plus brachytherapy vs brachytherapy alone	EPIC	External beam therapy resulted in worse EPIC scores at 24 mo compared with brachytherapy monotherapy
NSABP B-39/RTOG 0413: Phase III trial of WBI vs PBI in stage 0, I, or II breast cancer	Whole breast irradiation vs partial breast irradiation	BCTOS and 36-item Short Form Health Survey vitality scale	PBI associated with less fatigue in subjects not receiving chemotherapy Less pain with PBI
PIVOTAL: Phase 2 Trial of Prostate and Pelvic LN vs Prostate only RT in Advanced Prostate Cancer	Prostate-only radiation vs prostate and nodal radiation	Inflammatory Bowel Disease Questionnaire (IBDQ) and Vaizey ICIQ, and IPSS	Minimal change in questionnaire scores in both groups

Abbreviations: IPSS, international prostate symptom score; LN, lymph node; PBI, partial breast irradiation; WBI, whole breast irradiation.

recurrence, and treatment-related toxicity affect the cost-effectiveness of implementing new treatments.[34] In such a model, patients are assumed to be in 1 of a finite number of states of health, referred to as Markov states. Each state of health is assigned a utility (HRQoL), and the contribution of this HRQoL to overall HRQoL depends on the time a patient spends in each state of health. For example, a patient will have a different HRQoL assigned for the states of alive without evidence of cancer, alive with local cancer recurrence, alive with metastatic disease, and death.

CHALLENGES

A major challenge with the use of patient-centered outcome data in the research setting has been dealing with missing data, and the possible bias that these missing data can introduce. Missing data can result from failure to administer a survey, patient completion noncompliance, disease progression, and death. To deal with missing data, a technique called imputation, in which missing values are replaced by a set of plausible values, has been studied.[35] Patient compliance with PRO reporting can be enhanced when patients believe that PRO data are reviewed by their oncology team and that this enhances communication with their team. Integrating PROs into the oncology clinical workflow has the potential to improve data collection.[36] Such integration into the clinical workflow ideally involves reviewing worrisome PRO responses with patients and creating care plans to address such concerns.

Integration of PRO and HRQoL data collection and engagement with patients into a busy radiation oncology practice represents an additional challenge. An infrastructure to collect PRO and HRQoL survey results must be designed. In a radiation oncology clinic, PROs electronically captured on a tablet could be completed weekly before on treatment visits. Such a paradigm is currently used in the radiation oncology department at the University of Pennsylvania. Results should be incorporated into a patient's electronic medical record for physicians to see before treatment and follow-up visits. Although not all electronic medical record systems support PROs storage automation, such a feature would allow for real-time monitoring and trending of PROs by members of the care team.

Finally, in a busy clinic with varying patient needs, a radiation oncologist must buy into PROs and believe that PROs provide valuable information regarding the patient experience that can help provide personalized optimal care to patients.

SUMMARY

PROs and HRQoL have the potential to engage patients and providers, and allow for better communication and shared decision-making regarding care. When monitored longitudinally, such measures allow for earlier interventions that can help with symptom management and may improve traditional outcome metrics, including survival. The use of PROs as outcomes in clinical trials has allowed for changes in guidelines in the management of different cancers. The voice and experience of the patient, captured by such scales, enable providers to better detail the journey patients can expect to experience during treatment. Efforts to optimize the integration of these metrics into radiation oncology clinics are underway at some institutions, and lessons from such departments will be fundamental in allowing for the widespread uptake of such programs.

REFERENCES

1. Kemp R, Prasad V. Surrogate endpoints in oncology: when are they acceptable for regulatory and clinical decisions, and are they currently overused? BMC Med 2017;15:134.
2. Bentzen SM, Parliament M, Deasy JO, et al. Biomarkers and surrogate endpoints for normal-tissue effects of radiation therapy: the importance of dose-volume effects. Int J Radiat Oncol Biol Phys 2010;76:145–50.
3. Ganz PA. Quality of care and cancer survivorship: the challenge of implementing the Institute of Medicine recommendations. J Oncol Pract 2009;5:101–5.
4. Institute of Medicine (U.S.). Committee on quality of health care in America. Crossing the quality chasm: a new health system for the 21st century. Washington, DC: National Academy Press; 2001.
5. US Department of Health and Human Services, Food and Drug Administration. Guidance for industry: patient-reported outcome measure-use in medical product development to support labeling claims. Available at: http://www.fda.gov/downloads/drugs/guidances/UCM193292.pdf.
6. Siddiqui F, Liu AK, Watkins-Bruner D, et al. Patient-reported outcomes and survivorship in radiation oncology: overcoming the cons. J Clin Oncol 2014;32:2920–7.
7. Basch E, Iasonos A, McDonough T, et al. Patient versus clinician symptom reporting using the National Cancer Institute Common Terminology Criteria for Adverse Events: results of a questionnaire-based study. Lancet Oncol 2006;7:903–9.
8. Di Maio M, Gallo C, Leighl NB, et al. Symptomatic toxicities experienced during anticancer treatment: agreement between patient and physician reporting in three randomized trials. J Clin Oncol 2015;33:901–15.
9. Oliver A, Greenberg CC. Measuring outcomes in oncology treatment: the importance of patient-centered outcomes. Surg Clin North Am 2015;89:17.
10. De Graeff A, de Leeuw JR, Ros WJ, et al. Sociodemographic factors and quality of life as prognostic indicators in head and neck cancer. Eur J Cancer 2001;37:332–9.
11. Fang FM, Liu YT, Tang Y, et al. Quality of life as a survival predictor for patients with advanced head and neck carcinoma treated with radiotherapy. Cancer 2004;100:425–32.
12. Kaasa S, Mastekaasa A, Lund E. Prognostic factors for patients with inoperable non-small cell lung cancer, limited disease: The importance of patient's subjective experience of disease and psychosocial well-being. Radiother Oncol 1989;15:235–42.
13. Langendijk H, Aaronson NK, de Jong JM, et al. The prognostic impact of quality of life assessed with the EORTC QLQ-C30 in inoperable non-small cell lung carcinoma treated with radiotherapy. Radiother Oncol 2000;55:19–25.
14. Quinten C, Coens C, Mauer M, et al. Baseline quality of life as a prognostic indicator of survival: a meta-analysis of individual patient data from EORTC clinical trials. Lancet Oncol 2009;10:865–71.
15. Basch E, Deal AM, Kris MG, et al. Symptom monitoring with patient-reported outcomes during routine cancer treatment: a randomized controlled trial. J Clin Oncol 2016;24:557–65.
16. Mooney KH, Beck SL, Wong B, et al. Automated home monitoring and management of patient-reported symptoms during chemotherapy: results of the symptom at home RCT. Cancer Med 2017;6:537–46.

17. Basch E, Dueck AC, Rogak LJ, et al. Feasibility of Implementing the patient-reported outcomes version of the common terminology criteria for adverse events in a multicenter trial: NCCTG N1048. J Clin Oncol 2018. https://doi.org/10.1200/JCO.2018.78.8620.
18. Basch E, Pugh SL, Dueck AC, et al. Feasibility of patient reporting of symptomatic adverse events via the patient-reported outcomes version of the common terminology criteria for adverse events (PRO-CTCAE) in a chemoradiotherapy cooperative group multicenter clinical trial. Int J Radiat Oncol Biol Phys 2017;98(2):409–18.
19. Bruner DW, Hanisch LJ, Reeve BB, et al. Stakeholder perspectives on implementing the National Cancer Institute's patient-reported outcomes version of the Common Terminology Criteria for Adverse Events (PRO-CTCAE). Transl Behav Med 2011;1(1):110–22.
20. Wilkins A, Mossop H, Syndikus I, et al. Hypofractionated radiotherapy versus conventionally fractionated radiotherapy for patients with intermediate-risk localised prostate cancer: 2-year patient-reported outcomes of the randomised, non-inferiority, phase 3 CHHiP trial. Lancet Oncol 2015;16:1605–16.
21. Skolarus TA, Dunn RL, Sanda MG, et al. Minimally important difference for the Expanded Prostate Cancer Index Composite Short Form. Urology 2015;85:101–5.
22. Morgan SC, Hoffman K, Loblaw DA, et al. Hypofractionated radiation therapy for localized prostate cancer: executive summary of an ASTRO, ASCO, and AUA evidence-based guideline. Pract Radiat Oncol 2018;8:354–60.
23. Donovan JL, Hamdy FC, Lane JA, et al. Patient-Reported Outcomes after Monitoring, Surgery, or Radiotherapy for Prostate Cancer. N Engl J Med 2016;375:1425–37.
24. Lukka HR, Pugh SL, Bruner DW, et al. Patient reported outcomes in NRG oncology RTOG 0939, evaluating two ultrahypofractionated regimens for prostate cancer. Int J Radiat Oncol Biol Phys 2018;102:287–95.
25. Klopp AH, Yeung AR, Deshmukh S, et al. Patient-reported toxicity during pelvic intensity-modulated radiation therapy: NRG oncology- RTOG 1203. J Clin Oncol 2018;36:2538–44.
26. Arthur DW, Winter KA, Kuerer HM, et al. NRG oncology-radiation therapy oncology group study 1014: 1-year toxicity report from a phase 2 study of repeat breast-preserving surgery and 3-dimensional conformal partial-breast reirradiation for in-breast recurrence. Int J Radiat Oncol Biol Phys 2017;98:1028–35.
27. Hartsell WF, Scott CB, Watkins-Bruner D, et al. Randomized trial of short- versus long-course radiotherapy for palliation of painful bone metastases. J Natl Cancer Inst 2005;97:798–804.
28. Conway JK, Yurkowski E, Glazier J, et al. Comparison of patient-reported outcomes with single versus multiple fraction palliative radiotherapy for bone metastasis in a population-based cohort. Radiother Oncol 2016;119:202–7.
29. Whitehead SJ, Ali S. Health outcomes in economics evaluation: the QALY and utilities. Br Med Bull 2010;96:5–21.
30. Amin NP, Sher DJ, Konski AA. Systematic review of the cost effectiveness of radiation therapy for prostate cancer from 2003 to 2013. Appl Health Econ Health Policy 2014;12:391–408.
31. Grosse SD. Assessing cost-effectiveness in healthcare: history of the $50,000 per QALY threshold. Expert Rev Pharmacoecon Outcomes Res 2008;8:165–78.
32. Muurinen J-M. Demand for health: a generalised Grossman model. J Health Econ 1982;1:5–28.

33. Ryen L, Svensson M. The willingness to pay for a quality adjusted life year: a review of the empirical literature. Health Econ 2015;24:1289–301.

34. Tumeh JW, Shenoy PJ, Moore SG, et al. A Markov model assessing the effective and cost-effectiveness of FOLFOX compared with FOLFIRI for the initial treatment of metastatic colorectal cancer. Am J Clin Oncol 2009;32:49–55.

35. Gomes M, Gutacker N, Bojke C, et al. Addressing missing data in Patient-Reported Outcome Measures (PROMS): implication for the use of PROMS for for comparing provider performance. Health Econ 2016;25:515–28.

36. Basch E, Iasonos A, Barz A, et al. Long-term toxicity monitoring via electronic patient-reported outcomes in patients receiving chemotherapy. J Clin Oncol 2007;25:5374–80.

Financial Toxicity and Cancer Therapy
A Primer for Radiation Oncologists

Samuel R. Schroeder, MD, MBA, Vijay Agusala, BS, MBA,
David J. Sher, MD, MPH*

KEYWORDS

- Cancer • Financial toxicity • Financial burden • Medical expenditures • Quality of life

KEY POINTS

- The financial implications of cancer are significant and affect a significant percentage of the patient population.
- Financial toxicity can lead to morbidity and potentially mortality, in addition to significant quality-of-life decrements.
- The concept of financial toxicity accounts for monetary and consequential health-related effects associated with health care expenditures.
- Solutions to FT include effective patient screening; transparent pricing; and provider commitment to delivering evidence-based, high-value care.

INTRODUCTION

Financial toxicity (FT) has been defined as the harmful personal financial burden faced by patients receiving cancer treatment.[1] Similar to treatment-associated toxicity, the severity of FT can vary and also predispose a patient to morbidity and mortality. FT has been shown to be present across many types of malignancies, income levels, and stages of disease.[1,2] Given the long potential timeframe between initial work-up, diagnosis, treatments (surgical, radiation, and systemic), and post-treatment surveillance, there exists great potential for a patient to experience financial hardship. The overall cost of treatment must consider more than treatment expenses, including other out-of-pocket (OOP) costs, such as copayments, transportation, childcare, and loss of income.[1] Furthermore, some cancer treatments, such as imatinib for chronic myeloid leukemia, have allowed once incurable cancers to now be managed as chronic disease, further increasing lifetime costs to the patient and health care system.[3] All

Disclosure Statement: The authors have nothing to disclose.
Department of Radiation Oncology, UT Southwestern Medical Center, 2280 Inwood Road, Dallas, TX 75390, USA
* Corresponding author.
E-mail address: David.Sher@utsouthwestern.edu

Hematol Oncol Clin N Am 33 (2019) 1117–1128
https://doi.org/10.1016/j.hoc.2019.08.013
0889-8588/19/© 2019 Elsevier Inc. All rights reserved.

patients with cancer have an increased risk of excess financial burden and potential FT, including bankruptcy. Patients with advanced cancer or metastases are more likely to be vulnerable, because of the cumulative treatment costs and required long-term multimodal and complex therapies, compounded by normal living expenses and potential loss of employment income. In general, the development of FT reflects a clear double-hit phenomenon in patients' lives: treatment costs are prohibitively high, and the disease and treatments frequently reduce active income, if not their future earning potential.

Health insurance coverage, alongside illness status, cancer stage, and income level, is strongly associated with FT. Over the last several years, the American health insurance system has experienced major changes, specifically with the implementation of the Patient Protection and Affordable Care Act (PPACA) in 2010. The PPACA increased health insurance accessibility, resulting in greater numbers of Americans having health insurance than before. Conversely, with more of the population now insured, there is greater cost-sharing present in the system, with major financial implications for patients with cancer. In this review, we provide a short overview of the American health insurance system and its influence on the prevalence of FT and then summarize the predominant methods of FT measurement used in the literature. Additionally, we discuss the health effects of excess financial burden on this patient population, followed by several proposed solutions.

INFLUENCE OF INSURANCE PLANS ON FINANCIAL TOXICITY

In the United States, most of the working population is covered through employer-provided health insurance.[4] The years before the implementation of the PPACA saw increasingly widespread adoption of the employer-provided health insurance model. Health care expenditures continued to increase steadily from year to year, from consisting of 4.6% of the Gross Domestic Product in 1950% to 16.8% in 2015.[5,6] These rising costs have triggered increasing concerns, as health insurance premiums have risen 239% from 1999 to 2018. During this period, employee contributions to premiums increased 259% in the same time despite worker wages only increasing by 68%.

Patient Protection and Affordable Care Act

The PPACA, signed by President Obama in 2010, sought to increase health care insurance accessibility and coverage to those previously uninsured or ineligible, and address and curtail rising health care costs. Most relevant of the provisions to patients with cancer is that the PPACA required all health insurance plans to have annual OOP spending limits. The OOP limit is the monetary amount that the health care insurance enrollee pays during a policy period, after which 100% of the costs are covered by the insurance provider. However, the impact of this rule on FT has been inconsistent. For example, in the 2 years following PPACA, the rise in premium cost has been more than offset by decreased OOP expense for individuals making 250% or less than the federal poverty level, leading to an overall decrease in total health care expenditures for this group.[7] However, for those making 251% or greater of federal poverty level, more patients have health care expenses that exceed an affordability threshold (defined as OOP plus premium expenditures >19.5% of family income), demonstrating that FT is a potential threat for Americans with a wide range of income levels after PPACA enactment. In 2019, the OOP spending limit has been increased to $7900 for individual plans and $15,800 for family plans.[8] Increases in health care costs have increased health care premiums, especially for those individuals who do not receive subsidies.

As a consequence, in a hypothetical analysis that Claxton and colleagues[9] conducted using estimates for middle and high OOP plans, they observed that nearly 40% of households did not have the liquid financial resources to meet the middle OOP limit, and 51% were not able to meet the high annual OOP limit. Therefore, the OOP limits added by the PPACA, although beneficial theoretically, have limited utility when combating FT in this population.

Medicare

Medicare is the largest health insurer in the United States, providing health care coverage to individuals greater than or equal to 65 years of age, individuals less than 65 years with certain disabilities, and individuals with end-stage renal disease.[10] It has grown exponentially since its establishment in 1965, now encompassing close to 60 million beneficiaries.[11] This population is particularly susceptible to FT, because many are in retirement and have no active income.

Medicare Part A covers hospital stays, specifically costs incurred during inpatient stays.[9] Medicare Part B covers physician services and outpatient visits including radiation treatment, most infusion chemotherapy, and some oral anticancer agents. For a beneficiary with Part B and no supplemental coverage, 20% coinsurance is required for all Part B services with no OOP maximum. There are several supplemental coverage options that limit absolute OOP maximum spending to varying degrees, including employer-sponsored plans, Medigap, and Medicaid; approximately 19% of all Medicare beneficiaries have no supplemental or Part C coverage.[12] Medicare Part C, also known as Medicare Advantage, is optional and provides all Medicare services through private insurance. Part C plans must also set a global OOP maximum (set as $6700 in 2019), thereby protecting beneficiaries from potentially high coinsurance expenditures that are otherwise uncapped through Part B. With regards to total OOP costs among Medicare beneficiaries with newly diagnosed cancer with different types of supplemental coverage, one study observed mean OOP spending of $5976 for those insured by Medicare health maintenance organizations (HMO), $5492 for those with employer-sponsored plans, $5670 for those with Medigap insurance, and $8115 for those with traditional Medicare without supplemental insurance.[13]

More than 70% of eligible Americans purchase Medicare Part D benefits for prescription drug coverage.[11] Increases in prescription drug spending are a cause of growing concern for financial sustainability of the current third-party health care payor model, with Medicare spending comprising 29% of national retail pharmaceutical purchases in 2016.[14] Furthermore, OOP drug costs for covered individuals are expected to continue rising over the next decade, with a projected increase of 4.7% per year.[15] In 2016, the last year of available data, Medicare Part D enrollees spent an average of $1569 OOP on medications, an increase from an average of $1469 spent the year before (**Fig. 1**).[16]

EMPLOYMENT

Patients with cancer also experience the risk of temporary and long-term unemployment. A multinational meta-analysis consisting of nonelderly cancer survivors demonstrated this population has a relative risk of 1.37 for unemployment compared with healthy control subjects.[17] A separate multinational meta-analysis characterized employment patterns for cancer survivors and found that only 63.5% of cancer survivors ultimately returned to work, at a mean time of 151 days.[18] Within this analysis, socioeconomic risk factors for not returning to work included low income and manual labor. Thus, those patients already at higher risk of not being able to afford treatment

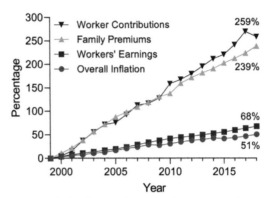

Fig. 1. Cumulative increases in family premiums, worker contributions to family premiums, inflation, and workers' earnings from 1999 to 2018. (*Modified from* 2018 Employer Health Benefits Survey. Henry J Kaiser Family Foundation. http://files.kff.org/attachment/2018-EHBS-Release-Slides.pdf; with permission.)

may experience a second potentially fatal financial blow of the two-hit model described previously. The impact of cancer diagnosis on employment income has also been assessed through the Panel Study of Income Dynamics.[19] Personal earnings decreased by 40% within the first 2 years of cancer diagnosis and did not recover over a 5-year period. Total household income decreased by 20% in the same period but did begin to increase at the end of study period, so even if a patient can maintain employment after treatment there may still be great potential for financial strain.

MEASURES OF FINANCIAL TOXICITY

A systematic review by Gordon and colleagues[20] characterized 25 studies involving FT, and demonstrated that the metrics used to measure FT vary dramatically. One commonly used metric was monetary measures (ie, absolute OOP cost compared with income); large population databases, such as Medicare claims, can provide OOP cost for specific services or medications that may predispose a patient to FT. Functional measures (ie, ability to secure a short-term loan) constitute another important way to measure FT. Within this domain, patient surveys are generally used to capture an overall financial snapshot at the time of diagnosis and treatment.[21] Finally, patient-reported, subjective measures (ie, patient perceptions on financial impact) represent another distinct FT metric. Such tools as the comprehensive score for FT (COST) and patient financial wellness scale patient-reported cost outcome measure have been created specifically to measure FT.[22,23] Additionally, other commonly used health-related quality of life (HRQoL) instruments, such as EORCT-QLQ-C30 or FACT-G, include limited assessment of financial burden that has been thoroughly reviewed elsewhere.[23] These domains are interrelated but also important to characterize individually. As the measure of FT has evolved, modern studies now tend to examine multiple domains of FT to gain new insights.

PREVALENCE OF FINANCIAL TOXICITY

The incidence of financial distress for patients with cancer has been reported as high as 49% from large meta-analyses.[20,24] Narang and Nicholas[13] analyzed health and retirement study data for Medicare beneficiaries enrolled in fee-for-service or HMO coverage and identified 1409 participants who were newly diagnosed with cancer during the study period. Yearly mean OOP expenditure was $3737 and at the 90th percentile of expenditure, annual spending was $8048 with financial burden of 29.6% (OOP expense/total household income). When beneficiaries were further divided by supplemental insurance status (no additional coverage, Medicaid, HMO, Medigap, or employer-sponsored insurance), the patients with no supplemental coverage incurred the highest mean OOP expenditure of $8115 despite having annual income ($44,767) lower than all other groups except Medicaid. The ubiquitous nature of Medicare for Americans aged 65 or greater allows for characterization of financial burden that would be more difficult in younger, privately insured individuals. The impact of age and financial hardship have been investigated and those aged 18 to 64 were significantly more likely to face material financial hardship compared with Medicare beneficiaries.[25] Additional studies give further support that younger age is a risk factor for FT.[26,27]

Zafar and colleagues[1] performed a survey assessing financial burden in patients with solid tumor diagnosis who received treatment with chemotherapy and/or hormonal therapy. The rate of underinsurance (defined as spending more than 10% of annual income on health care) was 55% and nearly all (98%) patients who requested copayment assistance used at least one form of financial coping strategies (ie, borrowing money). Subjective attributes were also analyzed and 82% of respondents requesting copayment assistance identified OOP expenditure as causing a moderate, significant, or catastrophic financial burden (36%, 35%, and 11%, respectively). Importantly, 64% of those not requesting assistance also reported moderate or higher financial burden, suggesting that OOP expenditures may dramatically affect those not thought to be at highest risk for FT.

Bona and colleagues[28] analyzed a cross-sectional study of survey results from the families of pediatric patients with progressive, recurrent, or nonresponsive cancers. A total of 94% of parents reported either cutting back on work hours or quitting their job entirely. Although OOP costs were not explicitly calculated, the median financial burden (defined as income loss/total income) for all families was 20%, and 15% of previously nonpoor families dropped lower than the 200% federal poverty level because of decreased ability to work. To obtain financial assistance, more than half of all families depended on fundraising, and dependence on fundraising did not vary across income levels.

Many studies have also characterized financial burden for specific cancer types. Shankaran and colleagues[29] looked specifically at patients with stage III colon cancer who underwent surgical resection and at least one cycle of adjuvant chemotherapy and found that 38% of patients reported financial hardship. Medicaid status was a significant risk factor for financial hardship, and 12% of patients reported insurance coverage denials that were significantly more prevalent for Medicaid enrollees (21% vs 6.8%). Arozullah and colleagues[30] analyzed financial burden among women diagnosed with breast cancer within the last 24 months, with a life expectancy greater than 6 months. OOP and lost income costs were observed to be an average of $1455/month in this study. Monthly cancer-related financial burden varied between different levels of household income, with risk of high financial burden increasing with lower monthly income. Cancer-related costs comprised 98%, 41%, and 26% of monthly income for patients with income levels of less than or equal to $30,000, $30,001 to $60,000, and greater than $60,000, respectively. Finally, 1-year OOP expenditures for private insurance beneficiaries treated for oropharynx cancer (surgery or radiation) were found to be approximately $5000.[31] Thus for cancer diagnoses requiring intense and/or multimodality therapy, there may be predisposing factors that can predict for financial hardship.

There is also evidence that cancer diagnosis predisposes patients to more permanent forms of personal FT, including bankruptcy. Ramsey and colleagues[32] linked Surveillance, Epidemiology, and End Results data with US Bankruptcy Court records and determined that patients with cancer were 2.65 times more likely to declare bankruptcy compared with patients without cancer. Additionally, younger patients tended to file bankruptcy at much higher rates compared with older individuals. In a continuation study, home foreclosure rates were found to be 156% and 96% higher for stage I and more advanced patients with cancer, respectively.[33] Furthermore, increased home equity levels significantly decreased mortgage defaults and foreclosures, suggesting that home equity serves as a buffer for FT.

HEALTH EFFECTS

The financial burden imposed by a cancer diagnosis may have downstream effects that negatively affect care delivery and HRQoL, especially in a population for whom financial difficulties predate their cancer diagnosis. The lack of financial stability presents another barrier to adequate care or preventative care. It has been shown that a preexisting financial burden, compounded by increasing OOP costs, can lead to delaying or completely forgoing recommended care.[34] This can have catastrophic effects including less effective treatment, disease recurrence, and higher morbidity and mortality.

The study by Zafar and colleagues[1] assessed specific coping mechanisms associated with financial burden and identified that 27% of patients requesting copayment assistance did not fill prescribed medications. Another study investigated the impact of cancer diagnosis and changes in prescription drug use and found that nonelderly recently and previously diagnosed patients with cancer were significantly more likely to change prescribed medication use for financial reasons.[35] Analysis of the 2010 National Health Interview Survey noted that individuals with cancer-related financial difficulties were significantly more likely to delay (18.3% vs 7.4%) or forgo (13.8% vs 5%) general medical care, not fill drug prescriptions, and not seek mental health care.[34] Another study of patients with chronic myeloid leukemia found that higher copayments (>$53/month) led an almost 70% greater chance of discontinuing the prescribed medication (imatinib) within the first 6 months of treatment.[36] This trend is growing more common in the context of increasing costs of chemotherapy.[37] This self-imposed limited access to health care and adequate treatment caused by financial constraints, combined with cost-related nonadherence to treatment plans leads to an overall lower quality-of-care.

Park and colleagues[38] analyzed the relationship between objective FT and HRQoL. Objective FT was defined as OOP medical expenditures greater than 10% or 20% of family income, which represented 15% and 6% of the study population, respectively. The HRQoL was measured using the Physical Component Summary (PCS) and Mental Component Summary (MCS) scores from the SF-12v2 questionnaire. On adjusted multivariable analysis, there was a significant negative association between financial burden exceeding 20% of family income and PCS/MCS scores. Financial burden exceeding 10% of family income was negatively associated with PCS but not MCS scores. This study included patients with a wide variety of cancer types but did not analyze potential linkages in FT by cancer type or stage. Nonetheless it provides insight regarding the global impact of financial strain. Analysis of the 2010 National Health Interview Survey further noted that increased financial hardship was an independent predictor of lower HRQoL.[34] Such an association has a significant implication for patients with cancer in that lower HRQoL has been shown to be independently associated with a negative prognosis in patients with cancer, with an increased chance of shorter survival.[39] The associated effects of cancer diagnosis and personal bankruptcy were compared with patients with cancer who did not file for bankruptcy.[40] Patients who filed for bankruptcy were more likely to be younger, female, nonwhite, and have locoregional versus distant disease. After propensity score matching was used to account for imbalances between the two groups, the hazard ratio for death in bankrupt patients was 1.79, which reached statistical significance.

Finally, because one may argue that FT may be particularly acute in the United States given the lack of a national health care system, a secondary analysis of 16 prospective clinical trials performed in Italy assessed the effect of financial burden on global quality of life in their public health care system.[41] Twenty-six percent of patients reported some type of financial burden, and there was a significant decrease in global quality of life for patients reporting a financial burden.

STARTING THE CONVERSATION

The administrative, financial, and treatment aspects of a cancer diagnosis are complex. Patients face many barriers to financial assistance with medical bills, based on citizenship status, socioeconomic status, availability of financial assistance, and complexity and heterogeneity of financial assistance applications.[34] Additionally, limited provider and patient knowledge of availability of assistance programs, combined with low referral rates to these programs, all contribute to the high prevalence of FT observed among patients with cancer.[42]

Although the American Society of Clinical Oncology has made efforts in the past to help providers and patients discuss costs of treatment, studies reveal that fewer than 20% of patients report talking about finances with their oncologist.[43] The most common reason why patients hesitate to discuss finances with their oncologist, per survey, is because they believe it is not the oncologist's job to discuss finances.[44] Patients fear bringing up costs and personal financial standing may cause the oncologist to prescribe a treatment regimen that has been adjusted according to cost rather than maximum efficacy.

From the perspective of the oncologist, although most recognize the negative effects of FT, many still feel discomfort when bringing up the topic of costs. Providers cite several barriers to making financially informed treatment decisions with input from patients. First, understanding total OOP cost for patients is difficult to nearly impossible, because different insurance reimbursements and drug pricing affect costs.[45] It can also be challenging to predict costs associated with the complications of different treatment options. However, providers should understand that therapeutically equivalent alternatives may exist that differ greatly in cost, and patient preference for the lower cost plan should be taken into account when making treatment decisions.[45] Better patient and provider communication in these instances can help prevent FT, help lower health care costs overall, with greater potential conservatory effects in health care systems with limited resources.[45]

Cancer navigators are individuals that help support and guide patients through their treatment plans, and are often the patient's first point of contact for any issue regarding their illness, especially with respect to financial assistance or toxicity.[46,47] Navigator's primary roles include scheduling and coordinating appointments, facilitating patient/provider communication regarding treatment preferences and options, and providing psychosocial support to patients and families.[48] A survey of 81 navigators revealed that three out of four patients experience FT as a result of cancer treatment, with more than 25% of navigators reporting that patients were unable to secure any financial assistance with their medical bills.[49] Given that navigators work closely with patients throughout the process and are members of the health care team with significant insight into the patients' personal lives and financial standing, they are in the ideal place to help screen for and combat FT. Instituting programs that provide financial training to current navigators may help with identifying patients who are at risk of FT.[49]

ACTIONABLE SOLUTIONS

Based on the increased understanding of risk factors that may predispose a patient to FT, it is imperative to identify the optimal time and method to screen patients for pre-existing or potential FT. Unfortunately, the optimal timing of screening has not been established, but patients could potentially benefit at multiple points throughout work-up and treatment.[50] Ideally, a financial screening instrument should be brief, integrated into routine clinical workflow, and assess financial risk in the short and long term. Thus, questions used in general and financial-specific patient-reported cost outcome measure batteries may serve as a starting point for initiating a screening program where at-risk patients can then be identified for earlier intervention. Given the complex nature of payment and reimbursement in the American health care system, there is growing interest in improving financial transparency. Starting in 2019, Centers for Medicare and Medicaid Services began mandating that hospitals provide a comprehensive list of charges online.[51] Because the charges are listed individually and rarely paid in full, this is not a practical way for patients to estimate expected cost. Additionally, the rates negotiated between hospitals and private insurance companies remain proprietary and vary dramatically. If realistic prices become available to providers and patients alike, the discussion of financial concerns would likely become more prevalent.

Currently, many medical costs are passed down to the patients, regardless of the necessity of the diagnostic test or treatment plan. For example, one disease site that may benefit from increased scrutiny is prostate cancer. For low-risk prostate cancer, there is level 1 evidence that prostatectomy and radiation do not improve prostate cancer–specific survival or overall survival compared with active surveillance.[52] Trogdon and colleagues[53] examined treatment of prostate cancer in elderly patients (age 70 or greater) and found that Medicare expenditures totaled $1.2 billion over a 3-year period and costs were primarily driven by treatment. Within this example, the principle of value-based care (defined as care quality and service/cost) can characterize treatments beyond survival end points. Combining high-value care with effective financial screening and price transparency allows providers and patients to begin to combat FT.

IMPLICATIONS FOR RADIATION ONCOLOGY

Within radiation oncology specifically, the progressive increase in hypofractionation holds the greatest promise for reducing FT. There is robust evidence for short-course treatments in common cancers (ie, breast and prostate), and increased diffusion of these regimens into routine practice should not only limit the time patients are not working but also minimize other unappreciated costs, such as child care and transportation costs.[54,55] A recent analysis compared the cost-effectiveness of conventionally fractionated, hypofractionated, and intraoperative treatment in early stage breast cancer.[56] Hypofractionated treatment was the most favorable option from quality-adjusted life-year and cost perspectives. Similarly, the financial implications of hypofractionated treatment of prostate have been analyzed and suggest that the use of moderate hypofractionation could save the US health care system $360 million annually.[57] Thus, hypofractionation has the potential to decrease costs throughout the health care system, which theoretically could translate into lower costs to the patients, although the impact on patient expenditures is unclear. However, any increase in the use of proton therapy may have the opposite effect on patient-borne costs, because particle therapy is significantly more expensive to deliver, and any reduction in reimbursement may be translated into more financial burden on treated patients.

In February 2019, Centers for Medicare and Medicaid Services issued a statement regarding bundled payments specifically designed for radiation oncology.[58] Within this plan, 17 cancer types (further specifics are unknown at time of publication) would receive a diagnosis-based payment according to the Medicare Physician Fee Schedule that would cover all care delivered within a 90-day period. How an alternative payment model will be implemented in radiation oncology has led to great uncertainty in the field, but the major thrust of this initiative is to reduce costs while maximizing value. In principle, such savings may be passed down to Medicare-eligible patients, but much like the alternative payment model itself, such downstream effects are impossible to predict.

SUMMARY

As cancer care continues to evolve and increase in cost, FT represents a real and growing risk for many patients. For oncologists, evidenced-based practice should guide treatment decisions to maximize value, not just to the health care system, but to patients themselves. Clinician awareness and sensitivity are mandatory to mitigate this risk in susceptible patients, and they must recognize that FT influences not just financial decision-making but also quality-of-life and potentially even overall survival.

REFERENCES

1. Zafar SY, et al. The financial toxicity of cancer treatment: a pilot study assessing out-of-pocket expenses and the insured cancer patient's experience. Oncologist 2013;18(4):381–90.
2. Khera N. Reporting and grading financial toxicity. J Clin Oncol 2014;32(29):3337–8.
3. Druker BJ, et al. Five-year follow-up of patients receiving imatinib for chronic myeloid leukemia. N Engl J Med 2006;355(23):2408–17.
4. Enthoven AC, Fuchs VR. Employment-based health insurance: past, present, and future. Health Aff 2006;25(6):1538–47.
5. Fuchs VR. Major trends in the U.S. health economy since 1950. N Engl J Med 2012;366(11):973–7.
6. Current health expenditure (% of GDP). 2019. Available at: https://data.worldbank.org/indicator/SH.XPD.CHEX.GD.ZS?year_high_desc=true. Accessed September 25, 2019.
7. Goldman AL, et al. Out-of-pocket spending and premium contributions after implementation of the affordable care act. JAMA Intern Med 2018;178(3):347–55.
8. Out-of-pocket maximum/limit. Available at: https://www.healthcare.gov/glossary/out-of-pocket-maximum-limit/. Accessed September 25, 2019.
9. Claxton G, Rae M, Panchal N. Consumer assets and patient cost sharing. San Francisco: Kaiser Family Foundation; 2015.

10. Hoffman ED Jr, Klees BS, Curtis CA. Overview of the Medicare and Medicaid programs. Health Care Financ Rev 2000;22(1):175–93.

11. CMS fast facts. 2019. Available at: https://www.cms.gov/research-statistics-data-and-systems/statistics-trends-and-reports/cms-fast-facts/index.html. Accessed September 25, 2019.

12. Cubanski J, et al. Sources of supplemental coverage among Medicare beneficiaries in 2016. 2018. Available at: https://www.kff.org/medicare/issue-brief/sources-of-supplemental-coverage-among-medicare-beneficiaries-in-2016/. Accessed September 25, 2019.

13. Narang AK, Nicholas LH. Out-of-pocket spending and financial burden among Medicare beneficiaries with cancer. JAMA Oncol 2017;3(6):757–65.

14. Kaiser Family Foundation analysis of National Health Expenditure Account data from the Centers for Medicare & Medicaid Services, O.o.t.A., National Health Statistics Group, Table 16, retail prescription drugs expenditures; levels, percent change, and percent distribution, by source of funds: selected calendar years 1970-2016.

15. Pauwels B, et al. Combined modality therapy of gemcitabine and radiation. Oncologist 2005;10(1):34–51.

16. Cubanski J, Neuman T, Damico A. Closing the Medicare Part D coverage gap: trends, recent changes, and what's ahead. Henry J Kaiser Family Foundation; 2018.

17. de Boer AG, et al. Cancer survivors and unemployment: a meta-analysis and meta-regression. JAMA 2009;301(7):753–62.

18. Mehnert A. Employment and work-related issues in cancer survivors. Crit Rev Oncol Hematol 2011;77(2):109–30.

19. Zajacova A, et al. Employment and income losses among cancer survivors: estimates from a national longitudinal survey of American families. Cancer 2015; 121(24):4425–32.

20. Gordon LG, et al. A systematic review of financial toxicity among cancer survivors: we can't pay the co-pay. Patient 2017;10(3):295–309.

21. Jagsi R, et al. Long-term financial burden of breast cancer: experiences of a diverse cohort of survivors identified through population-based registries. J Clin Oncol 2014;32(12):1269–76.

22. de Souza JA, et al. The development of a financial toxicity patient-reported outcome in cancer: the COST measure. Cancer 2014;120(20):3245–53.

23. Meisenberg BR, et al. Patient attitudes regarding the cost of illness in cancer care. Oncologist 2015;20(10):1199–204.

24. Altice CK, et al. Financial hardships experienced by cancer survivors: a systematic review. J Natl Cancer Inst 2016;109(2):djw205.

25. Yabroff KR, et al. Financial hardship associated with cancer in the united states: findings from a population-based sample of adult cancer survivors. J Clin Oncol 2016;34(3):259–67.

26. Landwehr MS, et al. The cost of cancer: a retrospective analysis of the financial impact of cancer on young adults. Cancer Med 2016;5(5):863–70.

27. Knight TG, et al. Financial toxicity in adults with cancer: adverse outcomes and noncompliance. J Oncol Pract 2018;14(11):e665–73.

28. Bona K, et al. Economic impact of advanced pediatric cancer on families. J Pain Symptom Manage 2014;47(3):594–603.

29. Shankaran V, et al. Risk factors for financial hardship in patients receiving adjuvant chemotherapy for colon cancer: a population-based exploratory analysis. J Clin Oncol 2012;30(14):1608–14.

30. Arozullah AM, et al. The financial burden of cancer: estimates from a study of insured women with breast cancer. J Support Oncol 2004;2:271–8.

31. Sher DJ, et al. Commercial claims–based comparison of survival and toxic effects of definitive radiotherapy vs primary surgery in patients with oropharyngeal squamous cell carcinoma. JAMA Otolaryngol Head Neck Surg 2018;144(10):913–22.

32. Ramsey S, et al. Washington State cancer patients found to be at greater risk for bankruptcy than people without a cancer diagnosis. Health Aff 2013;32(6):1143–52.

33. Gupta A, Morrison ER, Fedorenko C, et al. Leverage, default, and mortality: evidence from cancer diagnoses. Law and Economics Working Paper 2017;(514):15–35.

34. Kent EE, et al. Are survivors who report cancer-related financial problems more likely to forgo or delay medical care? Cancer 2013;119(20):3710–7.

35. Zheng Z, et al. Do cancer survivors change their prescription drug use for financial reasons? Findings from a nationally representative sample in the United States. Cancer 2017;123(8):1453–63.

36. Dusetzina SB, et al. Cost sharing and adherence to tyrosine kinase inhibitors for patients with chronic myeloid leukemia. J Clin Oncol 2014;32(4):306–11.

37. Bach PB. Limits on Medicare's ability to control rising spending on cancer drugs. N Engl J Med 2009;360(6):626–33.

38. Park J, Look KA. Relationship Between Objective Financial Burden and the Health-Related Quality of Life and Mental Health of Patients With Cancer. Journal of Oncology Practice 2018;14(2):e113–21.

39. Efficace F, et al. Validation of patient's self-reported social functioning as an independent prognostic factor for survival in metastatic colorectal cancer patients: results of an international study by the Chronotherapy Group of the European Organisation for Research and Treatment of Cancer. J Clin Oncol 2008;26(12):2020–6.

40. Ramsey SD, et al. Financial insolvency as a risk factor for early mortality among patients with cancer. J Clin Oncol 2016;34(9):980–6.

41. Gimigliano A, et al. The association of financial difficulties with clinical outcomes in cancer patients: secondary analysis of 16 academic prospective clinical trials conducted in Italy†. Ann Oncol 2016;27(12):2224–9.

42. Harris JK, et al. Referrals among cancer services organizations serving underserved cancer patients in an urban area. Am J Public Health 2011;101(7):1248–52.

43. Bestvina CM, et al. Patient-oncologist cost communication, financial distress, and medication adherence. J Oncol Pract 2014;10(3):162–7.

44. Meisenberg BR, et al. Patient attitudes regarding the cost of illness in cancer care. Oncologist 2015;20(10):1199–204.

45. Ubel PA, Abernethy AP, Zafar SY. Full disclosure: out-of-pocket costs as side effects. N Engl J Med 2013;369(16):1484–6.

46. MacReady N. The climbing costs of cancer care. J Natl Cancer Inst 2011;103(19):1433–5.

47. Bestvina CM, Zullig LL, Zafar SY. The implications of out-of-pocket cost of cancer treatment in the USA: a critical appraisal of the literature. Future Oncol 2014;10(14):2189–99.

48. Cantril C, Haylock PJ. Patient navigation in the oncology care setting. Semin Oncol Nurs 2013;29(2):76–90.

49. Spencer JC, et al. Oncology navigators' perceptions of cancer-related financial burden and financial assistance resources. Support Care Cancer 2018;26(4): 1315–21.

50. Khera N, Holland JC, Griffin JM. Setting the stage for universal financial distress screening in routine cancer care. Cancer 2017;123(21):4092–6.

51. Fiscal Year (FY) 2019 Medicare Hospital Inpatient Prospective Payment System (IPPS) 2019. Available at: https://www.cms.gov/newsroom/fact-sheets/fiscal-year-fy-2019-medicare-hospital-inpatient-prospective-payment-system-ipps-and-long-term-acute-0. Accessed September 25, 2019.

52. Hamdy FC, et al. 10-Year outcomes after monitoring, surgery, or radiotherapy for localized prostate cancer. N Engl J Med 2016;375(15):1415–24.

53. Trogdon JG, et al. Total Medicare costs associated with diagnosis and treatment of prostate cancer in elderly men. JAMA Oncol 2019;5(1):60–6.

54. Lee WR, et al. Randomized phase III noninferiority study comparing two radiotherapy fractionation schedules in patients with low-risk prostate cancer. J Clin Oncol 2016;34(20):2325–32.

55. Whelan TJ, et al. Long-term results of hypofractionated radiation therapy for breast cancer. N Engl J Med 2010;362(6):513–20.

56. Deshmukh AA, Shirvani SM, Lal L, et al. Cost-effectiveness analysis comparing conventional, hypofractionated, and intraoperative radiotherapy for early-stage breast cancer. J Natl Cancer Inst 2017;109(11).

57. Moore A, et al. The financial impact of hypofractionated radiation for localized prostate cancer in the United States. J Oncol 2019;2019:8.

58. HHS, editor. Continued analysis calls for prospective bundled payments for radiation oncology (RO) model transmittal 2256. Washington, DC: CMS Manual System; 2019.

Moving?

Make sure your subscription moves with you!

To notify us of your new address, find your **Clinics Account Number** (located on your mailing label above your name), and contact customer service at:

Email: journalscustomerservice-usa@elsevier.com

800-654-2452 (subscribers in the U.S. & Canada)
314-447-8871 (subscribers outside of the U.S. & Canada)

Fax number: 314-447-8029

Elsevier Health Sciences Division
Subscription Customer Service
3251 Riverport Lane
Maryland Heights, MO 63043

*To ensure uninterrupted delivery of your subscription, please notify us at least 4 weeks in advance of move.

Printed and bound by CPI Group (UK) Ltd, Croydon, CR0 4YY

03/10/2024

01040402-0003